P9-CPZ-490

$11.50

Epidemiology

Epidemiology

MAN and DISEASE

JOHN P. FOX, M.D., Ph.D., M.P.H.,

Professor of Preventive Medicine, School of Medicine, University of Washington, Seattle

CARRIE E. HALL, R.N., M.P.H.,

Assistant Professor, Schools of Medicine and Nursing, University of Washington, Seattle

LILA R. ELVEBACK, Ph.D.,

Professor of Biostatistics, Mayo Graduate School of Medicine, University of Minnesota, Rochester

THE MACMILLAN COMPANY
COLLIER-MACMILLAN LIMITED, LONDON

Library of Congress catalog card number: 76–80305

THE MACMILLAN COMPANY
866 THIRD AVENUE, NEW YORK, NEW YORK 10022
COLLIER-MACMILLAN CANADA, LTD., TORONTO, ONTARIO

Printed in the United States of America

Preface

Like other biomedical sciences, including clinical medicine itself, epidemiology deals with problem solving. As the subtitle "Man and Disease" suggests, epidemiologic problems are concerned with explaining the occurrence of disease in human populations and with exploiting explanations discovered for the development of methods to protect man against disease. Because of this latter natural byproduct of epidemiologic investigations, epidemiology is the basic science of preventive medicine.

As a discipline, epidemiology evolved in relation to the study of acute infectious diseases. However, in developed countries the most dangerous of these have been largely controlled and other diseases, chiefly chronic in nature and commonly presumed to be noninfectious, have increased in both relative and absolute importance. This change has resulted in a corresponding shift in the principal concern of many epidemiologists and in important modifications of the methods used in epidemiologic investigations. Indeed, it is usual today to distinguish epidemiologists according to their area of special interest, i.e. infectious or noninfectious disease epidemiology. Similarly, the currently available epidemiology textbooks can be characterized by whether they give major emphasis to acute infectious or to chronic and noninfectious disease problems.

The present book is intended to introduce the reader in a systematic way to the entire scope of epidemiology, relying heavily on the liberal use of specific disease problems to illustrate both principles and methods. The exposition of principles, it may be noted, is chiefly contained in Chapters 1 through 6, the remaining chapters being devoted largely to the description of methods. The considerable predominance of examples based on infectious diseases is in no way intended to diminish the importance of noninfectious disease epidemiology. In part, it reflects a natural tendency to draw heavily on the personal investigative experience of the authors for examples. More importantly, many concepts are more clearly

v

illustrated by infectious disease examples because, as a class, the occurrence of such diseases is more completely understood.

The book has been designed to appeal to a broad class of readers. For the benefit of the many potential readers (beginning students in medicine or nursing) who will have little knowledge of either epidemiology or biomedical science beyond that commonly acquired from the current news media, we have provided a summary of important concepts and a glossary at the end of each chapter when appropriate. At the same time we have hoped that our systematic coverage of epidemiology and the relative abundance of illustrative material documented by key references will be helpful to readers whose interest in the field has already developed. To provide a sense of continuity for all readers, a certain few diseases have been used to provide illustrative examples whenever appropriate throughout the book.

Although we have tried to make our presentation interesting enough to attract even casual readers, it is intended primarily as a textbook. How then can it best be used? While it would be presumptuous to tell other teachers of epidemiology how to conduct their courses, they may be interested in knowing how we have been using it. In brief, we use it to replace formal lectures which, we are convinced, constitute an ineffective method of teaching epidemiology. We prefer the seminar method in which a portion of each period is devoted to discussion of a preassigned portion of the text and the remaining larger portion to discussion of appropriate problem material since, as stated at the onset, epidemiology deals with problem solving.

As a final note, we are indebted to many individuals for assistance in the development and final preparation of this book. This help took many forms, including the suggestion of pertinent examples and constructive comments on both organization and expression of concepts. In particular we owe our thanks to Professor Morton D. Schweitzer, who criticized the entire text in late draft form, to Dr. Donald R. Peterson, who also read the entire manuscript and who contributed the final chapter, to Professor Donovan J. Thompson for constructive criticism of Chapters 7 and 8, and to Mrs. Thelma Shaw, our secretary, who assumed the role of production engineer and transformed an endless succession of rough drafts into a well-organized final manuscript.

J. P. F.
C. E. H.
L. R. E.

Contents

9 Patterns of Disease Occurrence—Person   185

10 Patterns of Disease Occurrence—Place   209

11 Patterns of Disease Occurrence—Time   239

1

Introduction to Epidemiology

1-1 The Concern of Epidemiology

Human curiosity is the fundamental motivation of epidemiology, as it is of any scientific discipline. Epidemiologic curiosity centers about the causation of disease in human populations. In its elemental form, such curiosity often is aroused by a particular illness—measles, poliomyelitis, a peptic ulcer, a heart attack, or cancer—occurring in yourself, a member of your family, a close friend, a patient in your care, or the President of the United States. Whatever the disease and whoever the person, you may well wonder why the particular victim was chosen from the vast number of other people, seemingly equally eligible, so many of whom somehow escaped attack.

The idea that illness depends upon chance alone becomes untenable with the knowledge that the occurrence of each type of illness follows a fairly characteristic pattern. Such patterns suggest that individual illnesses are determined in some part by the selective operation of one or more influences which should be susceptible to definition. The question is how to define or discover them. The complexity of our environment is such that study of the circumstances relating to illness in a single person may contribute very little. When contact with other similar illness is revealed, as with measles, the circumstance assumes meaning only when repeatedly discovered in similar studies related to other patients. To satisfy his ultimate curiosity, therefore, the epidemiologist must examine cases of measles or polio or coronary heart disease as they occur throughout a population, seeking to discover the circumstances or influences that distinguish those afflicted from the rest of the population and which, accordingly, may be the essential determinants of disease occurrence. Thus, the

1

discovery of factors essential or contributory to the occurrence of any particular disease is the most important concern of epidemiology.

Simple satisfaction of idle curiosity is not in itself a socially acceptable goal. However, satisfaction of scientific curiosity which leads to more complete understanding of the occurrence of natural phenomena is accepted as socially justifiable because such understanding, often with complete unpredictability, may lead to highly practical applications. Modern antibiotics, for example, constitute the practical outcome of efforts to understand the original observation by Sir Alexander Fleming that colonies of staphylococci on an agar plate had been dissolved in a zone around a colony of a penicillium mold (1). In epidemiology, increased understanding of the natural occurrence of disease may be followed, with more than usual predictability, by the development of effective methods for disease prevention by interception of the action of causative factors.

Smallpox, rabies, and cholera are particularly interesting to the student of epidemiology because they demonstrate that only partial understanding of factors influencing disease may lead to highly effective preventive measures which, in these examples, were developed long before the microbial nature of the causative agents had been demonstrated. At the end of the eighteenth century, Edward Jenner validated a belief prevalent among rural people in parts of England that human infection with cowpox induced resistance to smallpox; his scientific study initiated one of the most successful preventive measures of all time (2). Working only with the knowledge that rabies could be transmitted by means of the saliva of rabid dogs, a rabies control program instituted in Scandinavia had rid the entire area of that justly feared disease by 1825 (3). Finally, in the mid-nineteenth century an English anesthesiologist by the name of John Snow became curious about cholera. His subsequent extensive observations led him to a high level of understanding of the occurrence of cholera upon which he based a remarkably complete list of specific recommendations (Table 1-1) as to how its transmission could be prevented (4).

TABLE 1-1
The measures which are required for the prevention of cholera and all diseases which are communicated in the same way as cholera

A. Those which may be carried out in the presence of an epidemic:

  1. Strictest cleanliness should be observed by those attending the sick.
  2. Soiled bed and body linen of the patient should be immersed in water immediately to prevent transmission through the air of contaminated particles; nonwashable articles should be exposed to temperature of 212° F or more.
  3. Water not contaminated with the contents of cesspools or boiled water should be used for preparation of patient's food and for his drinking water.

4. When cholera prevails very much in the neighborhood all provisions which are brought into the house should be well washed with clean water and exposed to 212° F temperature, or at least they should undergo one of these processes and be purified either by water or by fire.

5. When a case of cholera occurs among persons living in a crowded room, the healthy should be removed to another apartment, leaving only those who are useful to wait on the sick.

6. As it would be impossible to clean out coal-pits, and establish privies and lavatories in them, or even to provide the means of eating a meal with anything like common decency, the time of working should be divided into periods of four hours instead of eight, so that the pitmen might go home to their meals, and be prevented from taking food into the mines.

7. The communicability of cholera ought not to be disguised from the people, under the idea that knowledge of it would cause a panic, or occasion the sick to be deserted.

B. The measures which can be taken beforehand to provide against cholera and other epidemic diseases, which are communicated in a similar way, are:

1. To effect good and perfect drainage.

2. To provide ample supply of water free from contamination from sewers, cesspools, house drains, or refuse of people navigating rivers.

3. To provide model lodging houses for the vagrant class and sufficient house room for the poor.

4. To inculcate habits of personal and domestic cleanliness in people everywhere.

5. Some attention should undoubtedly be directed to persons and especially ships arriving from infected places, in order to segregate the sick from the healthy. In the instance of cholera, the supervision would generally not require to be of long duration.

"I feel confident, however, that by attending to the above-mentioned precautions, which I consider to be based on a correct knowledge of the cause of cholera, this disease may be rendered extremely rare, if indeed it may not be altogether banished from civilized countries. And the diminution of mortality ought not to stop with cholera. . . ."

Source: Adapted from *Snow on Cholera*, being a reprint of two papers by John Snow, M.D., together with a biographical memoir by B. W. Richardson and an introduction by Wade Hampton Frost. New York: The Commonwealth Fund, 1936. pp. 133–137.

1-2   The Scope of Epidemiology

Despite increasingly great professional and lay interest in epidemiology, certain misconceptions as to its meaning and scope of interest are very common. The epidemiologist who so identifies himself in response to polite inquiry often finds himself in an embarrassing dilemma. Either he must permit the inquirer to retain his possible misconception or he must give a brief private lecture to explain that diseases of the skin (epidermis) are not his specialty or that epidemics of infectious diseases and their control do not constitute his exclusive interest.

Historically, epidemiology was born in relation to the study of the great epidemic diseases (especially cholera, plague, smallpox, yellow fever, and typhus) which, until the twentieth century, were the most obviously important threats to human life and health. The term *epidemic*, incidentally, is simply defined as the unusually frequent occurrence of a disease. To understand unusual disease occurrence, it soon was realized that the usual, or *endemic*, occurrence also must be studied. The methods developed for such study were readily applicable to the study of all important infectious disease, whether epidemic or not, e.g., diphtheria, scarlet fever, measles, infant diarrhea, syphilis, and tuberculosis. Especially in relation to these latter more chronic diseases, the importance of cultural patterns and environmental factors depending on social and economic status became apparent.

Today, influenza outbreaks excepted, major epidemics no longer seriously threaten the United States and other more highly developed countries, and most of the more important infectious diseases, such as diphtheria, whooping cough, typhoid, tuberculosis, and syphilis, are reasonably under control. However, keeping such diseases in check and seeking to understand more fully and to control influenza, other minor and major respiratory infections, viral hepatitis, and a fascinating variety of newly emerging infectious diseases continue to provide abundant challenges for the infectious disease epidemiologist. Further, if he is willing to sojourn outside his homeland, the epidemiologist from a highly developed country can help to resolve major health problems posed in the less developed countries by such historic "friends" as smallpox, malaria, cholera, and typhoid.

Meanwhile, diseases of other types have assumed importance as the current major health problems of advanced Western civilization. The new importance of these diseases stems in part from major changes in environment and way of life imposed by industrialization of the economy and the related migration of people to the cities. It also relates to the great numerical and proportional increase in older age groups in the population which has resulted from the withdrawal of infection as a common cause of early death. This withdrawal was forced by prevention (infant diarrhea, whooping cough, diphtheria, and tetanus) and by vastly improved means of treatment with the so-called "miracle drugs" (sulfonamides and antibiotics) which can cure most of the possibly fatal bacterial infections (scarlet fever and other streptococcal infections, meningitis, pneumonia, and tuberculosis). Cancer of nearly all types, high blood pressure, coronary artery disease, diabetes, and arthritis are among the lethal or chronic crippling diseases associated with older age. Cancer of several specific types (lung, bladder, and leukemia), peptic ulcer, accidents, and mental disorders are related in some part to changes in environment. With little or no modification, the principles and methods developed to explore causes for the occurrence of infectious diseases are proving applicable to the study of these increasingly important and presumably noninfectious diseases. Investigation of causal factors of the latter represents the new epidemiologic frontier.

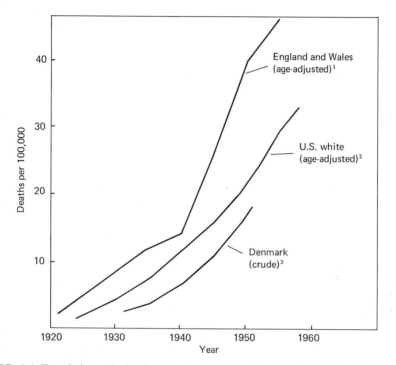

FIG. 1-1 Trends in male death rates (per 100,000) from cancer of the lung and bronchus in England and Wales, the United States, and Denmark. (1. Registrar General's Reports; 2. U.S. National Office of Vital Statistics; 3. Clemmesen, J., Nielsen, A., and Jensen, E., *Acta Un. Con. Cancer.* **9**:603, 1953.)

Some may argue that the forced withdrawal of infection as a major cause of death has simply left us to face the ultimate and sometimes less merciful alternate causes of death from which no escape is possible. If this be true, why should we waste our time in the study of these diseases? While death itself is admittedly inevitable, there are good reasons to think that certain important causes of death can be eliminated or greatly reduced when their causation is fully understood and that in other cases, death may be delayed. Cancer is one example. Figure 1-1 illustrates the recent world-wide increase in lung cancer which almost certainly indicates the increasing activity of some potent environmental influence (best current bet is cigarette smoking) which, if recognized, may be effectively neutralized. This and other instances in which an environmental cause of cancer has been clearly identified (radiation in leukemia, aniline dyes in bladder cancer) afford a reasonable basis for expecting that environmental influences susceptible to control may be important causes for many forms of cancer.

Coronary heart disease is another important example. Although sex and familial or genetic factors are partial determinants, this disease has become increasingly frequent in middle-aged men in the United States. The sex-selective change in frequency and the much better experience of men in many other countries clearly point to the operation of environmental influences. The business of the epidemiologist is to identify these influences and develop means for counteracting them.

1-3 Epidemiologic Investigations

An essential first step in the study of a particular disease is to describe accurately its occurrence in the population. This description requires that the specific disease can be recognized with reasonable reliability. Basic data as to disease occurrence that must be collected for each patient include time (day, month, season, year), place (country, political subdivisions thereof, urban or rural residence), and various personal attributes (age, sex, race or ethnic group). Desirable supplementary data, usually obtainable only by intensive study of selected patients, include information as to educational status, occupation, income level, contact with similarly ill persons, various aspects of the household and neighborhood environment (including presence of insects or other animals, plants, and, sometimes, geologic features), dietary habits, and recent unusual activities. Careful analysis of such data for patients with reference to the populations in which they reside should reveal the general patterns of disease occurrence and recognition of groups that are at greatest risk of disease.

Clues as to causative (or etiologic) factors in a particular disease may derive from analogies with known diseases of similar pattern of occurrence or from the recognition of factors commonly affecting members of high-risk groups. Simple examples include diseases which, like measles, are dependent on contact for transmission of the infectious agent or diseases related to special occupations, such as the bone cancers of the lower jaw which evolved in persons employed in applying radium paint to the hands and dials of watches in a New Jersey factory (5). Somewhat more subtle was the association of yellow fever with a particular mosquito vector (*Aedes aegypti*) which was first suggested by Carlos Finlay of Cuba (6).

Each of these associations formed the basis of a hypothesis as to a causative influence, the testing of which constitutes the next step in epidemiologic investigation. A basic principle to be stressed here is that an ultimately acceptable hypothesis must be consistent with the known facts regarding disease occurrence.

Testing methods vary with the hypothesis but have in common the principle of observation under controlled conditions which is inherent in the scientific method. Investigation may center about experimental disease in the laboratory, with interest in factors that increase or lessen susceptibility, in methods for specific diagnosis, or in possible mechanisms of transmission. More characteristically, investigation will take the form of field studies centered about the natural occurrence of disease. Whatever the setting, field or laboratory, the methods employed are of two main types, observational and experimental.

Observational studies are particularly characteristic of epidemiology and, when directed toward testing hypotheses, are usually analytic. "Observational" implies that the investigator does not manipulate the population studied but simply observes circumstances and events in the normal pattern of life. "Analytic" implies a search for association between disease occurrence and possible causative influences. In seeking such association the population studied is classified according to absence or presence (or future development) of specific disease and according to "attributes" which may influence disease occurrence. These may include age, sex, race, economic status, occupation, place and nature of residence, the occurrence of similar illness in close relatives or associates, and various aspects of personal behavior such as dietary preferences or cigarette smoking.

A common initial approach is to look backward from illness (the retrospective or "case history" study). A modern but already classical example is the study by N. M. Gregg, an ophthalmologist in Sydney, Australia, who noted an unusual occurrence of congenital cataracts in children born in 1941, many of whom also had serious cardiac defects. By interviewing mothers of 78 defective children, he discovered that 68 (87 per cent) had experienced rubella early in the related pregnancy (7). This coincidence so impressed him that, even without exploring the disease experience of mothers producing normal infants during the same period (the conventional and necessary control group), he became convinced that maternal rubella was responsible for the defects he had observed. This hypothesis received quick support from the results of several more complete retrospective studies and was established beyond reasonable doubt by studies utilizing a forward-looking (prospective) approach.

The more convincing, but usually much more difficult, prospective approach begins with groups selected from persons still free of the disease being investigated. In the presently considered problem, such groups should consist of pregnant women selected without knowledge of the outcome of pregnancy (preferably before it could be known) and divided into those who had rubella during pregnancy and those who escaped. The earliest example of such a prospective study of Gregg's hypothesis was sponsored by the Australian National Health and Medical Research Council (8). A search was instituted for women in southern Australia who had experienced an acute rash disease during pregnancy from 1939 to 1943. This produced a total of 49 women who had contracted rubella. The relationship between the time of onset of rubella during pregnancy and the occurrence of congenital defects in the infants born subsequently is shown in Table 1-2. Like Gregg's retrospective study, this study also

TABLE 1-2

Relationship between the time of contraction of rubella during pregnancy to the occurrence of congenital defects in the infants born subsequently

Month of Pregnancy	Number of Infants with Congenital Defects	Number of Healthy Children	Total
0 to 1	8	—	8
1 to 2	17	—	17
2 to 3	4	4	8
3 to 4	1	2	3
4 to 5	—	3	3
5 to 6	1	3	4
6 to 7	—	3	3
7 to 8	—	1	1
8 to 9	—	2	2

Source: Charles Swan, A. L. Tostevin, Brian Moore, Helen Mayo, and G. H. Barham Black. Congenital Defects in Infants Following Infectious Diseases During Pregnancy. *Med. J. Aust.* ii: 201–210, 1943.

lacked a formally designated control group (in this case, women who had escaped rubella). Fortunately, distribution of the women according to the month of pregnancy in which rubella occurred provided a particularly significant internal control group composed of those whose rubella occurred after the third month. This permitted the conclusion that the risk of congenital defect was high if rubella occurred during the first trimester but negligible if rubella was experienced later in pregnancy. Several later prospective studies have provided more precise (and somewhat lower) estimates of the risk of abnormal outcome (highest if rubella occurs in the first eight weeks) and have revealed that early spontaneous abortion is an important additional form of abnormal outcome (9, 10).

At this point, one may ask whether maternal rubella has been causally related to the congenital defects observed later in the infants. The evidence cited is clearly compatible with the hypothesis and is regarded as so convincing that various measures based on it are widely recommended or practiced (although so far with little effort to measure their success). These measures include: (1) the "rubella party" at which a lucky girl with newly acquired rubella attempts to share her good fortune with other susceptible girls so they may become immune prior to bearing children; (2) liberal use of gamma globulin (presumed to contain antibody to rubella) when a susceptible pregnant woman has been inadvertently exposed; and (3), if not contravened by religious scruples, "therapeutic" abortion when rubella does occur early in pregnancy. Despite the wide acceptance of the hypothesis, it cannot be regarded as established in a rigorous sense by the evidence cited so far, because all the evidence of association, both retrospective and prospective, is of the observational type.* Unlikely as it may seem in this particular instance, some as yet unrecognized factor might be responsible for both the occurrence of rubella in pregnant women early in pregnancy and for the development of the congenital defects. As a rather improbable but still possible mechanism, some abnormal hormonal activity during pregnancy may increase susceptibility to rubella and also interfere with normal embryonic development.

"Scientific proof" of a causal relation is an illusory and virtually unattainable goal, the nearest approach to which is association demonstrated in rigorously designed experimental studies. Subjects to be observed (laboratory animals or human volunteers) are formed into two or more groups by the investigator who then imposes the factor under study on one of them. Assignment of subjects to the experimental groups is a critical step which is properly done only by using some formal method of randomization. This insures exclusion of any prejudice (conscious or unconscious) on the part of the investigator in the selection process. Hopefully, it will also yield study groups similar to one another with respect to factors other than that under test which may influence the outcome of the experiment.

Experiments involving deliberate attempts to produce disease in man are limited by obvious ethical considerations. In a crucial but necessarily small-scale experiment (because of the danger to human life), the Walter Reed Commission in 1900–1901 assigned human volunteers to groups which were subjected to various types of possible exposure to yellow fever (11). This epic study confirmed the hypothesis of Carlos Finlay, since the disease developed only in those volunteers who were bitten by

---

*Recently it has been shown that rubella virus infects the fetus and that aborted fetuses or live-born defective children harbor the virus (10). Although still observational in nature, this direct linkage of the suspected agent with the "disease site" is a most compelling argument for a causal relation.

Aedes aegypti mosquitoes which had fed previously on patients in the early stages of yellow fever.

When human subjects are involved, experimental attempts to prevent disease are much more readily accepted than attempts to produce disease and, fortunately, may have equal significance. The 1954 field trial of the Salk vaccine, involving nearly two million children, was conducted in two distinct parts (12). The better planned but smaller portion of this experiment involved 750,000 first-, second-, and third-grade children of consenting parents in many parts of the United States. By a formal method of randomization they were divided into vaccine and placebo-control groups of equal size, similar, hopefully, with respect to pre-existing natural immunity and risk of future exposure to poliovirus infection. In the less well-controlled part of the experiment vaccine was given to second-graders, while first- and third-grade children served as uninoculated controls. In this trial, very large numbers of subjects were necessary to ensure meaningful results because clinical poliomyelitis occurs with relative infrequency. If the causal relation of poliovirus to clinical poliomyelitis had not been established already, the success of this trial would have helped to demonstrate the relation. Indeed, crucial demonstration of suspected causal relations often can be obtained by the successful experimental application of preventive measures based on such suspected relations. Returning to yellow fever, the work of General William Gorgas, in successfully controlling the disease in Cuba and Panama by attacking the suspected mosquito vector, should have erased any lingering doubts as to the validity of the mosquito hypothesis.

1-4   The Foundations of Epidemiology

It must be clear by now that epidemiology is not the proprietor of a well-defined and homogeneous body of knowledge, as is the case with a basic or pure science such as chemistry. Rather, epidemiology is a discipline which has evolved relatively specialized methods for investigating disease causation and bringing to bear, according to the needs of the moment, specific knowledge and special skills from many other sciences. With some justice, epidemiology has been called a method rather than an independent science. The array of other disciplines upon which epidemiology may draw is too large to permit their complete enumeration here. However, some examples will suggest the extent to which epidemiology relies on other sciences.

It is almost axiomatic that the ability to identify or diagnose a specific disease with reasonable reliability is a prerequisite to its epidemiologic study. For example, the clinically somewhat similar diseases typhus and typhoid fever were commonly confused in the pre-Pasteur era. Only when the clinical differences were recognized did it become possible for William Budd to demonstrate the key role of human feces in typhoid (13) and for Nicolle to determine the dependence of typhus upon the human body louse (14). Specific recognition of disease (diagnosis) is in the domain of clinical medicine but, in itself, depends on a variety of other disciplines. Physics provides various diagnostic tools, including the X ray. From biochemistry comes a variety of tests useful in detecting metabolic disturbances such as diabetes and gout. From the broad area of microbiology come methods for recovering and recognizing viral, bacterial, fungal, and larger parasitic agents of disease and for detecting the development of specific antibodies stimulated by the infecting agent. Finally, diagnosis based on recognition of characteristic gross and microscopic tissue changes induced by disease (for example, cancer) is the contribution of pathology.

A second large area relates to the study of specific disease agents. For the moment we can state that there are many categories of known agents (for example, chemical, physical, and microbial), that knowledge of certain basic properties of such agents is important to epidemiology, and that such knowledge is provided by other appropriate disciplines. As a single example we may consider the virus which causes yellow fever and about which much important information has been provided by the branch of microbiology known as virology. This knowledge was of special importance after 1930 when it became apparent that the Finlay hypothesis of man-to-man spread via the *Aedes aegypti* mosquito did not explain the occurrence of yellow fever in many rural and forested areas. Of basic import was the knowledge that yellow fever virus can remain alive under ordinary conditions for only a brief period in the free state and that its longer survival and multiplication can occur only within suitable cells of susceptible living hosts. This meant that the long-term persistence of the virus in nature and its transmission could not be mediated by simple environmental contamination but must depend on periodic transfer from one host to another, in this instance an alternating series of vertebrate and arthropod (vector) hosts. Determination of which species of hosts participated in the newly recognized sylvatic cycle of yellow fever required a combination of laboratory and field studies. The former were concerned with the susceptibility of potential vertebrate and arthropod hosts to infection and the ability of susceptible arthropods to transmit the infection. The studies in the field represented efforts to trace the virus in nature and depended on methods for recovering virus from currently infected hosts, for identifying that recovered as yellow fever virus, and for detecting antibody to yellow fever virus in previously infected vertebrates, both man and lower animals. The rural occurrence of yellow fever in man was found to result from a spillover of virus from a transmission cycle in the forest canopy. This cycle involves tree-dwelling mosquitoes and monkeys, the particular species of each varying from one region to another in South America and Africa. Man becomes infected only when he intrudes, chiefly for occupational reasons, into the realm of the sylvatic vectors (15).

The physical and biological setting in which disease occurs and disease agents are harbored is another important area for study. The field study of sylvatic or jungle yellow fever, for example, depended heavily on knowledge of the flora and fauna of the affected regions. Entomologists were needed to determine which blood-sucking arthropod species were sufficiently abundant to play a significant role and what were their individual preferences as to habitat and feeding. To obtain similar information regarding birds and lower animals, ornithologists and mammalogists were required. Because since the earliest times many diseases have been thought to be influenced by weather conditions, meteorology has long been an ally of epidemiology. The most important role of meteorology at present, however, is in relation to respiratory and possibly other illnesses deriving from industrial and motor vehicle pollution of the urban atmosphere.

Possibly the most important area of common interest in epidemiology is the human population. Demography provides information as to the distribution of the population with respect to many characteristics such as age, sex, race, geographic distribution, and occupation which are basic to describing the relative frequency of diseases in population segments defined by these attributes. A key aspect of the jungle yellow fever story provides a simple illustration. In 1932 yellow fever was definitely observed to occur in the absence of *Aedes aegypti* mosquitoes in the Valle do Canaan in Esperito Santo state in Brazil. The tip-off that the source of the virus was in the adjacent forests was the fact that the population most affected was the adult male who worked in the forests cutting wood and building roads (15).

Existing information and special survey methods for acquiring needed additional information concerning economic status, habits, customs, attitudes, and other social factors that may influence health are the special contribution of the social sciences, particularly cultural anthropology and sociology. Examples of such influences range from grossly obvious to relatively subtle relationships. The Oriental practice of using night soil (human feces) to fertilize crops which are consumed without cooking greatly assists various species of higher parasites and smaller intestinal pathogens such as the typhoid bacillus and hepatitis virus to transfer to previously uninfected human hosts and so to perpetuate themselves. The Hindu scruple against taking the life of any lower form of living being necessitates a vegetarian diet (inadequate protein intake is a hazard) and makes difficult the control of diseases spread by flies and other insects (e.g., typhoid and malaria) or by animals (e.g. rabies). The habit of cigarette smoking, widespread in Western civilizations, appears to influence such disparate diseases as lung cancer and coronary heart disease. On the more subtle side, the practice of circumcision of males, in the light of recent evidence, may account in part for the low incidence of cervical cancer among Jewish women (16).

Finally, regardless of the type of disease, the nature of the influences or factors under investigation, and the approach (experimental or observational) to be utilized, the epidemiologist is confronted with problems of study design and of collection, tabulation, analysis, presentation, and interpretation of data. Because it provides guidance in resolving these problems, basic training in statistics is essential to the epidemiologist and consultation with statisticians is frequently desirable. The important role of statistics can be illustrated in part by indicating two important types of question relating to the 1954 nationwide trial of Salk vaccine which can be answered only by employing statistical methods. First, in plans for this trial a key decision was necessary regarding the size of the study population. How many children should be included in each group, vaccine or control, to ensure that decisive results would be obtained? Second, the relative incidence of paralytic poliomyelitis was substantially lower in the vaccinated children than in the unvaccinated controls; was the difference large enough that it could be attributed with confidence to the influence of the Salk vaccine rather than to chance variability in sampling from two populations with the same disease incidence?

1-5   Some Everyday Uses of Epidemiology

In the foregoing sections, emphasis has been largely on the role of epidemiology in providing new information concerning disease causation and, as an important by-product, developing and testing methods for prevention. Although there is no likelihood of exhausting important unresolved problems of causation and, correspondingly, no end to the need for research epidemiology, that discipline plays important roles in everyday application of established knowledge. These center about both the individual and the community.

In this day of relative scientific sophistication, much information concerning the epidemiologic aspects of disease is widely disseminated and nearly all educated parents have something of the epidemiologist in them. In the extreme instance, they may try earnestly to contribute to new understanding of causation. Thus, the father of a child dying of leukemia dedicated his spare time and substantial money during a two-year period to collecting data, unfortunately in an unguided and fruitless manner, which he considered to support the not unreasonable hypothesis that leukemia is infectious. More commonly, the parental epidemiologist limits his concern to efforts to protect his family against influences adverse to health. These efforts include providing proper nutrition, avoiding exposure to contagious diseases and other known hazards, and seeking available prophylaxis when exposure has occurred. Thus, when a sick insectivorous bat attacked and bit a Florida boy without provocation in 1953 (17), the father captured the animal and turned it over to the proper health authorities to be examined for rabies infection. In 1953 transmission of rabies by bats was believed limited to the Vampire species and the captured insectivorous bat was examined only to allay the anxiety of the father. Demonstration that it was indeed rabid led not only to providing timely prophylaxis (Pasteur treatment) to the boy but also to the discovery that rabies is widely endemic in bats of all species, a finding that profoundly altered existing concepts regarding wild life reservoirs of rabies virus.

Epidemiologic understanding also is of importance to the private practitioner in managing individual patients in his care. It is most obvious in the preventive aspects of practice, for example, the routine infant and childhood immunizations, guidance as to diet and activities during pregnancy, and the protection of prospective travellers by prophylactic immunizations and advice as to other measures needed to guard against the disease hazards peculiar to the regions to be visited. Such understanding, however, is no less important to the proper management of actual illness. Knowledge of the patient's usual pattern of living (including occupation), of his recent unusual activities (trips, visitors, eating), and of locally prevalent infectious diseases can assist greatly in establishing a correct diagnosis upon which specific treatment can be based. If the illness is infectious, knowledge of incubation period, duration of communicability, and mechanisms of transmission are essential to protecting others in the family. And in certain chronic illnesses such as peptic ulcer, hypertension, and coronary heart disease, proper management includes the recognition of and efforts to minimize various environmental influences believed to contribute to disease persistence and progression.

It is in relation to the community as a whole that epidemiology plays its best-known work-a-day roles. In effect, the public health epidemiologist serves as both diagnostician and therapist for the community as an aggregate. He maintains continuing surveillance to recognize problems as they emerge, investigates to determine their immediate causes, recommends the preventive measures needed to "cure" the problems, and evaluates by periodic or continuing surveillance the extent to which the "cure" is achieved. Although completely new disease may confront him on rare occasions, as when rickettsialpox first burst on the scene in 1946 in the Borough of Queens in New York City (18), disease "friends" of long standing most often challenge the epidemiologist. Typhoid fever, for example, periodically comes to life from its reservoir of known (registered) and unknown chronic carriers when an undefended pathway opens up between the infected feces of the carrier and the mouths of susceptible members of the population. Finding this pathway may be simple, as in an outbreak in 1957 involving residents of many different states who had in common recent attendance at a summer conference in the Ozarks of a small religious sect (19). In this instance, because of inadequate sanitary provisions the water supply became polluted. In other instances, as in 1946 in the Washington Heights district in New York City, the pathway may be more elusive. On this occasion a stopped-up sewer line in an apartment building housing a known carrier resulted in contaminated sewage dripping on the produce of a small vegetable store located in the same building. Because the store fronted on a different street from that of the apartment house entrance, recognition of its relation to the residence of the carrier was long delayed (20). Currently, viral hepatitis is increasingly important throughout the United States. In 1961, in New Jersey, an uncommonly high incidence in well-to-do business men suggested the operation of an unusual mode of spread. Investigation incriminated raw clams dug from the fecally polluted waters of Raritan Bay (21).

The foregoing examples suggest a final analogy with which we may summarize the role of applied epidemiology in the community. The police department normally is responsible for maintaining law and order, and the health department has a similar charge in respect to health. Within the latter, the epidemiologic unit, customarily manned by specially trained physicians, nurses, and other personnel, is in many ways the counterpart of the detective bureau. Each problem of importance, whether posed by an old or new disease, requires painstaking investigation. Except for the usual preclusion of the experimental approach, the methods are the same as those used in epidemiologic research. Indeed, they not infrequently lead to truly new information, since even well-known diseases occasionally find new ways of manifesting themselves.

1-6   Summary

Major concerns of epidemiology are: (1) discovery of factors essential to or contributing to disease occurrence; and (2) development of methods for disease prevention.

Epidemiology originated in relation to the great epidemic diseases. However, its scope now embraces all diseases. Because of their increasing relative importance, chronic and noninfectious diseases are progressively more frequent subjects of epidemiologic study.

Epidemiology is more method than a body of knowledge. In investigating disease causation, it depends heavily on knowledge and skills drawn as needed from many other sciences. These include clinical medicine, microbiology, pathology, zoology, demography, anthropology, sociology, and, almost universally, statistics.

Investigation of a disease begins with description of its occurrence in terms permitting recognition of that population at greatest risk. The pattern of occurrence, by analogy with other diseases of known causation or by associations suggested, provides the basis for hypotheses as to disease causation. To be fully acceptable, any hypothesis must be consistent with the known facts regarding disease occurrence. Hypotheses are tested by controlled studies of observational or experimental nature. For the former, two basically different but analytic approaches may be employed. The retrospective approach involves a search for some significant difference in the past experience of groups of patients and comparable nonpatients. The prospective approach involves the search for significant differences in the occurrence of a specific disease among comparable groups exposed and not exposed to a suspect causative factor. Experimental studies also are prospective, but exposure (to potentially causative or preventive factors) is imposed on or withheld from groups chosen by some randomizing method, use of which excludes possible prejudice in selection of groups and helps assure their comparability.

Epidemiology also has work-a-day roles in applying existing knowledge in disease prevention and investigation of disease occurrence. The epidemiologist is, in effect, a disease detective.

GLOSSARY

Carriers (chronic)   Healthy persons harboring and excreting an infectious agent (for a long period or indefinitely).

Communicability (period of)   Time during which a patient with an infectious disease is a potential source of infection for other persons.

Endemic   Usual frequency of disease occurrence.

Epidemic   Unusually frequent occurrence of disease in the light of past experience.

Epidemiology   The study of the factors determining the occurrence of disease in populations.

Etiology (etiologic)   Cause (causative).

Incubation period   Interval between effective exposure to an agent (usually infectious) and onset of related disease.

Pathogen   Agent capable of causing disease.

Placebo   In present usage, an inactive preparation given to control subjects in trials of a similar-appearing active preparation (vaccine, drug, etc.); traditionally, the inactive "pink pills" given by physicians to please or satisfy patients for whom no active medication is indicated.

REFERENCES

1. Maurois, André. *The Life of Sir Alexander Fleming*. London: Jonathan Cape, 1959, pp. 124–125.
2. Jenner, Edward. An inquiry into the causes and effects of the variola vaccinae, a disease discovered in some of the western counties of England, particularly Gloucestershire, and known by the name of cow pox. 1798. Reprinted by Cassell & Company, 1896. Available in Pamphlet Vol. 4232, Army Medical Library, Washington, D.C.
3. Johnson, Harold N. Rabies Virus in *Viral and Rickettsial Infections of Man*, 4th ed., Frank L. Horsfall and Igor Tamm, eds. Philadelphia: J. B. Lippincott, 1965, Chap. 38.
4. *Snow on Cholera*, being a reprint of two papers by John Snow, M.D., together with a biographical memoir by B. W. Richardson and an introduction by Wade Hampton Frost. New York: Commonwealth Fund, 1936.
5. Castle, William B., Drinker, Katherine R., and Drinker, Cecil K. Necrosis of the jaw in workers employed in applying a luminous paint containing radium. *J. Indust. Hyg.* **7**:371–382, 1925.
6. Finlay, Carlos. El mosquito hipotéticamente considerado coma agente de transmission de la fiebre amarilla. *An. r. Acad. de cien. med. de la Habana* **18**:147–169, 1881.
7. Gregg, N. McAlister. Congenital cataract following German measles in the mother. *Trans. Ophthal. Soc. Aust.* **3**:35–46, 1941.
8. Swan, Charles, Tostevin, A. L., Moore, Brian, Mayo, Helen, and Black, G. H. Barham. Congenital defects in infants following infectious diseases during pregnancy. *Med. J. Aust.* **ii**:201–210, 1943.
9. Siegel, Morris and Greenberg, Morris. Fetal death, malformation and prematurity after maternal rubella—results of a prospective study, 1949–1958. *New Eng. J. Med.* **262**:389–393, 1960.
10. Dudgeon, J. A. Maternal rubella and its effect on the foetus. *Arch. Dis. Child.* **42**:110–125, 1967.
11. Reed, Walter. The propagation of yellow fever: observations based on recent researches. *Med. Record* **60**:201–209, 1901.
12. Francis, Thomas Jr., *et al.* An evaluation of the 1954 poliomyelitis vaccine trials. *Amer. J. Public Health* **45**:(5) Part 2, 1955.
13. Budd, William. *Typhoid Fever: Its Nature, Mode of Spreading, and Prevention* (London, 1873). Reprinted by Delta Omega, New York, 1931.
14. Nicolle, C., Comte, C., and Conseil, E. Transmission experimentale du typhus exanthematique par le pou du corps. *C. R. Acad. Sci.* **148**:486–489, 1909.

15. Warren, Andrew J. Landmarks in the Conquest of Yellow Fever in *Yellow Fever*. George K. Strode, ed. New York: McGraw-Hill, 1951, Chap. 1.
16. Terris, Milton and Oalmann, Margaret. Carcinoma of the cervix. An epidemiologic study. *J. Amer. Med. Ass.* **174**:1847–1851, 1960.
17. Venters, Homer D., Hoffert, Warren R., Scatterday, James E., and Hardy, Albert V. Rabies in bats in Florida. *Amer. J. Public Health* **44**:182–185, 1954.
18. Huebner, Robert J. Rickettsialpox—General Considerations of a Newly Recognized Rickettsial Disease in *Rickettsial Diseases of Man*. F. R. Moulton, ed. Washington D.C.: American Association for the Advancement of Science, 1948, pp. 113–117.
19. Neill, William A., Martin, J. D., Belden, E. A., and Trotter, W. Yates. A widespread epidemic of typhoid fever traced to a common exposure. *New Eng. J. Med.* **259**:667–672, 1958.
20. Rouché, Berton. A Game of Wild Indians in *Eleven Blue Men*. New York: Berkley Publishing Company, 1953, pp. 30–43.
21. Dougherty, W. J., and Altman, R. Viral hepatitis in New Jersey 1960–1961. *Amer. J. Med.* **32**:704–716, 1962.

2

The Roots of Epidemiology

2-1 Prehistoric Understanding of Disease Causation

As noted in the previous chapter, epidemiology was born of the study of the great epidemic diseases such as bubonic plague, cholera, and smallpox which occured in periodic waves associated with high mortality. These dramatic events understandably attracted the first serious efforts to explain disease occurrence. The evolution of man's understanding of the causation of such diseases is a fascinating story which merits at least brief recapitulation here.

We can only speculate as to man's beliefs concerning the origins of disease in prehistoric times. Unquestionably, traumatic causation of disease, often fatal, was quite clearly understood from the beginning, and such understanding was exploited in personal and intertribal combat in the evolution of both weapons and protective devices. Poisoning also must have been recognized at a relatively early stage, since, as illustrated by the story of Socrates and the cup of hemlock, it was a widely recognized selective method of individual destruction from the beginning of written history. However, diseases resulting from more subtle causes such as infection probably were explained, if at all, on the basis of relatively primitive *post hoc ergo propter hoc* reasoning which was heavily influenced by prevailing superstitions and religious beliefs. Chance association of prominent events such as the increasing prevalence of rabies in relation to the rising of the dog star (Sirius) or outbreaks of dysentery in relation to flooding of the Nile led to concepts of causal relations of divine or supernatural forces.

19

2-2 The First Epidemiologist

Hippocrates (*c.* B.C. 460–377) is regarded as the father of clinical medicine because of his accurate descriptions of syndromes on the basis of characteristic symptoms and findings and his belief that, for syndromes so characterized, rational prognoses and systems of treatment could be developed. However, Hippocrates also was the first person to attempt to explain disease occurrence on a rational rather than a supernatural basis. Since he recognized disease as a mass phenomenon as well as one affecting individuals, he deserves recognition as the first true epidemiologist. He dealt with epidemiology in three of his books, Epidemic I, Epidemic III, and Airs, Waters and Places (1). Of special significance, he differentiated between endemic disease which differed from one locality to another and epidemic disease which varied in point of time. His major contribution was one of method, namely to make and record observations in a roughly quantitative manner and, largely by intuition, to attempt to draw conclusions from them. Although he lacked the basic statistical concepts so essential to modern epidemiology, he did recognize the association of disease of certain types with such factors as place, water conditions, climate, eating habits, and housing. His admittedly primitive efforts to formulate an overall hypothesis for disease occurrence were founded on the basic idea that matter was made up of four elements: earth, air, fire, and water. These elements had the corresponding qualities of being cold, dry, hot, and moist, and were carried in the body by the four humors, phlegm, yellow bile, blood, and black bile. As Hippocrates viewed it, the root of disease lay in disturbances in Constitution, a term which to him embraced meteorologic and climatologic phenomena. In this concept and in his efforts to associate disease with more specific aspects of the environment, he foreshadowed many currently accepted beliefs in epidemiology.

The next figure of importance was Galen (*c.* 129–199 A.D.). His important contributions to medicine were in experimental physiology and comparative anatomy. In the area of epidemiology, unfortunately, he rendered only what must be construed as a major disservice. As perhaps the original "armchair epidemiologist," he wore out little shoe leather in making observations of his own. Rather, he contented himself with elaborating on Hippocrates' theories. For him, disease resulted from the interaction of three sets of factors. These included temperament, which he construed as the innate qualities of the body; procatarctic factors, which he defined as deriving from the way of life; and constitutions of the atmosphere, which apparently represented an ill-defined concept of environmental influence. His authority was such that his rigid concepts as to disease causation were imposed on medical thinking for 1600 years; for his disciples and their successors all problems of causation had been solved (2).

2-3   The Concept of Contagion

The first to give voice to the theory of contagion was a sixteenth-century Italian physician and poet who practiced in Verona. Hieronymus Fracastorius (1478–1553) was most renowned in his own time for his medical poem entitled *Syphilidis, sive Morbi Gallici, libri tres* in which he somewhat glamorized syphilis and dubbed it the "French disease." However, in a book published in 1546 and entitled *De Res Contagiosa* he expressed essentially the complete idea of the transfer of infection via minute, invisible particles (3). Although this concept was respected enough in his time that he prevailed upon Pope Paul III to transfer the Council of Trent to Bologna because of the prevalence of a contagious disease in Trent, this work and its vitally important concept were virtually forgotten for the next two hundred years. While Fracastorius must be credited with the first formal expression of the concept of contagion, the idea had long been implicit in the attitudes towards sufferers from at least one dread disease, leprosy. Ramses II and Moses were among the early lepraphobes and, by 1200 A.D., the Christian church was sanctioning such practices as the conduct of antemortem funeral services for the leper who was then provided with his bell and cup and prohibited from further contact with his fellow man or who, in more extreme circumstances, might actually be buried alive or burned at the stake (4).

2-4   Epidemic Constitutions of the Atmosphere

Thomas Sydenham (1624–1689), an English physician, has been regarded as the English Hippocrates. His contemporaries recognized him for his successful cooling treatment of smallpox, his introduction of the use of laudanum (an opium derivative) as a pain killer, and his observation of the efficacy of Peruvian bark, the original quinine, in malaria. He also revived the Hippocratic idea of epidemic constitutions and industriously studied variations in epidemics of different diseases with respect to season, year, and age of sufferer. In particular, he was insistent that observation should have precedence over theory in the study of the natural history of disease. Unfortunately, despite this laudable approach, his ultimate conclusions contributed little to the true understanding of disease causation. Apparently he considered that undefined atmospheric changes resulted in "epidemic constitutions" which, by grafting themselves onto any existing illness, gave to all concurrent illness a common character determined by the particular "constitution" (5).

The Sydenham views persisted in colonial America. Noah Webster (1758–1843), compiler of the first American dictionary, also was the most important early American epidemiologist. Educated as a lawyer, he became interested in epidemics of influenza, scarlet fever, and yellow fever which occurred in cities along the Atlantic Coast during the last decade of the eighteenth century. Armed with information obtained during extensive correspondence with physicians, including Benjamin Rush in Philadelphia, he entered into the controversy between the contagionists and anti-contagionists, siding with the latter. In 1799 he published a two-volume work, *Epidemic and Pestilential Diseases*, in which he concluded that the epidemics occurred when multiple special environmental factors combined to affect a large number of people at the same time (6). American medical men, including the influential Dr. Rush (1745–1813), subscribed to this theory for the next fifty years (7).

2-5   The Birth of Vital Statistics

Perhaps more important to epidemiology than Sydenham was a London tradesman by the name of John Graunt (1620–1674). The systematic recordings of deaths, known as *Bills of Mortality*, had been initiated in London in 1603. By 1629 this recording had become reasonably complete for the city of London and provided such information as name, sex, date of death, and type of illness. Although certain enterprising citizens previously had exploited the periodically issued numbers of dead as the basis for wagers, Graunt was the first to see in the accumulating information the basis for the earliest vital statistics. An example of his analysis of deaths in the year 1632 is provided in Table 2-1. He was able to point out the extremely high infant mortality rate and to call attention to the usual excess of male births. In addition, he utilized the mortality information for estimating the rate of population die-off and so, in effect, created the first life tables (8). Graunt's contribution is perhaps the more remarkable because it was not until nearly two hundred years later that Sir William Farr (1807–1883), then the Registrar-General, further exploited the information available with respect to fatal illness, by developing systematic statistics with reference to specifically diagnosed disease (9). We may also note that at almost the same time in the United States Lemuel Shattuck (1793–1859) in Boston began moving in the same direction (10).

2-6   Infection and Immunity

Despite failure to recall specifically the work of Fracastorius, there was, by the middle of the eighteenth century, general acceptance of the theory of contagion in particular diseases such as measles, syphilis, and smallpox.

TABLE 2-1

Excerpts from "Natural and Political Observations Mentioned in a Following Index, and Made Upon the Bills of Mortality," John Graunt, London, 1662

The Diseases, and Casualties This Year Being 1632

Abortive and Stillborn	445	Jaundies	43
Afrighted	1	Jawfaln	8
Aged	628	Impostume	74
Ague	43	Kil'd by Several Accident	46
Apoplex, and Meagrom	17	King's Evil	38
Bit with a mad dog	1	Lethargie	2
Bleeding	3	Livergrown	87
Bloody flux, Scowring, and Flux	348	Lunatique	5
Brused; Issues, Sores, and Ulcers	28	Made away themselves	15
Burnt and Scalded	5	Measles	80
Burst, and Rupture	9	Murthered	7
Cancer, and Wolf	10	Over-laid, and starved at nurse	7
Canker	1	Palsie	25
Childbed	171	Piles	1
Chrisomes, and Infants	2,268	Plague	8
Cold, and Cough	55	Planet	13
Colick, Stone, and Strangury	56	Pleurisie, and Spleen	36
Consumption	1,797	Purples, and Spotted Fever	38
Convulsion	241	Quinsie	7
Cut of the Stone	5	Rising of the Lights	98
Dead in the street, and starved	6	Sciatica	1
Dropsie and Swelling	267	Scurvey, and Itch	9
Drowned	34	Suddenly	62
Executed, and prest to death	18	Surfet	86
Falling Sickness	7	Swine Pox	6
Fever	1,108	Teeth	470
Fistula	13	Thrush, and Sore Mouth	40
Flox, and Small Pox	531	Tympany	13
French Pox	12	Tissick	34
Gangrene	5	Vomiting	1
Gowt	4	Worms	27
Grief	11		

	Males	4,994		Males	4,932	
Christened	Females	4,590	Buried	Females	4,603	Whereof, of
	In All	9,584		In All	9,535	the Plague—8

Increased in the Burials in the 122 Parishes, and at the Pesthouse this year—993

Decreased of the Plague in the 122 Parishes, and at the Pesthouse this year—266

Source: Wilcox, W. F., ed. *Natural and Political Observations made upon the Bills of Mortality by John Graunt* (a reprint of the first edition, 1662). Baltimore: Johns Hopkins Press, 1937.

Indeed, contagion is said to have been exploited by the Massachusetts colonists in their dealings with the Indians; if true, it constituted possibly the first instance of biological warfare. The story has it that the blankets of smallpox patients were presented to the Indians as gifts, with the result that a severe and decimating epidemic spread through the Indian tribes (11).

It is clear that concepts of immunity in relation to smallpox also existed at about this time. Indeed, they probably existed as early as the eleventh or twelfth century among the Chinese who are said to have practiced variolation (the specific inoculation of young persons with smallpox lesion material to give them, hopefully, a modified form of disease). Variolation had been introduced with apparent success into England in the early eighteenth century and was first practiced in the Massachusetts colony during the smallpox epidemic of 1721 by a physician named Zabdiel Boylston. Cotton Mather, a noted Massachusetts minister, gave strong support to Boylston during the storm of opposition this practice aroused. Thus, he shares with Boylston the earliest recorded advocacy of preventive medicine in the American colonies (12).

In Gloucestershire, England in the early eighteenth century cowpox was widely prevalent and, among farm folk, it was frequently recognized that the disease was transmitted to man in the form of minor vesicular lesions. Many believed that this gave immunity to smallpox. In 1774 Benjamin Jesty, a farmer, is said to have inoculated his wife and children with cowpox material and to have subsequently challenged them with smallpox lesion material without inducing disease (13). This incident was unknown to Jenner (1749–1823) when he repeated essentially the same experiment using material from a vesicle on the hand of a dairymaid. His detailed description, published privately in 1798 after being rejected by the Royal Society of Medicine, led to the general acceptance of vaccination with cowpox as a reliable method for protection against smallpox (14).

Another dread disease, rabies, also was partially understood as early as 1806 when it was shown in Scandinavia that it could be transmitted by the saliva of a rabid dog. This information was exploited so effectively that, by 1825, rabies was under complete control in Scandinavia and apparently has never returned since (15).

John Snow (1813–1858) was another pioneer in the field of epidemiology. In his own time he was particularly noted as the anesthesiologist who used chloroform to assist Queen Victoria in the delivery of two of her children. As an avocation, he developed an interest in cholera, investigating many instances of its occurrence in sporadic cases and outbreaks in the period between 1848 and 1854. Snow's published monograph (1855) describing his observations is a remarkable example of closely reasoned inferences from careful observations which led to concepts of the nature of the cause of cholera and its modes of transmission. His findings have stood the test of time and permitted the development of effective recommendations for the control of that disease (cf. Table 1-1) (16). Ten years before Pasteur's refutation of the theory of spontaneous generation, Snow argued that cholera was communicable from man to man, and that its cause was a living cell which multiplied with great rapidity but was too small to be seen under the primitive microscopes then in use. Transmission, he hypothesized, resulted from the ingestion by a susceptible person of minute amounts of infectious fecal material conveyed by direct contact, by food, or, perhaps most important of all, by contaminated water. Although Snow is popularly known for his detailed study of the Broadstreet pump (Golden Square) epidemic of cholera in London in 1854, his greatest contribution was probably what he called his "Grand Experiment." By counting deaths from cholera in the neighborhoods in which houses were served randomly by the Southwark and Vauxhall and the Lambeth water companies, he was able to show clearly the difference in the incidence of cholera among two populations that were alike except for the difference in the source of their water supply. As shown in Table 2-2, those whose water came from the sewage-polluted basin of the Thames River (Southwark and Vauxhall Company) had a far higher mortality from cholera than their next-door neighbors whose faucets were linked to a supply originating much further upstream (Lambeth Company).

2-7   The Germ Theory

Although Snow had forcefully postulated the existence of a specific microorganism as the cause of cholera, his concept was not generally accepted in his time. Then prevailing beliefs concerned themselves with mysterious miasmas in the air which were thought to derive from decaying organic matter or even from stardust or earthquakes. However, the germ theory of disease was just around the corner. Louis Pasteur (1822–1895) had demonstrated the dependence of fermentation upon microorganisms by 1857, and by 1864 he showed that organisms causing fermentation were not spontaneously generated but came from similar organisms present in ordinary air (17). This observation so impressed the famous English surgeon, Lord Lister, that in 1865 he virtually revolutionized surgical practice by utilizing carbolic acid to combat atmospheric germs and so minimize "putrefication" in setting compound fractures and in other surgical procedures (18). Pasteur's later work concerned itself for the most part with problems of economic importance and began with the study of a disease of silkworms that was threatening the French silk industry. He demonstrated that there were two distinct diseases caused by different bacilli and was able to show how infected stocks of worms

TABLE 2-2

Deaths in the population supplied by the Southwark and Vauxhall Water Company and the Lambeth Water Company, London 1853

	NUMBER OF HOUSES	DEATHS FROM CHOLERA	DEATHS IN EACH 10,000 HOUSES
Southwark and Vauxhall Company	40,046	1,263	315
Lambeth Company	26,107	98	37
Rest of London	256,423	1,422	59

Source: Snow on Cholera being a reprint of two papers by John Snow, M.D., together with a biographical memoir by B. W. Richardson and an introduction by Wade Hampton Frost. New York: The Commonwealth Fund, 1936, p. 86.

could be recognized. From this, Pasteur went on to the study of anthrax, for which he again was able to isolate the causative agent and to cultivate an attenuated form which could be used to induce immunity in cattle. He referred to this artificial immunization as "vaccination," a term intended as homage to Jenner. Pasteur is best known today for his work with rabies, in relation to which he utilized the term "virus" to describe a type of pathogenic microorganism which he believed to exist but which he could not cultivate. Once again he was able to demonstrate the effectiveness of immunization in preventing disease (19).

During this period of dramatic progress toward the understanding of infectious diseases Patrick Manson (1844–1922) in 1878 demonstrated the role of an arthropod vector in the transmission of the widely distributed tropical disease, filariasis, which is caused by a parasitic worm (20). This observation foreshadowed the tremendously important later observation, made jointly by Manson and Ronald Ross, of the role of mosquitoes in the transmission of malaria (21).

2-8   Proof of Disease Causation

The example of Pasteur in recovering various bacteria from disease situations led many other workers to follow in his footsteps. Among the more noted of these was Robert Koch (1843–1910) who was the first to isolate the agents responsible for tuberculosis and Asiatic cholera. Although these contributions were more than substantial, Koch's most lasting contribution was the introduction of scientific rigor to the proof of primary causation. This rigor was urgently needed, because bacteria were being cultured everywhere and all too often erroneously related to diseases. Koch described certain postulates which, he insisted, must be met before a causative relation could be accepted between a particular bacterial parasite and the disease in question. First, the parasite must be shown to be present in every case of the disease by isolation in pure culture. Second, it must not be found in cases of other disease. Third, once isolated, the agent must be capable of reproducing the disease in experimental animals. Fourth, the agent must be recovered from the experimental disease produced (22). For his contributions in the field of bacteriology, Koch received the Nobel prize in 1905.

With the stimulus supplied originally by Pasteur's early work and the discipline dictated by Koch, understanding of the primary causation of infectious diseases expanded with tremendous rapidity. However, great difficulties were encountered with those diseases now known to be caused by viruses. Problems arose largely from the fact that viruses are obligate intracellular parasites (i.e., can multiply only within cells of suitable hosts) and cannot be cultivated in pure culture as Koch demanded. Also, they often are quite host specific. Thus measles virus readily infects man but can infect dogs only as young puppies, whereas the closely related virus of canine distemper causes serious disease in dogs but apparently is unable to infect man. Because of such host specificity, it has frequently been impossible to successfully reproduce a virus disease of man in experimental animals. Consequently, certain additional considerations have entered into the elements of proof when one considers viral infections. These include the importance of the recovery of the agent from the diseased tissues themselves, the demonstration of increase in amount of serum antibody to the agent in question coincident with the period of disease, and, perhaps of most practical importance, the specific preventive effect of vaccines known to contain the viral antigen (23).

The problems of proof of causation are further complicated by a fact which Koch apparently did not recognize, namely, that infection with a potential pathogen does not inevitably lead to disease. We now recognize that healthy people frequently are infected with viruses or other potentially disease-producing microbial agents. This makes it essential that undue significance not be given to the simple fact of isolation of a potential pathogen from a diseased individual. Although modified to meet the problems posed by viruses, Koch's postulates still provide a central guideline to the rigorous proof of causation we must constantly demand. An analogy suggested by the noted British epidemiologist Major Greenwood bears particularly on the desirability of experimental reproduction of disease. Pointing out that all known facts suggest that, if one were to hold a mouse under water for five minutes, the mouse would drown, Greenwood went on to note: "But, if you wish to carry emotional conviction, you must actually drown a mouse" (24).

2-9 Expanding Scope of Epidemiology

The foregoing discussion has been almost completely concerned with concepts relating to diseases of communicable nature. This is understandable, because the study of diseases in populations developed almost entirely with respect to infectious diseases, particularly those of epidemic nature. However, as was noted in the opening chapter, epidemiology has expanded tremendously in scope. Epidemiologists are no longer concerned only with epidemics of infectious disease but have recognized that the study of potentially epidemic diseases in the inter-epidemic interval is essential to understanding the epidemic manifestations. They also have moved on to study infectious diseases that normally are not epidemic, such as diarrheal diseases of infants, whooping cough, syphilis, and tuberculosis. Finally, epidemiology has ventured far into the study of diseases that are not believed to be infectious at all. An early precedent for such concern can be found in a study of the eighteenth-century outbreak of Devonshire colic in England, a disease that turned out to be a result of lead poisoning (25). Modern epidemiology retains its interest in infectious diseases, because many, such as infectious hepatitis, remain incompletely understood, and old friends such as typhoid and smallpox and even cholera have a disconcerting way of reappearing from time to time. However, a much greater amount of epidemiologic effort is going into the study of presumably noninfectious diseases, among which coronary heart disease, diabetes, accidents, cancer of all types and mental illnesses are included.

2-10 Summary

Hippocrates stands as the first epidemiologist for his observation of the association of disease with environmental factors. The concept of contagion was voiced in 1546 by Fracastorius but was then overlooked for many years. Vital statistics were born when John Graunt, a London tradesman, exploited the "Bills of Mortality." Before Pasteur, Jenner gave practical demonstration of immunity and Snow propounded the infectious nature of cholera. The germ theory gained acceptance with the work of Pasteur and the discipline of Koch whose famous postulates introduced scientific rigor in proof of causation. Presently, the purview of epidemiology has broadened to include diseases of all types.

GLOSSARY

Communicable   As applied to disease, one resulting from spread or transmission of an infectious agent.

Contagion Literally, transmission of infection by direct contact; liberalized to include short-range airborne spread and transmission by freshly contaminated fomites (clothes and objects closely associated with the person).

Immunity Insusceptibility; biologically, immunity is usually to a specific infectious agent and is one result of infection.

Incidence Number of new cases of a disease within a specified period of time.

Infection Lodgment and multiplication of a microbial agent in intimate relation to a host.

Parasite A form of life (often microbial) which lives at the expense of a living host (not always harmful to the host).

Pathogen(ic) An agent, usually infectious, capable of causing disease (capable of causing disease).

Prognosis Outlook with regard to the outcome of an illness, e.g., complete recovery, partial recovery, or death.

Vector The "vehicle" by which an infectious agent is transferred from an infected to a susceptible host.

Vital statistics Data relating to birth, death, marriage, divorce and illness (morbidity).

REFERENCES

1. *The Genuine Works of Hippocrates*. Francis Adams, trans. Baltimore: Williams and Wilkins, 1939, pp. 19–41, 98–141.
2. Sigerist, Henry E. *The Great Doctors*. New York: W. W. Norton, 1933, pp. 68–77.
3. *Ibid*, pp. 100–108.
4. Rosen, George. *A History of Public Health*. New York: MD Publications, 1958, pp. 62–64.
5. Dewhurst, Kenneth. *Dr. Thomas Sydenham* (1624–1689). Berkeley and Los Angeles: University of California Press, 1966.
6. Winslow, C. E. A. The Colonial Era and the First Years of the Republic (1606–1799)—The Pestilence That Walketh in Darkness. No. 1 in *The History of American Epidemiology*, Franklin H. Top, ed. St. Louis: C. V. Mosby, 1954. pp. 36–44.
7. *Ibid*, pp. 31–36.
8. Wilcox, W. F., ed. *Natural and Political Observations made upon the Bills of Mortality by John Graunt* (a reprint of the first edition, 1662). Baltimore: Johns Hopkins Press, 1937.
9. Greenwood, Major. *Medical Statistics from Graunt to Farr*. Cambridge, England: Cambridge University Press, 1948, pp. 69–73.
10. Rosen, George, *op. cit.*, pp. 241–243.

11. Fothergill, LeRoy D. Biological Warfare and Its Defense. *Public Health Rep.* **72**:865–871, 1957.
12. Winslow, C. E. A., *op. cit.*, pp. 19–21.
13. Clendening, Logan. *The Romance of Medicine.* Garden City, N.Y.: Garden City Publishing Co., 1933, pp. 218–219.
14. Jenner, Edward. Vaccination Against Smallpox in *Scientific Papers.* Charles W. Eliot, ed. New York: P. F. Collier & Son, 1910, pp. 153–231.
15. Johnson, Harold N. Rabies Virus in *Viral and Rickettsial Infections of Man*, 4th ed. Frank L. Horsfall and Igor Tamm, eds. Philadelphia: J. B. Lippincott, 1965, Ch. 38.
16. *Snow on Cholera* being a reprint of two papers by John Snow, M.D. together with a biographical memoir by B. W. Richardson and an introduction by Wade Hampton Frost. New York: Commonwealth Fund, 1936.
17. Pasteur, Louis. The Physiological Theory of Fermentation in *Scientific Papers.* Charles W. Eliot, ed. New York: P. F. Collier & Son, 1910, pp. 289–381.
18. Sigerist, Henry E., *op. cit.*, pp. 375–379.
19. Pasteur, Louis. Prevention of Rabies in *The Founders of Modern Medicine* by Elie Metchnikoff. New York: Walden Publications, 1939, pp. 379–387.
20. Faust, Ernest C., Beaver, Paul C., and Jung, Rodney C. *Animal Agents and Vectors of Human Disease*, 3rd ed., Philadelphia: Lea and Febiger, 1968, p. 278.
21. Ross, Ronald. *The Prevention of Malaria.* New York: E. P. Dutton, 1910.
22. Frobisher, Martin. *Fundamentals of Microbiology.* 7th ed. Philadelphia: W. B. Saunders, 1962, p. 354.
23. Huebner, Robert J. The virologist's dilemma. *Ann. N.Y. Acad. Sci.* **67**:430–438, 1957.
24. Greenwood, Major. *Epidemics and Crowd-Diseases.* London: Williams and Norgate Ltd., 1935, p. 59.
25. Baker, George. *An Inquiry concerning the cause of the Endemial Colic of Devonshire.* Medical Transactions, Vol. 1, 3rd ed. London: College of Physicians, Printed for J. Dodsley, P. Elmsly, and Leigh and Sotheby, 1785, pp. 175–256.

3

Disease Causation:
General Concepts and the
Nature and Classification
of Disease Agents

The history of epidemiology is really the story of the evolution of our ideas as to disease causation. The high points in this story undoubtedly deal with the work of Pasteur and his immediate successors in identifying specific microbial or parasitic agents as the apparent causes of many specific diseases and the work of Koch in formalizing the rigorous criteria to be fulfilled in satisfactory proof that a specific infectious agent was indeed the primary or true cause of a specific disease.

3-1   Primary Cause and Contributing Factors

It is common to overemphasize the importance of the primary or true cause of disease, in part because it is conceptually simple and even more because of wishful thinking based on the comparatively few instances in which knowledge of the primary cause has led to a specific and effective preventive method such as the Enders vaccine against measles. Care of the public health would be simplified greatly if, for every specific disease entity, we could establish a specific cause, be it a virus or an unbalanced component of the diet, which could be attacked specifically, directly, and effectively. In a delightful attempt to put the importance of the primary cause in better perspective, Major Greenwood recounted the fable of Dr. Crookshank, whose civilian role as a London police surgeon involved him in studying the causes of death in murdered persons and who did his bit during World War I by studying the causes of death among British troops in combat. Since Dr. Crookshank regarded war as nothing more than mass murder, he saw clearly that the causes of death he observed were the true causes of war. Thus he emerged from the war with the conviction that prevention of future wars required finding some method for circumventing the various types of bullets and poison gas which constituted the primary or true causes of death and, hence, of war (1). To a certain extent, we acknowledge the cogency of his reasoning by our continuing interest in the success of disarmament conferences.

Another way to dispel the illusion that the primary cause is the only important cause of disease is to consider a specific example such as tuberculosis. In a very superficial way, we might say that man contracts the disease because he becomes the involuntary host of the tubercle bacillus which multiplies within him and overwhelms his defenses. The tubercle bacillus is indisputably the primary agent and all too commonly it does exist in man's environment. However, even when present in the environment, it may not reach the individual man or if it does, it may not multiply and infect him. Finally, even if the bacillus succeeds in infecting man, the infection may not result in active disease or tuberculosis. The several possible outcomes of exposure are illustrated by an episode in Denmark during World War II in which more than 300 students were exposed in a poorly ventilated classroom to a teacher who developed open tuberculosis (2). This episode, described more fully in Chapter 12, provided a unique chance to measure the effectiveness of BCG vaccine* which had been administered to a third of the students prior to the exposure. Present interest, however, centers in the group of 94 students who had escaped both vaccination and natural infection (indicated by their lack of skin sensitivity to tuberculin) prior to the period of exposure. Twenty-four of these escaped infection and remained tuberculin-negative; 29 experienced only subclinical infection; and, of the remaining 41 students who showed evidence of primary tuberculosis, only 14 developed progressive pulmonary disease. Quite evidently, simply pointing to the tubercle bacillus as the primary cause does not fully answer the question "Why does man have tuberculosis?" There must be important additional factors (or causes) which help to determine that disease occurs.

We will do well to re-examine each of the steps in the development of disease. First, does the tubercle bacillus in fact reach man? The likelihood of this occurring, much smaller in the United States now than fifty years

*BCG vaccine contains living but attenuated tubercle bacilli derived from the original strain of Calmette and Guérin.

ago, depends on several factors. These include the number of sources of the bacillus in man's environment, their proximity to the individual, and (closely related to level of education) the actions he may take to avoid exposure. Open cases of disease constitute the principal sources which, in order of decreasing proximity, may exist in a family member, in a classmate, or teacher, or in a casual contact within the community. Even in the Danish classroom situation the degree of exposure probably varied in relation to class seating arrangements.

If the bacillus reaches man, we may next ask whether it actually infects him. For a variety of reasons, including variation in the abundance of bacilli in the sputum source and the influence of sunlight and other factors in the physical environment adverse to the tubercle bacillus, the number of viable organisms received may be too few to cause infection. Also, even with a potentially infective dose, the portal of attempted entry may not give access to susceptible tissues, i.e., it may be dermal rather than respiratory or oral; or the individual host mechanisms may prevent multiplication of the bacilli. In the case of the exposed Danish students who had received BCG vaccine, it is tempting to assume that defense mechanisms enhanced by specific immunity prevented infection in most cases.

Finally, admitting that infection has been established, we may ask whether clinical disease actually ensues. Again, many factors shape the answer, including dosage or number of viable organisms introduced, their special capacity to produce disease (the pathogenicity of different strains of tubercle bacilli varies), and characteristics of the human host which affect his resistance or susceptibility. These last include genetic influences, nutritional state, possible intercurrent infection, and specific immunity as induced by prior natural infection or the BCG vaccine. Only as we are able to answer these subsidiary questions do we begin to approach an answer to the basic question of why man has tuberculosis.

In general, as illustrated by tuberculosis, causation is rarely single or simple. The whole complex of causes is constantly at work in the individual, in the group, and in man's environment. Causes within the individual may include a latent infecting agent, perhaps acquired early in childhood, various stress factors that affect resistance, genetic determinants of susceptibility or resistance, and the individual's own habits and pattern of life. Within the group, cases and carriers must be considered as sources of infection, as must the mingling in children of parental genes related to susceptibility and resistance, the degree of cooperative action to combat adverse environmental influences as reflected in social structure, and the overall density of population as it affects the frequency and extent of human contact. Finally, in the environment we have mechanisms such as infection of cattle which nurture and perpetuate tubercle bacilli and many influences that affect both human exposure and susceptibility. In summary, the tubercle bacillus as a species; its strain-determined pathogenicity; the genetic character of the host; his age, sex, and state of nutrition; the operation of various stress phenomena; the extent of human contact in homes and places of work; the inadequacy of ventilation and sunlight; the lack of medical care and proper nutrition, are just a few of the determinants of tuberculosis.

3-2   Classes of Contributing Factors and Their Interaction

Health is best visualized as an equilibrium state in which multiple and diverse factors are balanced. Disease occurs when the balance is disturbed by change in the force with which one or more factors operate. As illustrated above for tuberculosis, factors of importance usually operate in concert, rather than singly, and their interaction constitutes what has been aptly described as "the web of causation" (3). Logically, a cause precedes an effect. Epidemiologically, association of a potential cause with a disease effect is suggested (but far from proved) when an increase in activity of the "cause" is followed by an increase in occurrence of a specific disease. Recognition of such association and evaluation of the relative contribution to disease occurrence of a single potential cause (factor) obviously is complicated when multiple causes are operating. Full analysis of the causation of tuberculosis or any other specific disease, nonetheless, requires that each important cause or contributing factor be identified and its importance evaluated independently.

Three classes of contributing factors are commonly recognized and are discussed separately in the immediately succeeding chapters. These deal with factors relating, respectively, to the agent, the host, and the environment. As here employed, "agent" is synonomous with the primary or true cause without which a specific disease cannot occur. Agent factors derive from those innate properties of agents which help determine mechanisms of transmission and reservoir and ability to cause disease in man. For microbial agents, these contributing factors include: (1) ability to survive in the free state (to resist temperature, sunlight, and other environmental influences); (2) the capability and requirements for multiplication outside the human host (bacteria can multiply in nonliving media such as food or milk, whereas viruses can multiply only within living cells of vertebrate or arthropod hosts); and (3) the capacity to cause disease (pathogenicity), an attribute that may vary from strain to strain of the same microbial species.

The term "host" here refers to man and, more specifically, the particular man or group of men of immediate concern. Host factors are biologic (age, sex, race, specific immunity, and other attributes that relate to susceptibility or resistance) or behavioral (as governed by habits and customs).

"Environment" embraces all that is external to the agent and the human host(s) immediately in question, including fellow men. Environmental factors, thus, are very numerous and are commonly subdivided into three classes which relate, respectively, to the physical, biologic, and socio-economic segments of the environment.

To illustrate graphically the interaction of agent, host, and environmental factors, Dr. John Gordon has employed the analogy of a lever balanced over a fulcrum (the environment) by weights at either end, representing respectively the agent and the host as shown in Figure 3-1.

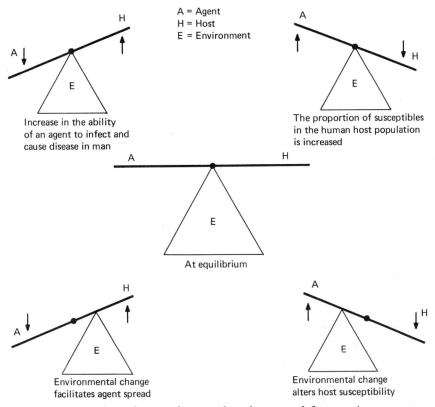

FIG. 3-1 Interaction of agent, host, and environmental factors. A = agent, H = host, E = environment.

When the system is in balance (the equilibrium state), health prevails. When any of the forces change, the balance is disturbed and disease increases. Four simple examples of change are illustrated. Increase in the weight of the agent could result from the emergence of a mutant strain of influenza virus with its antigenic character so altered that pre-existing host immunity becomes ineffective. The weight of the host could increase as the result of gradual population turnover owing to births and deaths or more rapid change in composition as a result of war-motivated population shifts. Either of these changes would increase the proportion of persons susceptible to specific microbial agents. The leverage of the agent also would be increased by an environmental change that facilitated agent spread. A dramatic example of this occurred in 1954 in Delhi when a flood-induced reversal of the flow of the Jamuna River made the sewage outfall temporarily lie upstream of the water intake (4). This resulted only in a massive epidemic of infectious hepatitis, because other sewage-borne disease agents succumbed to the heroic chlorination of the water that was promptly begun. Finally, an environmental change which alters host susceptibility would increase the leverage of the host. This can be illustrated by the increasingly common phenomenon in industrial urban areas of the sudden buildup of air pollutants during atmospheric inversions to levels which are believed to increase the susceptibility of the human respiratory tract to infection. These few and overly simple illustrations should suggest how readily balance (health) is disturbed by changes in the force of contributing factors.

3-3 Nature and Classification of Disease Agents

Agent defined "Agent" has so far been conceived of in a general sense as *the* factor without which the related disease cannot occur. More precisely, "agent" can be defined as a substance, living or inanimate, or a force, sometimes rather intangible, the excessive presence or relative lack of which is the immediate or proximal cause of a particular disease. For many diseases, including such important ones as arteriosclerosis, coronary heart disease, hypertension, peptic ulcer, and schizophrenia, the agent as so defined is still unrecognized. Although each instance in which satisfactory understanding of disease causation has been achieved has included identification of a specific agent, we must be prepared to discover that, in future cases (including some of the diseases just named) a complex of two or more factors acting in concert may be required and, even further, that no single member of the complex is in itself indispensable.

With this reservation clearly in mind, we now can undertake a survey of known or potential disease agents, classifying them systematically according to their basic natures.*

Nutritive elements Nutritive elements include not only fats, carbohydrates, and proteins as sources of energy and body-building materials,

*The classification scheme described represents a modification of one originally proposed by Perkins (5).

but also very specific substances such as the essential amino acids present in many types of protein, numerous vitamins which are widely distributed in foods, minerals (including many needed only in trace amounts), and even water. Although man has wide tolerance in his requirements for almost all nutritive elements, overabundance or relative lack of a specific food substance or class of substances may result directly in disease. Although not popularly considered a disease except in its extreme manifestations, obesity resulting from the simple overabundance of caloric intake is probably the most prevalent single disease entity in the United States.

More commonly accepted examples of nutritional disease are represented by numerous specific deficiency states which, although common in the underdeveloped portions of the world, are relatively infrequent in most segments of the United States population. Use of the term "limey" for British sailors commemorates one of the earliest recognitions of a deficiency disease. Although scurvy had long been recognized as a clinical disease entity, it was not until the middle of the eighteenth century that Dr. James Lind demonstrated that citrus fruits were a specific preventive (6). On the basis of his work, the British navy in 1795 made the inclusion of limes or lime juice a compulsory part of the shipboard diet of sailors. The specific vitamin involved in this case is known as vitamin C or, chemically, as ascorbic acid, a substance which is readily synthesized. A much more recent but equally classic example of deficiency disease is pellagra. Associated with neurologic manifestations and a prominent skin rash, this disease manifested a particularly high incidence in the late spring and early summer among the families of cotton mill workers in the southeastern part of the United States. The classical epidemiologic investigations by Goldberger and his associates led to the clear demonstration that pellagra is not an infectious disease (as had previously been supposed) but is due to deficiency in the niacin component of the B 12 vitamin complex (7).

Currently, there is a great interest in the possibility that the quality of one class of foods may be important in determining the occurrence of arteriosclerosis. As a class of foods, fats come in two forms: saturated (meaning that the carbon atoms of the contained fatty acids are bound to a full complement of hydrogen atoms) and unsaturated (the carbon atoms can bind to additional hydrogen atoms). Saturated fats come chiefly from animal sources such as eggs, dairy products, pork, and prime beef; unsaturated fats are of vegetable origin. As the United States has become more affluent, consumption of foods rich in saturated fats has increased. The underlying hypothesis is that high intake of saturated fats often gives rise to abnormally high levels of blood cholesterol which is then deposited on the walls of blood vessels as the first step in the development of arteriosclerosis (hardening of the arteries). It is further contended that unsaturated fats, which are equally nutritious calorically, are not converted into cholesterol and may in fact serve to depress serum cholesterol levels if included in the diet in proper proportions (8).

Exogenous chemical agents The group of exogenous chemical agents includes those irritants, poisons, and allergens which arise outside of the host and are capable of producing disease when they come in contact with or enter the host. They range in nature from chemical poisons such as arsenic (well known, at least to the mystery story fan) to the common allergens such as ragweed and might be construed to include even water. Inhalation of too much water results in death by drowning, but the question, albeit a bit academic, is whether the agent of disease in this instance is water (too much) or air (too little). In general, whether or not disease is produced and the type of disease if it is produced are governed by the portal of entry and the nature of the agent itself. Poisonous mushrooms, for example, can be handled with safety but induce characteristic and often fatal disease when eaten. One basis for classifying exogenous chemical agents depends on the usual mode of transmission and portal of entry.

Noxious substances that are borne in the air and produce their harmful effects when inhaled are referred to as inhalants. These include gases such as carbon monoxide, vapors from commercial or household solvents of which carbon tetrachloride is very familiar, fumes that arise from molten metals, and an array of airborne particles including pollens and irritating dust. Two problems of great current interest revolve about agents that fall in the general class of inhalants. One of these is the problem of pollution of the air with noxious gases and fumes deriving from industrial processes and automobile exhausts. These pollutants are suspected of playing a role in the excess mortality from lung cancer in urban areas, in the evolution of emphysema and other chronic respiratory diseases, and also in triggering epidemics of severe and often fatal asthmatic attacks when atmospheric inversions lead to the development of heavy smog as has happened periodically in London or in a notorious episode in Donora, Pennsylvania in 1948 (9). A second problem is the increasing use of aerosolized toxic insecticides with a resulting hazard to the user and to others who may be close by. This reawakening of interest in the disease-producing potential of the air around us is more than faintly reminiscent of the ancient concern about "miasmas."

Other exogenous chemical agents usually gain entrance into the human host when ingested with food or beverages. These often are accidental adulterants such as boric acid or ordinary table salt mistakenly used for powdered or granulated sugar in the preparation of infants' feeding formulas. Rachel Carson's popular book *Silent Spring* (10) has led to increased concern about inclusion in foods of trace amounts of the newer and highly poisonous insecticides. The concern here is not with immediate consequences but with possible long-term effects resulting from the gradual accumulation in the human body of these stable and hard-to-eliminate compounds. Particularly dramatic was the nearly complete absence of cranberries for Thanksgiving in 1960. The great bulk of the cranberry crop was withheld from the market because it had been sprayed with an insecticide which had just been reported to produce cancer in rats. Whether or not such a carcinogenic effect would have occurred in man was and is not known.

Even medicines are a source of very great concern. The ordinary aspirin tablet in usually recommended dosage can lead to the depression of bone marrow activity and resulting hemorrhagic disease in occasional sensitive individuals. Overdosage can be lethal, especially in small children, who may mistake specially flavored aspirin for candy and consume the entire contents of a bottle. The most difficult problem of all, the possible long-term harmful effects of medicines, has been a continuing concern of our federal Food and Drug Administration. In 1964 this agency earned the well-deserved plaudits of the President and the nation by withholding a license for a new tranquilizer, thalidomide. In other countries, particularly in Germany, this drug proved to have a highly developed ability to interfere with the normal development of fetuses when taken by women in the early months of pregnancy.

A final group of exogenous agents is made up of those which ordinarily exert their harmful effect by simple skin contact. Many of these are contacted in the course of normal occupations and lead to characteristic skin eruptions over exposed surfaces, including the well-advertised entity known as "dishpan hands." Others represent such natural hazards as poison ivy and poison oak which also affect exposed skin surfaces (sometimes extensively when exposure of persons wearing bathing suits occurs). Still other substances, including some of the newer insecticides, can actually invade the body through the skin, although they do not cause obvious dermal disease.

Endogenous chemical agents   Human bodily functions, if not properly regulated, may give rise within the body to chemicals which work to produce disease. These may be abnormal products such as those resulting from the breakdown of tissue in extensive burns. More often they are normal products of metabolic activity which are in relative excess or deficiency. Normal breakdown products of tissue metabolism may accumulate abnormally when impaired kidney function interferes with their elimination, a condition referred to as uremia. Serum bilirubin (a product of the breakdown of hemoglobin) may accumulate to abnormally high levels, causing yellowing of the eyeballs and skin (jaundice) when the normal excretory function of the liver is impaired in certain types of liver disease. Lipids in the blood serum, particularly cholesterol, have already been mentioned in relation to the development of arteriosclerosis.

Hormones, produced by the glands of internal secretion (endocrine), comprise an especially important class of endogenous chemical agents. The more common diseases associated with over- or undersecretion of particular hormones are generally well known. Thus, in the case of thyroxin, we are familiar with the popeyed expression and highly nervous disposition of the victim of hyperthyroidism and with the contrasting placidity and tendency to overweight observed in persons with hypo-thyroidism. Over- or underproduction of pituitary growth hormone is infrequent but leads to the well-known growth disturbances, of giantism and dwarfism, respectively. Similar illustrations could be cited for every endocrine gland and its associated hormones. In each case, the immediate cause of disease (the agent) is the chemical hormone produced endo-genously by the host. Less well understood but of great interest is the apparent relation of certain sex hormones to cancers of such organs as the breast in women and the prostate in men. Progression of these cancers often can be slowed in women by removal of the ovaries or injection of male hormones and in men by removal of the testes or injection of female hormones. For his pioneering work in this field Charles Huggins was awarded the Nobel Prize in Medicine in 1966.

Physiologic factors   This heading is paradoxical since, by definition, physiologic factors are those that determine the normal physiology of the body. Nonetheless, events and changes that evolve in the "normal" life span have relation to specific disease conditions in certain individuals. One of these events is pregnancy. When the developing fetus is abnormally located, as in a fallopian tube, pregnancy (or the fetus) is clearly the agent of potentially serious disease. Although its role as an agent of disease otherwise is less clear, pregnancy also is a condition which is necessary and essential to a series of disease conditions known as toxemias of pregnancy. These range from somewhat aggravated morning sickness (hyperemesis gravidarum) to the very serious complication known as eclampsia.

Aging is another phenomenon in the general category of physiologic factors. However, it is more readily visualized as a contributing cause of disease than as a primary or necessary cause. For example, our ability to deal effectively with infection in the absence of specific immunity tends to decrease with age after early childhood. In the case of very common infections this phenomenon is masked by the rapid increase with age in the prevalence of specific immunity. Thus, the frequency of poliomyelitis decreases sharply with age because the number of nonimmunes also decreases. However, among those nonimmune both the proportion of infections that result in paralytic disease and the proportion of individuals who die of the disease increase with age. More directly, we may think of degenerative changes which seem to be inevitably associated with aging. The loss of elasticity of the lens and changes in the ocular muscles often result in a serious visual handicap in older individuals. Loss of the elasticity of the walls of small arteries in the brain can result in significant impairment in mental capacity. These and other similar changes obviously interfere with function and hence do result in disease. For this reason, according to strict definition, we should qualify them as "agents of disease."

Genetic factors Although the concept of genetically determined susceptibility to diseases is important, our immediate concern at this point is the situation in which the gene or combination of genes itself is the direct cause of the disease. Conditions in which this is believed to be the case range from that extremely prevalent disease of males, alopecia or baldness, through diabetes and gout to more infrequent but dramatic conditions such as Tay-Sachs disease (amaurotic family idiocy), progressive muscular dystrophy, and hemophilia. The current general concept is that these and many other diseases, some of which perhaps have yet to be recognized as belonging to this category, cannot occur unless the requisite genetic pattern exists. For some, it is perhaps sufficient that the genetic pattern exist. For others, the evolution of disease may require some additional environmental stimulus. This is the general concept underlying the term "penetrance," 100 per cent penetrance being the situation in which only the gene is required. Most of these genetic abnormalities are so subtle that morphologic examination of the genetic material reveals no abnormality. However, increasing knowledge concerning the chromosomal pattern of man has revealed a number of situations in which morphologically evident chromosomal abnormalities, particularly the number of chromosomes, are associated with specific diseases such as mongolism, Klinefelder's syndrome,* and Turner's syndrome.† The problems of demonstrating gene causation are particularly difficult when the penetrance is low and when there is no association with a clear morphological abnormality in the chromosomal pattern (11). Nonetheless, the whole area of gene relationship to disease is being re-examined in the light of newer knowledge concerning nucleic acid chemistry and the genetic codes contained within these nucleic acids.

Psychic factors Psychic factors describe the somewhat intangible forces and influences that pertain to the "psyche," the conscious and subconscious mental state of the individual. Further, it is assumed that psychic factors largely derive, at least indirectly, from human relationships. With such an intangible disease agent to concern us, we need not be surprised that there is a dearth of concrete evidence that psychic factors are chiefly

---

*Affecting about 2 per 1,000 males, associated with an extra X chromosome and characterized by feminization, sterility, tallness, and, in some cases, reduced intelligence.

†Seen in 1 per 3,000 females who possess only a single X chromosome and characterized by nondevelopment of secondary sex characteristics, sterility, short stature, webbed neck, and mild deafness.

responsible for either physical or mental illness. Nonetheless, there is a strongly established clinical impression that such is the case and a serious effort has begun to mobilize valid epidemiologic evidence to support this belief. Whether psychic factors will emerge in the role of true disease agents or simply as contributing factors it is still too early to predict. There is a strong belief that some psychic element is associated with almost every physical illness. There is also an increasingly strong conviction that some organic explanation must exist for any disease state, despite, for example, our inability to explain the deaths of primitive people who have been placed under an "evil spell."

It is of some interest to mention a few of the more common situations in which psychic factors are believed to play a major role. On the minor side, headache, nausea and vomiting, or diarrhea are common manifestations obviously brought on by anticipation of a trying experience such as an examination or a football game. The signs and symptoms, it may be added, are no less real than if they were induced as the result of a specific viral infection. Somewhat more serious are conditions such as peptic ulcer and hypertension, which are quite prevalent in our modern society and are believed to have a strong psychic or emotional causative factor even though the specific mechanisms have not yet been delineated for either disease.

Physical factors   Most of us through personal experience, like the proverbial infant putting his finger in the flame of a candle, have learned at first hand of the harmful effects of the more obvious physical forces and energies such as fire, sunlight, and mechanical forces including those resulting from gravity. Somewhat more subtle, because the effects are not so immediately evident, are changes in atmospheric pressure which at one extreme may produce altitude sickness or at the other the dread disease of divers known as the "bends." Even more subtle, because the forces themselves are imperceptible and the effects may be very long delayed, are ionizing radiations deriving from the universe outside us, the geologic formations beneath us, the X-ray machines in the doctors' and dentists' offices, or from fallout from atom bombs. This last class is a matter of special concern, and we still are without definitive answers as to the magnitude of the related hazard. We know that in proper dosage irradiation of this type is tumorigenic, that it greatly depresses bone marrow activity and thereby renders the host hypersusceptible to various infectious agents, and that, by action on gonadal cells, it induces latent harmful effects manifest by mutations in succeeding generations. Factors of dosage and the degree of risk under specified conditions of dosage are problems for which we have not yet found answers. Concern about ionizing irradiation also enters heavily into our thinking about life in outer space and our program for exploring the moon.

Invading living parasites   Parasites comprise one of the best understood and largest groups of disease agents. Members of this group belonging to the animal kingdom are referred to as higher parasites (parasites, for short) and are either metazoa (multicellular animals) such as the arthropod mites of scabies and helminths (intestinal worms), or protozoa (single-celled animals) such as ameba and the malarial parasites. The remaining classes of invading parasites are usually assigned to the plant kingdom and include fungi, bacteria, rickettsiae, and viruses. Philosophically, one may boggle at considering viruses as "living," because these agents replicate by perverting the host-cell metabolic mechanisms over which control is assumed by the chemically definable molecules of nucleic acid which constitute the essence of life of viruses. Nonetheless, by whatever the mechanism, viruses do replicate and, with this as the criterion, should be considered as living agents.

Diseases caused by the higher parasites (metazoa and protozoa) are commonly referred to as parasitic and, as a class, are most important in underdeveloped areas. Pot bellies and serious anemia are caused by hookworms. Hugely swollen legs and scrotums result when lymph channels are obstructed by filarial worms. Infection with a pathogenic ameba, *Endamoeba histolytica*, can result in acute dysentery with bloody diarrhea and in serious abscesses of the liver. On a global scale the most important parasitic disease, in terms of both morbidity and mortality, is malaria which causes intermittent debilitating bouts of fever, chronic anemia, enlargement of the liver and spleen, and, on occasion, serious cerebral disease.

The terms "communicable" and "infectious" are employed to describe the diseases caused by the other invading parasites. Those caused by fungi also are referred to specially as mycotic diseases, or mycoses. Examples include such serious systemic mycoses as histoplasmosis (characterized by localization of the agent, *Histoplasma capsulatum*, in the lungs) and the widely prevalent superficial infection commonly known as "athletes foot." Important bacterial agents include streptococci (scarlet fever, rheumatic heart disease), pneumococci (lobar pneumonia), *Salmonella typhosa* (typhoid fever), *Treponema pallidum* (the spirochetal cause of syphilis), and *Mycobacterium tuberculosis* (the agent of tuberculosis). Rickettsiae form a small but important group which includes the causes of epidemic (louse-borne) and murine (flea-transmitted) typhus and of tick-transmitted Rocky Mountain spotted fever. Viruses come in many sizes and shapes (as seen with the electron microscope) and include the well-established causes of disease such as measles, mumps, and chickenpox which are part of the usual childhood experience; poliomyelitis; most acute upper respiratory illnesses; several serious forms of encephalitis, including rabies; and a number of more exotic diseases such as yellow fever. Viruses also are blamed by practicing physicians for most apparently infectious illnesses for which no other cause is obvious (many patients are told "it's the virus").

Although knowledge concerning invading parasites has grown fantastically since the days of Pasteur and Koch, there remain two problems of great current interest. One is the possibility that some of the important diseases heretofore presumed to be noninfectious may prove to be of infectious origin after all. Of special interest in this connection are the many forms of cancer. Certain cancers of lower animals, particularly acute leukemias which have exact counterparts in man, are clearly caused by viruses. We also know that some viruses that commonly infect man (certain of the adenoviruses, most notably) are able to induce cancers when inoculated into baby hamsters. Further, certain viruses which are not tumorigenic by themselves may act in concert with chemical carcinogens (cancer-inducing substances) to induce cancers following exposures to otherwise noneffective doses of the carcinogens (12). Thus, we have the possibility opening before us that viruses may be the true etiologic agents for certain cancers and, whether essential or not, may play contributory roles in the causation of still other cancers.

A second general problem has to do with deciding which microbial agents are really agents of disease in man. Many amebas and a whole host of known bacterial species are saprophytes (nonpathogenic for man). For the most part, those bacteria that are pathogens have now been well identified. However, new viral species are being recognized with great rapidity, and many of them are coming from nonhuman sources such as arthropods or, if from human sources, from apparently healthy individuals. Because of the intimate relationship between viruses and their hosts (viruses are obligatory intracellular parasites), there is a greater presumption that viruses will be pathogens than is the case with bacteria. Hence, it is common to consider at least those viruses that have come from human sources as "agents in search of disease."

3-4 Summary

Causation of disease is typically complex. Even when the primary cause or specific agent is known, many contributing factors or secondary causes influence disease occurrence in important ways. Analysis of causation requires evaluation of these contributing factors which, for convenience, are categorized as relating to the agent, the host, or the environment.

Health is viewed as an equilibrium state, departure from which results in disease and occurs when forces in the agent, host, or environmental sectors are changed.

Agents of disease are defined as substances or forces the excess presence or relative absence of which is essential to the occurrence of disease. Insofar as known or suspected, they fall into one or another of eight broad classes: nutritive elements, exogenous chemicals, endogenous chemicals, physiologic factors, genetic factors, psychic factors, physical forces, and invading living parasites. The possibility is recognized that, for some diseases, there may be no single agent but a complex of two or more factors acting in concert, perhaps with no single factor being indispensable.

GLOSSARY

Allergen A specific substance which induces allergy (hypersensitivity), e.g., plant pollens which cause hay fever.

Disease State of dysfunction, subjectively or objectively apparent.

Endogenous (exogenous) Arising within (or without) the host.

Latent (infection) Persistence of an infectious agent within the host without symptoms (and often without demonstrable presence in blood, tissues, or bodily secretions of host).

Pathogenicity Ability to cause disease.

REFERENCES

1. Greenwood, Major. *Epidemic and Crowd-Diseases*. London: Williams and Norgate, 1935, p. 61.
2. Hyge, Tage E. The efficacy of BCG vaccination. *Acta Tuberc. Scand.* **32**:89–107, 1956.
3. MacMahon, Brian, Pugh, Thomas F., and Ipsen, Johannes. *Epidemiologic Methods*. Boston: Little, Brown, 1960.
4. Melnick, Joseph L. A Water-Borne Urban Epidemic of Hepatitis, in *Hepatitis Frontiers*. F. W. Hartman *et al.*, eds. Boston: Little, Brown, 1957, pp. 211–225.
5. Perkins, W. H. *Causes and Prevention of Disease*. Philadelphia: Lea and Febiger, 1938.
6. Lind, James. A Treatise on Scurvy. Edinburgh, 1753. Quoted in Clendening, Logan. *Source Book of Medical History*. New York: Paul B. Hoeber, 1942, pp. 465–468.
7. Terris, Milton, ed. *Goldberger on Pellagra*. Baton Rouge: Louisiana State University Press, 1964.
8. Stamler, Jeremiah. Current status of the dietary prevention and treatment of atherosclerotic coronary heart disease. *Progr. Cardiovasc. Dis.* **3**:56–95, 1960.
9. Schrenk, H. H., Heimann, H., Clayton, G. D., Gafafer, W. M., and Wexler, H. Air Pollution in Donora, Pa.: Epidemiology of the Unusual Smog Episode of October, 1948. Public Health Bull. No. 306. Washington: Federal Security Agency, 1949.

10. Carson, Rachel. *Silent Spring.* Boston: Houghton Mifflin, 1962.
11. Neel, James V., Shaw, Margery W., Schull, William J., eds. *Genetics and the Epidemiology of Chronic Diseases.* Public Health Service Pub. No. 1163. Washington: U.S. Department of Health, Education, and Welfare, 1965.
12. Martin, Christopher M. Virus-carcinogen interactions. *Bact. Rev.* **28:**480–489, 1964.

4

Agent Factors Important to Disease Occurrence

As gross as the impact of a fall, as subtle as human emotions, as evident as a burning flame, as invisible and mysterious as the most minute virus, disease agents have as one common property the fact that, in their excessive presence or relative lack, they are directly noxious to man. Utilizing the group of agents designated as "invading living parasites," this chapter will explore the additional properties of agents that are important to disease occurrence and consider the general problem of reservoir and transmission mechanisms.

4-1 Properties of Living Parasites Important to Disease Occurrence

The properties of a living parasite that are directly important to disease occurrence are those that relate to its perpetuation as a species, that govern the type of contact it has with the human host, and that determine the production of disease following such contact. Also important epidemiologically are characteristics which are useful in the classification and specific identification of living agents. Important attributes such as size, structural details, and chemical composition are intrinsic characteristics, that is, they can be described after appropriate direct examination of the agent. Other attributes are described only on the basis of the behavior of the parasites in their hosts and can be classed as "host-related" properties.

47

4-2 Intrinsic Properties of Living Parasites

The most obviously intrinsic properties of microorganisms are chemical composition and morphology (size, shape, and structure). The former embraces the genetically crucial nucleic acids, enzyme systems that play a role in self-replication and perhaps in attack on hosts, and the proteins which determine antigenic character. Morphology and chemical composition provide the basis for the classification and specific identification of living agents. In the case of newly encountered agents, classification alone may be helpful for predicting important properties by analogy with known agents similarly classed. Morphology alone commonly provides the principal basis for species identification as well as classification of the higher parasites such as roundworms, hookworms, tapeworms, and the several species of malarial parasites. For bacteria and viruses, morphology

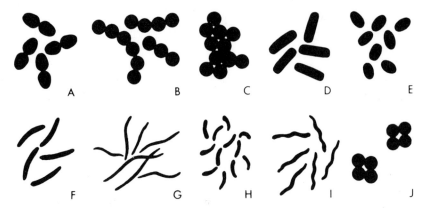

FIG. 4-1 Bacterial forms: *A*, diplococci; *B*, streptococci; *C*, staphylococci; *D*, bacilli; *E*, coccobacilli; *F*, fusiform bacilli; *G*, filamentous bacillary forms; *H*, vibrios; *I*, spirilla; and *J*, sarcinae. (Bernard D. Davis; Renato Dulbecco; Herman N. Eisen; Harold S. Ginsberg; W. Barry Wood, Jr. *Microbiology*. New York: Hoeber Medical Division, Harper and Row, 1967.)

is important to grouping but almost never is adequate for species identification. Figure 4-1 shows schematically some of the bacterial forms as seen with the light microscope. More specific identification depends on growth requirements, type of colonies formed, and, as described later, antigenic character. As shown in Figure 4-2, the electron microscope reveals that viruses differ greatly in size and also take a variety of forms. With special staining procedures and use of even greater magnification (up to 300,000 ×) fine structural details of viruses can be seen and provide a further basis for classification. Certain features of the chemical composition of viruses also aid in their classification, for example, whether their

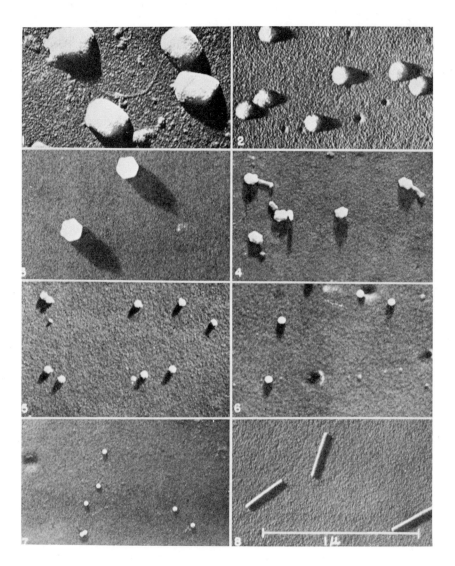

FIG. 4-2 Electronmicrographs of eight viruses shown at the same magnification ($\times$ 50,000): (*1*) vaccinia virus; (*2*) PR8 influenza virus; (*3*) cytoplasmic virus of *Tipula poludosa* (R. C. Williams and K. M. Smith, unpublished); (*4*) T4 bacteriophage; (*5*) T3 bacteriophage; (*6*) Shope papilloma virus; (*7*) poliomyelitis virus; (*8*) tobacco mosaic virus. Micrographs 3 to 7 show frozen-dried preparations. [Micrographs by R. C. Williams, unpublished; virus preparations: (*1*) by R. C. Williams; (*2*), (*6*), and (*8*) by C. A. Knight; (*4*) and (*5*) by D. Fraser; (*7*) by C. E. Schwerdt and F. L. Shaffer, all of the Virus Laboratory, University of California, Berkeley.] (Thomas R. Rivers and Frank L. Horsfall. *Viral and Rickettsial Infections of Man*, 3rd ed. © The National Foundation. Philadelphia: J. B. Lippincott, 1959.)

nucleic acid is DNA (desoxyribo- form) or RNA (ribo- form) and whether they have a lipoprotein envelope (inactivated by ether) or not (ether stable).

Their antigenic character, dependent upon both the chemical composition and the molecular configuration of their protein, lipoprotein, and polysaccharide components, is the most distinctive of all properties of microorganisms. The antigenic character is important in at least three ways. First, this distinctive property is the basis for the specificity of immunity to infection and disease. Because of this, infection with measles virus gives rise to immunity only to measles and not to chickenpox or mumps. Second, for agents similar in size, shape, and behavior in the laboratory (e.g., ability to cause disease in animals or changes in cell cultures), exact identification depends on tests with specific antisera to known agents for reaction between the agent and corresponding antibody contained in one of the antisera. With viruses, neutralization of the viral effect commonly results when agent and specific antibody react. Observation of such a result, for example, would make it possible to say that a virus from the feces of a patient with paralytic disease which causes poliovirus-like changes in cell culture is type 1 and not type 2 or type 3 poliovirus. Finally, antigens prepared from known agents can be used to demonstrate that an individual host has experienced infection with a specific microbial agent. Infection typically stimulates the production of specific antibody and the demonstration of its presence in a serum specimen is evidence that the specimen donor has been infected. In the case of our patient with paralytic poliomyelitis, examination of two serum specimens, one collected at disease onset and the second during convalescence, should have revealed a marked increase in antibody to type 1 poliovirus. This finding by itself would have been evidence that the infection had occurred recently and was the probable cause of the disease.

The long-term survival of a parasite depends on viability (ability to survive in the free state), on its growth requirements, and on its overall host range. The viability of microorganisms is a function of their ability to withstand adverse environmental influences such as increased temperature, loss of moisture, and both visible and invisible radiation. Polio and other enteroviruses are notably viable in moist environments, a fact which permits them to utilize many indirect modes of transmission. Other microbial agents such as the tetanus bacillus develop specially resistant forms known as spores which can contaminate the environment for many months or years.

The importance of growth requirements can be illustrated by comparing viruses with bacteria. Viruses can replicate only within suitable cells of their appropriate hosts and so can do no more than remain viable when in the free state. In contrast, most bacteria are able to multiply outside of their hosts if their nutrient requirements can be satisfied. The importance of nutrients to bacterial multiplication should become evident if we consider the typhoid bacillus in sewage-contaminated water or in food or milk. Given warm temperature and a little time, the bacilli multiply vigorously in food or milk. This means that the infecting dose will be large so that nearly all consumers will become infected and disease will follow after a short incubation period. In water no multiplication is possible, and the organism is subject to both dilution and gradual attrition owing to adverse environmental influences. Hence, water-transmitted doses are likely to be tiny, many exposed persons will escape infection, and the incubation period of resulting disease will be greatly prolonged.

Host range is the spectrum of animals and arthropods an agent can successfully parasitize or infect. The broader the range, the greater are the possibilities for successful links in the transmission and reservoir mechanisms. Among agents utilizing arthropod vectors we may compare St. Louis encephalitis virus with *Rickettsia prowazekii*, the cause of epidemic typhus. St. Louis virus infects many avian and mammalian species and also parasitizes a wide range of mosquitoes. The typhus agent, in contrast, has but one mammalian host, man, and but one arthropod vector, the human body louse. The viruses of poliomyelitis and rabies can be similarly contrasted. Whereas polioviruses can infect certain monkeys under laboratory conditions, they are restricted in nature to man. Rabies virus, on the other hand, can infect all known warm-blooded vertebrates.

Another important property is the vulnerability of the agent to chemotherapeutic or antibiotic substances. This may influence disease occurrence in two opposing ways. To the extent that treatment with these substances may shorten the period of infectivity, transmission of the disease agent will be curtailed. This is clearly the case in infection with beta hemolytic streptococci which cause such acute illnesses as tonsillitis and scarlet fever and such chronic and crippling illnesses as rheumatic fever and acute glomerulonephritis. In untreated infections streptococci may persist for long periods, whereas adequate treatment with penicillin usually terminates infection within one or two days. However, the availability of effective treatment can lead indirectly to increased occurrence of disease. An example is syphilis, the spirochetal agent of which also is highly vulnerable to penicillin. Because infection can be cured so easily, many individuals have abandoned precautions against infection and, for a while, health authorities relaxed their systematic attacks on the disease.

Populations (strains) of microbial species are subject to unpredictable changes in important genetically determined characteristics. Usually these result from changes in the microenvironment that require new qualities for parasite survival. This leads to the natural selection of forms, either arising by mutation or pre-existing as minority members of the population, which are capable of surviving and which often possess important new properties. The ways in which such changes may influence the occurrence of disease in man are various. One particularly vexing type of change is in vulnerability to chemotherapeutic agents which results in the evolution of drug-resistant strains of microorganisms. The gonococcus provides the most dramatic example of such change. This agent of a common venereal disease was uniformly susceptible to sulfonamides when they were introduced in the late 1930s. Within little more than a year after use of these drugs became widespread, virtually all strains had become resistant. Potentially more serious is the case with the tubercle bacillus. Prolonged treatment of tuberculosis with streptomycin or isoniazid commonly leads to the evolution of permanently resistant strains. Since other effective drugs are not available, this phenomenon is of major significance to the management of secondary infection deriving from treated patients.

At least some microbial agents can undergo change in antigenic character. The best-known example of this is influenza virus of group A. As far as now known, this virus depends for survival on a continuing chain of human infections. This it must maintain despite the fact that by about age ten most persons will have experienced infection and be immune. This resourceful virus, therefore, changes its antigenic coat sufficiently that it can maintain infection despite pre-existing immunity in the host. The normal pattern is of progressive minor changes in antigenic character over a period of years with periodic major changes so great that pre-existing immunity has no apparent influence on infection or disease. The worldwide pandemics of Asian influenza in 1957, and the Hong Kong variant in 1968, represented the results of such major changes. Such antigenic instability obviously poses a major obstacle to efforts to control influenza by vaccination.

Other examples involve changes in the interaction between agent and host and can be attributed with less certainty to changes in the agent. A number of diseases have shown a tendency to decline in severity over the years. In medieval times syphilis was a highly fatal disease known as the great pox. "Black" measles in Great Britain was an extremely serious disease as of 1800; in Glasgow it accounted for 10.8 per cent of all deaths during the period 1807–1812. As shown in Table 4-1, measles still caused many deaths in childhood a century later (1). Decline in the severity of scarlet fever is even more recent, having taken place since the 1930s. In none of these instances is it possible to decide whether the phenomenon resulted from changes in the agent or changes in the host or a combination.

The emergence of apparently new pathogens is another phenomenon that may indicate change in an agent. Presumably, such new agents of disease find their way to man from a pre-existing reservoir in the arthropod or lower vertebrate fauna. It is reasonably certain, for example, that the virus of St. Louis encephalitis did not cause disease in man prior to 1932 when a small outbreak occurred in Paris, Illinois. This outbreak was recognized in retrospect after the very extensive 1933 epidemic in St.

TABLE 4-1

Comparative mortality from measles in Great Britain

AGE (YEARS)	GLASGOW, 1908		ENGLAND AND WALES, 1960	
	NOTIFICATIONS PER 100,000 POPULATION	% MORTALITY	NOTIFICATIONS PER 100,000 POPULATION	% MORTALITY
Under 1	7,337	11.7	777	0.104
1–	14,177	14.2	2,126	0.045
2–	17,422	4.2	2,740	0.046
3–	16,643	1.7	3,041	0.010
4–5	16,560	1.2	3,242	0.005
Under 5	14,215	5.8	2,356	0.030

Source: Adapted from Morley et al., J. Hyg. (Camb.) **61**:118, 1963.

Louis (2). Since then, human infection and disease caused by St. Louis encephalitis virus have been widely recognized throughout the country. It is impossible now to say whether environmental changes opened new pathways to man for the virus or whether the virus somehow learned to infect and produce disease in man. Since human infection represents a blind end in the chain of infection for the virus, it seems more likely that some environmental change did take place.

Adaptation of a parasite to a new reservoir host also may reflect occurrence of a change in the agent. The long-established reservoir mechanism for the plague bacillus (*Pasteurella pestis*) is a continuing cycle of transmission involving domestic rats and their fleas. However, after being introduced into North America via the West Coast port San Francisco shortly after 1900, the plague bacillus established i.. sylvatic cycle involving various wild rodent species and their ectoparasites. In the past fifty years by means of this cycle the bacillus has spread progressively eastward until more than half of the continental United States is infected (3). It is not at all certain, of course, that this development resulted from an adaptive change by the plague bacillus. Indeed, the fact that similar sylvatic cycles (involving different wild rodent species) occur in South America, South Africa, Russia, and Asia suggests that a wide host range is an important intrinsic characteristic of *P. pestis*.

4-3   Host-related Properties of Living Parasites

Those attributes which describe the behavior of parasites in their hosts can be defined only with reference to specific hosts and are here referred to as host-related properties.

Infectivity is the property of being able to lodge and multiply in (to infect) a host. The basic measure of infectivity is the minimum number of infective particles required to establish an infection. For a given microbial agent (or strain of an agent) this number may vary substantially from one host to another and, within one host species, with the portal of entry, host age, and other host characteristics. Wild strains of yellow fever virus, for example, are one hundred times more infective for suckling mice than for developing chick embryos. In suckling mice they are equally infectious by all routes of inoculation (portals of entry). However, in adult mice demonstration of similar high infectivity requires direct intro-duction of the virus into the one organ containing highly susceptible cells, the brain. Such precise and direct comparisons of infectivity, usually involving animals, can be made only under experimental conditions. Except for agents such as rhinoviruses which cause trivial disease, direct measuring of infectivity is precluded in man and our estimates are based on the relative ease with which natural transmission occurs. With contact-transmitted agents one measure is the frequency with which infection occurs among susceptible persons within a reasonable incubation period following known exposure to an infectious patient (the *secondary attack rate*). On the basis of such evidence, we can order a number of familiar diseases according to the relative infectivity of their causative agents, as in Table 4-2. In this gradient of infectivity, we might use measles and chickenpox to illustrate near maximal infectivity, mumps or German measles (rubella) to illustrate intermediate infectivity, tuberculosis, as an example of relatively low infectivity, and leprosy, which may require as much as thirty years of intimate exposure for successful transmission, as illustrating the lowest possible degree of infectivity (this last may reflect, in part, a very long incubation period).

Pathogenicity refers to the ability of the microbial agent to induce disease. This ability depends, of course, on a variety of factors such as the rapidity and extent to which the agent multiplies in the host, the extent of tissue damage caused by agent multiplication, and whether or not the agent elaborates a specific toxin as do the diphtheria and tetanus bacilli. However, whatever the mechanism for disease production, the measure of pathogenicity is simply the proportion of infections which do result in disease. This measure ordinarily can be easily and directly determined by the study of naturally occurring infection and disease in man. As with infectivity, we can set up a gradient of pathogenicity utilizing an array of well-known microbial species (see Table 4-2). The agents of smallpox, rabies, measles, and chickenpox are highly pathogenic viruses in that nearly every infection in a susceptible individual results in characteristic disease. Rhinoviruses (common cold) also are fairly high in this scale, with about 80 per cent disease occurrence after infection. Mumps and German measles again fall in an intermediate spot, with from 40 to 60

TABLE 4-2

Some well-known infectious diseases ordered according to three host-related properties of their agents

Relative Degree	Infectivity BASIS: SECONDARY ATTACK RATE*	Pathogenicity BASIS: $\dfrac{\text{INFECTED WITH DISEASE}}{\text{TOTAL INFECTED}}$	Virulence BASIS: $\dfrac{\text{SEVERE (e.g., FATAL) CASES}}{\text{TOTAL CASES}}$
high	smallpox measles chickenpox poliomyelitis	smallpox rabies measles chickenpox common cold	rabies smallpox tuberculosis leprosy
inter-mediate	rubella mumps common cold	rubella mumps	poliomyelitis
low	tuberculosis	poliomyelitis tuberculosis	measles
very low	leprosy (?)	leprosy (?)	rubella chickenpox common cold

*Limited to contact-transmitted diseases.

per cent of infections yielding characteristic clinical expression. Near the bottom of the scale we find polioviruses, infection with which results in typical paralytic disease only once in 300 to 1,000 or more times. We may also point out that different strains of the same virus may vary in pathogenicity. Indeed, as demonstrated for polioviruses by Albert Sabin, this variation may be sufficient that essentially nonpathogenic strains can be found or produced which can be safely employed as living vaccines.

Although commonly offered in medical dictionaries as a synonym of pathogenicity, virulence can be usefully defined as referring to the severity of the disease which occurs. Criteria of severity may be permanent and serious sequellae (e.g., paralysis in poliomyelitis) or death. The measure of virulence is the number of severe cases over the total number of cases. When death is the criterion, this measure is the familiar *case fatality rate*. Although considerable variation in severity may be observed among illnesses caused by any particular agent (you may recall with some relish how much sicker than you your cousins were when you all had measles), we can once more construct an array of microbial agents to illustrate (as in Table 4-2) a gradient of virulence. Again let us stay with viruses, using those we placed in the pathogenicity gradient but now using case fatality as our measure of virulence. In this instance, rabies is at the very head of the list, because in man case fatality is believed to be 100 per cent. Smallpox, with a case fatality of 20 to 40 per cent, is a poor second. Polio, with 7 to 10 per cent mortality among cases of paralytic disease, might be third. Measles, with an occasional death resulting from encephalitis or bacterial complications, is far down the scale. Chickenpox, mumps, and German measles rank along with the common cold as having essentially zero case fatality.

The final host-related characteristic of importance is the ability of the microbial agent to induce specific immunity in the host, a property referred to as antigenicity or, perhaps more aptly, as *immunogenicity*. Agents may differ in this respect because their intrinsic antigens are more or less immunogenic or because the amount of antigen formed in the host during infection varies. Epidemic typhus and scrub typhus are both caused by rickettsiae. However, when incorporated into vaccines in equivalent amounts, *Rickettsia prowazekii* which causes epidemic typhus is a much better antigen than *Rickettsia orientalis* which causes scrub typhus. The importance of extent of agent multiplication can be illustrated by live-virus yellow fever vaccine. Certain passage lines of the 17D vaccine virus strain were more immunogenic than others because, it developed, they were better able to multiply in man (4). The site of agent multiplication and the extent of agent dissemination in the host also are relevant factors. Here we might contrast influenza virus, which multiplies only in the epithelial cells lining the tracheo-bronchial tree, with measles and yellow fever viruses, which spread through the blood stream and multiply in numerous sites throughout the body. Immunity to the latter viruses is much more effective and far more durable.

4-4   The Host–Parasite Relation

From the standpoint of the living invading parasite the importance of infection is not in any resulting disease in the host but that the infecting agent has found a suitable shelter in which to multiply and from which it may be disseminated. Key questions are how long the agent can persist in the host and how soon and by what avenues it can escape. The latter point relates particularly to modes of transmission and will be discussed in a following section. Present interest is in the time relations and the terms used to describe important phases of infection. Figure 4-3 illustrates these schematically.

Persistence in the host is important to the agent for as long as escape remains possible. The length of persistence (line showing agent present) varies greatly between agents and for some (certain higher parasites, tubercle bacilli, and a number of viruses and rickettsiae) may be virtually for the life of the host. During periods when the persisting agent is quiescent (perhaps hidden within host cells) and cannot be readily recovered, the infection is termed *latent*. Conversely, when the agent is being shed by the host (as in feces or respiratory secretions) or can be recovered from the blood or tissues, the infection is said to be *patent*. Infections typically are latent at first, becoming patent only when the agent has multiplied sufficiently. For many agents (especially common enteric and respiratory viruses and bacteria) infection is self-limited and the end of the patent period coincides with disappearance of the agent

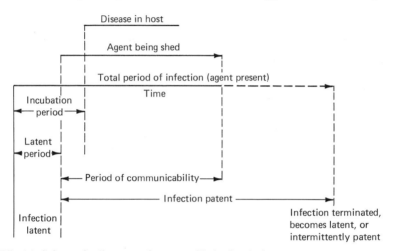

FIG. 4-3 Schematic diagram of stages of infection in host.

from the host. For others, the infection may again become latent, either permanently, as some have postulated for measles virus, or for variable periods of time. Infections with *R. prowazekii* (epidemic typhus) and varicella virus (chickenpox) may become patent and cause disease after years of latency, whereas herpes simplex and many adenovirus infections are intermittently patent over long periods.

Rapidity of disease spread is closely related to how soon the agent can escape from the host, that is, how soon the host becomes a source of infection. The time between initiation of infection and first shedding of the agent is called the *latent period*. This is almost always shorter (sometimes much shorter) than the more easily observed and better known *incubation period*, that is, the time until disease develops. The time during which the host is infectious for others is known as the *period of communicability*. It will not endure for the entire period of agent shedding if the amount excreted falls below that needed for transmission (broken line in Figure 4-3). Neither the period of communicability nor that of shedding has any necessary relation to the occurrence or duration of disease. This usual lack of correspondence between communicability of the host and presence of disease is responsible for the slight success of attempts to check disease spread by isolation of patients. Examples include measles in which communicability is greatest in the three or four days before rash appears and poliomyelitis and infectious hepatitis in which communicability also begins well before disease onset or, much more typically, occurs in infected persons who experience no disease at all.

4-5 Mechanisms of Reservoir for Living Parasites

Because it is used differently by different persons the term "reservoir" must be defined here. In many textbooks and other literature, man or some lower vertebrate is designated as the reservoir of a particular microbial agent, e.g., influenzavirus (man) or rabies virus (foxes, skunks, and so on). We prefer to define "reservoir" more comprehensively as the total mechanism responsible for the perpetuation of the microbial species. Although redundant in the light of this definition, the phrase "reservoir mechanism" is frequently employed to emphasize the foregoing basic concept. With the possible exception of agents such as the tetanus bacillus, which forms spores with almost indefinite powers of survival in the contaminated environment, perpetuation of any microbial species of necessity involves a continuing chain of transmission from one host to another—"host" in this sense including both invertebrate and vertebrate species. As a matter of generality, chains with very long links which require infrequent transmissions provide greater assurance that a particular microbial species will survive. One of the best-adapted parasites of man, in this sense, is herpes simplex virus, the cause of common fever blisters as well as a number of more serious conditions. Once man has become infected he remains infected throughout the rest of his life, with periodic recrudescence of infection. Thus, the basic perpetuating chain of transmission for herpes simplex virus may involve acquisition of infection during childhood (perhaps from one's parents) and transmission to the succeeding generation, represented most conveniently by one's own children.

It is important to note that the reservoir may consist of chains of transmission which involve alternating links representing host species of quite different types, particularly vertebrate and invertebrate. The plague bacillus, the viruses of yellow fever and St. Louis encephalitis, and the parasites of malaria are important agents which depend on such mechanisms. Such a chain is illustrated schematically for St. Louis encephalitis virus in Figure 4-4. In these instances we refer to the invertebrate host as the vector which, it should be noted, is biologically involved. The agent multiplies within the vector and in certain instances, including the malarial parasite, undergoes a necessary phase in its life cycle only in the vector.

The role of man in the reservoir and, hence, his importance to the survival of a microbial species vary greatly with the specific parasite. For many organisms, including measles, mumps, herpes simplex, and poliovirus, man—the only host—is essential to survival. For a few, such as yellow fever virus or paratyphoid bacilli, man is an important alternate host. Finally, many agents such as the bacillus which causes tularemia or the viruses of rabies and St. Louis encephalitis are pure zoonoses,

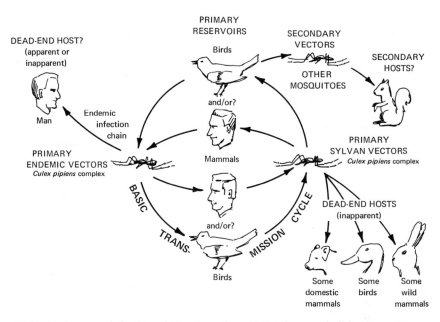

FIG. 4-4 Summer infection chains for urban St. Louis encephalitis. A. D. Hess and Preston Holden. The arthropod-borne encephalitides. *Ann. N.Y. Acad. Sci.* **70:**294-311, 1958.) Copyright The New York Academy of Sciences, 1958. Reprinted by permission.

having a reservoir which does not involve man at all. When man does become infected, he represents only a blind-end infection, as shown for St. Louis encephalitis virus in Figure 4-4.

It should be clear that participation of a human or lower vertebrate host in the reservoir mechanism requires excretion or shedding of the agent at some stage of infection but does not depend on the occurrence of disease. People with clinically silent poliovirus infections (comprising at least 75 to 80 per cent of all infection) are potentially better sources of infection than patients with "typical" paralytic disease, because the latter are restricted in activity and have limited possibilities of contact once disease develops. One might also repeat that the period of greatest infectivity for measles is during the two or three days before onset of the obvious rash.

The length of the link in the transmission chain provided by the individual infected vertebrate host varies with the agent. The most common situation involves acute infection with relatively brief excretion of the infectious agent. This is the case with the common cold, with influenza, and with such childhood exanthems as measles and rubella. The survival of the agents of these diseases depends on a continuing chain of transmission with relatively short links. In other instances, the infected host may excrete the agent for a longer but not indefinite period. Thus polioviruses are excreted on the average for about fifty days and may be excreted for three months or longer in individual instances (5). Similar prolongation of the link also results if a brief period of excretion follows an unusually long incubation period, as in rabies for which the incubation period in dogs (or man) may be as long as six months to a year. In a few instances the vertebrate host may remain infected for life. This is of greater importance when man, with his long life span, is the host than when other vertebrates are involved. The persistently infected host may be continuously infective as with the human typhoid carrier or intermittently infective as in the previously mentioned infection with herpes simplex virus. In some cases, recrudescent infection and renewed infectivity is relatively infrequent and may be long delayed. This is illustrated in man by herpes zoster (shingles) and Brill's disease which represent recrudescence of infection with varicella virus (chickenpox) and *Rickettsia prowazekii* (epidemic typhus), respectively. A final possibility is that persisting infections may be transmitted congenitally from generation to generation. This occurs with lymphocytic choriomeningitis virus in mice and may occur with serum hepatitis virus in man. Although the congenitally infected individual may not experience disease, he is a continuous source of infection for others.

Infections of invertebrate hosts also vary in ways important to the reservoir mechanism. Infection of invertebrate species ordinarily endures for the life of the arthropod and has no influence on the life span, except for infection with *R. prowazekii* (epidemic typhus) which inevitably kills the infected vector (the human body louse). Hence, if the adult arthropod hibernates over the winter, as do ticks and some mosquitoes, the stage of arthropod infection may represent a long link in the chain of transmission. Also, in the case of malaria and a number of other higher parasites, infection of the arthropod may be necessary for the completion of an essential stage in the developmental cycle of the parasite. Finally, the arthropod species itself constitutes a nearly complete reservoir mechanism when the agent is passed through the ovum from one arthropod generation to the next. This phenomenon has been observed in ticks infected with the rickettsial agent of Rocky Mountain spotted fever or the bacillus of tularemia and with mites infected with *R. orientalis*, the cause of scrub typhus. Indeed, transovarial passage of *R. orientalis* in the mite vector is essential to the cycle of transmission, because the individual mite feeds only once on warm-blooded hosts (during the larval stage). Hence, the mite acquiring the infection has no opportunity to directly infect another vertebrate host (6). This is illustrated in Figure 4-5. Fortunately, transovarial passage is incompletely efficient so that unless it is renewed by feeding on other infected vertebrates, infection may die out after three or four generations.

Finally, inanimate features of the environment may play a role in the

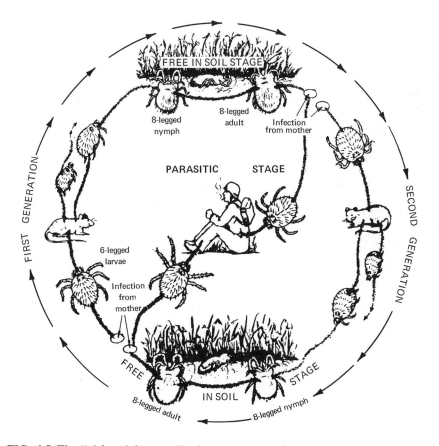

FIG. 4-5 The "rickettsial stream" of *R. tsutsugamushi* in nature through two generations of mites. Continuity through transovarial passage to parasitic larvae, transstadial passage to nonparasitic nymphs and adults is shown with new lines of infection from infected rats, and termination of other lines in accidental infection of man. (Army Med. Musuem No. 93587.) (C. B. Philip. Observations on Tsutsugamushi disease (mite-borne or scrub typhus) in northwest Honshu Island, Japan, in the fall of 1945. *Amer. J. Hyg.* **46**: 45-59, 1947.)

reservoir mechanism. Such occurs (1) when, as with some bacteria, the agent can multiply in the free state; (2) when, even without multiplication, the agent has an unusual survival capacity; or (3) when, as with some higher parasites, brief sojourn under proper environmental conditions is required for a necessary stage in the life cycle. Situation (1) is illustrated by "food poisoning," most episodes of which are caused not by a preformed poison but by multiplication of bacteria (usually staphylococci or salmonellae) in contaminated and unrefrigerated food. Staphylococci elaborate a potent poison (exotoxin) capable of rapidly inducing (within two to three hours) hyperperistalsis with acute diarrhea and vomiting. The many salmonella species produce similar effects after a longer incubation period (twelve to twenty-four hours) necessary for the further multiplication of these organisms within the human intestines. Situation (2) is typified by the spores of the tetanus bacillus or the fungus *Histoplasmosis capsulatum* which linger indefinitely in contaminated soil. Finally, situation (3) is illustrated by the infamous hookworm which must undergo a necessary state in its development cycle in the inanimate environment. Eggs deposited (in human feces) on soil of suitable composition, moisture, and temperature hatch into larvae which can penetrate the skin of the barefoot human host.

4-6   Mechanisms of Transmission of Living Parasites

Transmission involves transport of an agent from one vertebrate host to another. The sequential steps in the transmission cycle are escape from the source host and conveyance to and effective entry into the recipient host. In the following discussion we will see how the mechanisms utilized in one step help determine those operating in the next. This correspondence is illustrated in Table 4-3. Our concern, of course, is focused on transmission cycles in which man is a potential recipient host. Although man is also the most common source host for living agents of human disease, lower vertebrates may be common or, as with rabies virus, the only source hosts for some agents.

Escape means the emergence of the agent from an infected source host. The most obvious avenues of escape are in discharges from infected lesions such as carbuncles; saliva; mucous secretions of the respiratory tract, conjunctiva, and genital tract; and urine and feces, all of which correspond to sites of agent localization. Thus, typhoid bacilli are found in feces, tubercle bacilli or pneumococci in sputum, rhinoviruses in nasal and pharyngeal secretions, and the agents of trachoma and pinkeye in the conjunctival exudate. The urine may contain typhoid bacilli and in recent times has been found to harbor one or another of several viruses. Another important but less obvious avenue of escape is the bloodstream. The escape of agents circulating in the blood is usually engineered by

TABLE 4-3

Correspondence between escape, conveyance, and portals of entry

AVENUE OF ESCAPE	MODE OF CONVEYANCE	PORTAL OF ENTRY	TYPE OF DISEASE
Respiratory secretions	airborne droplets, fomites	respiratory tract	common cold, measles
Feces	water, food, fomites, flies	alimentary tract	typhoid, poliomyelitis
Lesion exudate	direct contact, fomites, sexual intercourse	skin, genital mucous membrane	carbuncles, syphilis, gonorrhea
Conjunctival exudate	fomites, flies	ocular mucous membrane	tachoma
Blood	blood-sucking arthropod vector	skin (broken as by insect bite)	malaria, yellow fever, epidemic typhus

blood-sucking arthropods that become infected while taking their usual blood meals.

Having escaped from an infected host, the agent is faced with the problem of conveyance, that is, reaching a new susceptible host. Direct contact describes the situation when no vector is involved and transmission occurs during direct contact between an infected host and a susceptible host. Most literally, direct contact occurs in kissing, shaking hands, or, most intimately, in sexual intercourse. In practice, the term is broadened to include short-range airborne spread and transmission by way of freshly contaminated fomites. This expanded meaning, indeed, is required to justify our use of the term "contagious" (meaning transmitted by contact) to describe diseases such as smallpox, measles, and chickenpox.

Indirect modes of conveyance involve the vector concept, the vectors often but not always being animate (usually arthropods). Among animate vectors it is important to distinguish between those that are mechanical and those that are biological. The former is illustrated by the filth fly which dirties its feet in the privy or on animal excrement and then wipes them off on exposed foods such as a peeled banana or slice of bread. The truly biological vector must experience infection, with multiplication of the microbial agent, before transmission can occur. Understandable ignorance of this distinction nearly defeated the Walter Reed Commission in its efforts to resolve the problem of transmission of yellow fever. After several unsuccessful trials with mosquitoes freshly fed on patients, transmission succeeded when mosquitoes fed more than ten days previously were inadvertently used (7). This experience led to recognition that infected arthropod vectors may be able to transmit only after a period of time (referred to as the *extrinsic incubation period*) during which the agent multiplies in the arthropod to a level sufficient for transmission to occur.

Indirect transmission also frequently involves inanimate vectors. The nature of these vectors and the length of the paths they may describe vary with the specific microbial agent, particularly with its ability to survive in the free state. Most common probably is airborne transmission, chiefly via infected droplet nuclei which hang in the air for relatively long periods. Fomites, meaning intimate personal articles such as a handkerchief, a drinking glass, or a well-chewed lead pencil, provide relatively direct mechanical mechanisms. Food, milk, and water provide potentially longer-range mechanical mechanisms which are usually employed by agents excreted in the feces and lead ordinarily to the oral portal of entry.

The essential requirement for an effective portal of entry into a susceptible host is that it provide ready access to a tissue in which the pathogen can lodge and multiply. Certain animal parasites and other agents transmitted by blood-sucking arthropods penetrate or are injected through the originally intact skin. Otherwise, a broken skin or mucous membrane, the respiratory tract, the alimentary tract, or the bloodstream serve as the usual portals of entry. Agents such as the rickettsia of epidemic typhus or the virus of yellow fever can utilize various portals under unusual circumstances, although both normally enter through the skin with the assistance of their appropriate arthropod vectors. Other agents, however, are extremely restricted. In particular, the influenza virus can lodge and multiply only in the columnar epithelium lining the tracheo-bronchial tree and so is noninfectious except when it enters by the respiratory route. Similarly selective are the spores of tetanus which are harmless when ingested but which multiply and produce their lethal toxin when introduced deeply into tissues where they are protected from air.

4-7   Transmission and Reservoir Mechanisms of Nonliving or Inanimate Agents

The foregoing discussion has centered entirely on living microbial agents, because this class has been longest known and is best understood. This group also provides analogies for many of the concepts and approaches we adopt in our efforts to understand other types of disease. Many of the factors relevant to nonliving agents will be considered further in a succeeding chapter on environmental factors. However, it may be useful to point out some of the analogies that exist between living parasites and inanimate agents of disease.

One example is provided by the toxic vapors that arise from a commonly used commercial solvent. The concepts of infectivity, pathogenicity, and virulence find their counterpart in the single concept of toxicity which is measured in terms of minimum effective dose. There is no problem with respect to mode of conveyance, which is airborne, or to portal of entry, which is respiratory. The term "reservoir" takes on a literal meaning, since it refers to the tank or container in which the solvent is kept.

A more difficult example takes an industrial accident as the disease. The reservoir in this instance would be the drill press or other machine tended by the injured worker. The agent might be considered physical force; its mode of transmission, direct contact (abetted perhaps by carelessness on the part of the host); and its portal of entry, the actual site of injury.

Although these analogies are somewhat forced, the main points to remember are that all disease agents possess properties which help to determine the occurrence of the disease and that, for every agent, there must be some counterparts to the mechanisms of transmission and reservoir just described for infectious agents.

4-8   Summary

Properties of living parasites important to disease occurrence are those governing perpetuation of the agent species, its contact with man, and how it produces disease. Some properties (intrinsic) can be defined directly, whereas others (host-related) must be defined with reference to the human or other host.

Intrinsic properties of importance include: morphology and chemical composition (related to classification and identification); viability in the free state, growth requirements, and host range (all important to long-term survival of the agent); antigenic character (important to specificity of immunity, identification of agent, and diagnosis of infection and disease); susceptibility to chemotherapeutic or antibiotic agents; and susceptibility to mutation (reflected in changes in ability to cause disease, host range, antigenic character, resistance to antibiotics).

Host-related properties include: infectivity (ability to infect a host); pathogenicity (ability to cause disease); virulence (ability to cause severe or fatal disease); and antigenicity or immunogenicity (ability to induce immunity in the host).

For the agent, infection of a host provides shelter in which to multiply and from which to spread. Persistence in the host is important only so long as opportunity remains for escape. When the agent is being excreted or is readily recoverable, the infection is patent; when the agent is hidden, the infection is latent. The time from initiation of infection until shedding of the agent is the latent period and is usually shorter than the time to disease onset (incubation period). The interval during which the host is an effective source of infection is the period of communicability and is unrelated to the occurrence or presence of disease.

The reservoir for living parasites is defined as the total mechanism for perpetuation of the microbial species. It comprises a continuing chain of transmission, the links of which commonly are made up of individual infected hosts (vertebrate or invertebrate). The links may be within one host species, such as man, or alternate between different species, as vertebrate and invertebrate hosts. Long persistence in one host means a link of longer duration and less frequent transmission to insure agent survival. For agents unusually viable or able to multiply outside of the host, persistence in the inanimate environment also may provide a link.

Transmission involves escape of an agent from a source host, conveyance to a susceptible host, and entry therein. Transmission may be direct (direct contact) or indirect, involving a vector (mode of conveyance). The avenue of escape from an infected host is related to the site of infection. The portal of entry must provide access to a susceptible tissue. Escape, conveyance, and entry are usually interrelated, for example, respiratory escape, airborne conveyance, respiratory portal or fecal escape, food or water conveyance, and oral portal.

Although applying strictly only to infectious agents, the foregoing concepts in some part can be applied by analogy to other classes of agents.

GLOSSARY

Antibody   A globulin, found in tissue fluids and blood serum, produced in response to stimulus by a specific antigen and capable of combining specifically with that antigen; often referred to as "immune substance."

Antigen   Substance capable of inducing specific immune response.

Antigenic character   Aspect of chemical arrangement unique to agent and responsible for specificity of immunity resulting from infection.

Antigenicity   Ability to stimulate immune response.

Antiserum   Serum containing specific antibody.

Enteric   Intestinal or alimentary.

Exanthem   Disease with skin rash.

Extrinsic incubation period   In arthropods, time necessary after acquisition of infection for agent to multiply sufficiently that it can be transmitted by arthropod.

Exotoxin   Toxin (poison) released by a microorganism into its microenvironment, e.g., tetanus toxin produced by the tetanus bacillus.

Fomites   Intimate personal articles, e.g., handkerchief, drinking glass, clothing, toys.

Host   Vertebrate or invertebrate species capable of being infected (or for noninfectious agents, affected) by an agent.

Host range   Array of hosts susceptible to infection with an agent.

Infectivity   Ability of an agent to infect.

Infectivity, period of (period of communicability)   Period during which an infected host is a source of infection.

Morphology   Structural configuration.

Mutation   Change in genetically determined character.

Portal of entry   Avenue by which parasite enters the host.

Recrudescence   Reactivation of infection.

Reservoir (mechanism)   Mechanism for perpetuating agent species.

Transmission   Transport of agent from a source to a susceptible host.

Viability   Ability to remain alive in the free state.

Virulence   Measure of severity of disease.

Zoonosis(es)   Disease(s) of lower vertebrate species.

REFERENCES

1. Morley, D., Woodland, Margaret, and Martin, W. J. Measles in Nigerian children. A study of the disease in West Africa, and its manifestations in England and other countries during different epochs. *J. Hyg. (Camb.)* **61**:115–134, 1963.
2. Clarke, Delphine H. and Casals, Jordi. Arboviruses: Group B, in *Viral and Rickettsial Infections of Man*, 4th ed. Frank L. Horsfall and Igor Tamm, eds. Philadelphia: J. B. Lippincott, 1965, p. 622.
3. Hirst, L. Fabian. *The Conquest of Plague*. Oxford: Clarendon Press, 1953, pp. 196–198.
4. Fox, J. P., Kossobudski, S. L., and Fonseca Da Cunha, J. Field studies on immune response to 17D yellow fever virus; relation to virus substrain, dose and route of inoculation. *Amer. J. Hyg.* **38**:113–128, 1943.
5. Gelfand, H. M., LeBlanc, D. R., Fox, J. P., and Conwell, D. P. Studies on the development of natural immunity to poliomyelitis in Louisiana. II. Description and analysis of episodes of infection observed in study group households. *Amer. J. Hyg.* **65**:367–385, 1957.
6. Philip, Cornelius B. Observations on Tsutsugamushi disease (mite-borne or scrub typhus) in northwest Honshu Island, Japan, in the fall of 1945. *Amer. J. Hyg.* **46**:45–59, 1947.
7. Reed, Walter. The propagation of yellow fever: observations based on recent researches. *Med. Record* **60**:201–209, 1901.

5

Factors Deriving from the
Human Host

5-1 Inherent and Acquired Characteristics

"Our nation," Lincoln stated in his Gettysburg address, "is dedicated to the proposition that all men are created equal." Biologically this is not true, even for newborn infants. In the course of the growth and development of individuals, further differences, both biological and in manner of living, become evident. These differences, whether inherent or acquired, between individuals and between groups have much to do with the occurrence of disease.

Truly inherent differences may contribute to susceptibility or resistance to various specific diseases such as tuberculosis, coronary heart disease, or cancer and may exist on an individual basis or between ethnic groups. A possible example of the latter is susceptibility to tuberculosis which some people believe is greater in Negroes than in Caucasians. Both individuals and groups may differ with respect to specific immunities, these differences depending upon prior infection experience. In a typical United States urban community, immunity deriving from previous infection operates to restrict measles chiefly to young children, among whom the build-up of susceptibles is such that periodic "epidemics" occur at intervals of about three years. However, in the Faroe Islands in 1846 measles was introduced after having been absent for sixty-five years, and virtually the entire population developed the disease because there was no herd immunity to restrict the virus spread (1). Customs and behavior also differ substantially between individuals and between groups. A personal taste for raw clams may lead to an increased risk of infectious hepatitis, or the common consumption of raw fish, as in Scandinavian and other ethnic groups, opens the door to an increased incidence of fish tapeworm. Finally, although differences are important, we should not forget the many attributes shared by all of mankind which bear on resistance and susceptibility to disease occurrence.

From the examples cited it is evident that some of the human factors that may influence disease occurrence in man are truly biologic, whereas others derive from man's behavior and may more properly be grouped under the heading "habits and customs." In the following discussion we will consider separately the biologic and behavioral influences on disease. Also, although much of the discussion will center about the individual human host, that individual ordinarily is part of a group, and factors which have an influence on him will also have an influence on the group of which he is a part.

5-2 Agent-Host Interaction

Before attempting to isolate specific factors for consideration, we may productively visualize the possible consequences of interaction between a disease agent and the human host. Although we will use a living invading parasite as a model, the principles illustrated are generally applicable to disease agents of other categories. A key principle to emphasize is the nearly universal existence of a gradient of response to exposure and infection. To state the principle in another way, fully developed, overt disease is never a reliable measure of the extent of activity of a disease agent.

The immediate results of contact with an agent may be resolved into three possibilities. First, because of inadequate dose, unsuitable portal of entry, or specific host immunity, the parasite may fail to lodge and establish an infection. Second, infection may be established but be subclinical. Third, infection may cause disease. The frequency with which disease follows infection varies with the pathogenicity of the agent. In the case of poliovirus, clinically inapparent infections predominate, whereas infections with measles virus (unless modified by administration of gamma globulin) nearly always result in characteristic disease. Further, the overt disease which occurs may range from minimal to most serious and the final outcome may vary from complete recovery to death of the host. This latter outcome is unsatisfactory not only to the host, but also to the many parasites whose survival as a species depends on the host.

Other than survival, three aspects of the outcome of infection remain of particular importance. The first is the clinical state of the host. Was recovery really complete or were there permanent sequellae? Such aftermaths may be either nonprogressive, as the paralysis following poliomyelitis, or potentially progressive. Examples of the latter include heart or kidney disease following streptococcal infections, progressive pulmonary disease caused by tuberculosis, or the slowly evolving sequence of changes in untreated syphilis leading to serious cardiovascular or neurologic disease.

Persistence of the disease agent is the second aspect. Whether silent or overt, infection almost inevitably renders the host infectious (i.e., a source of infection for others) for at least a brief period of time. The term "carrier" is used for the host who is infectious in the absence of disease, either because disease did not develop or because clinical recovery has occurred. In some instances, as in the case of Typhoid Mary, the carrier state may persist for a lifetime (2). More often, it endures for a few weeks or months as with carriers of polioviruses, diphtheria bacilli, streptococci and meningococci. Other infections become latent, meaning that the agent persists but is no longer being shed. Such latent infection may come to life later and the infected host again become an active source of infection. The viruses of herpes simplex and chickenpox illustrate these situations. The former may be intermittently shed with or without associated disease over a lifetime. The latter rarely and unpredictably recrudesces in association with an uncomfortable disease known as shingles, or herpes zoster.

The third important aspect is the state of post-infection resistance. Recovery usually is followed by some degree of immunity to reinfection. If this is incomplete, the recovered individual may experience reinfection, with or without disease, and again become a potential source of infection for others. In summary, the consequences of interaction between host and agent are extremely variable, and it now becomes important to consider those characteristics of the host which contribute to this variation.

5-3   Host Defenses

To use a military metaphor, the body of the host represents a citadel and the multiplicity of disease agents outside of the host form an army of besiegers attempting to gain entrance. Depending on the nature of the agent, one or more lines of defense are inherent in the structure or normal function of the human body.

Structural aspects   The intact skin and mucous membranes provide the body with an envelope which is impermeable to many living parasites and exogenous chemical agents. Since mucous membranes are more easily penetrated than the intact skin, the conjunctiva, the respiratory tract, and the gastrointestinal tract often serve as portals of entry for various living and chemical agents of disease. Accessory skin structures such as hair, sebaceous glands, sweat glands, and fat pads protect the body against certain physical forces and aid in the thermal regulation of the body. The anatomy of the upper respiratory tract is very cleverly designed to prevent the deep penetration of larger airborne particles into the small bronchi, bronchioles, and alveoli of the lungs. Unfortunately, the design also facilitates retention of the smallest particles, such as fine silica dust which gives rise to the chronic condition known as silicosis. The skeleton, itself, with the cranium, the bony thorax, and the wide-spreading pelvic bones, provides structural protection against physical force to vital organs such as the brain, the heart and lungs, the various abdominal viscera, and the gonads. Within the abdominal cavity, the well-lubricated surface of the peritoneum covers the abdominal viscera and facilitates their sliding out of the line of direct pressure and sharp penetrating objects.

Functional aspects Our several senses (pain, touch, smell, taste, sight, and hearing) activate evasive action when danger threatens, as when the smell of illuminating gas is perceived or an inconsiderate motorist touches his horn when you are halfway across the street. Many reflexes are important defensively. The cough and the sneeze represent efforts to rid the respiratory passages of harmful substances, the wink reflex protects our eyes from danger, and vomiting and diarrhea purge our gastrointestinal tract. Mucous secretions, as exemplified by tears, have a simple cleansing action and also may contain specific antibody against microbial pathogens. The columnar epithelial cells of the upper respiratory tract possess cilia whose beating keeps a sheet of mucous with its trapped particulate matter constantly moving towards the outside. The sweat glands of the skin are vital to our thermal regulation. Finally, when barriers such as the skin are breached or overt trauma occurs, the normal healing processes of the body commence to repair the damage and restore the defenses.

Several mechanisms aid in defense against exogenous chemical agents. For some poisons such as arsenic, nicotine, and perhaps even alcohol, the body develops a tolerance so that ever larger doses are needed to produce a toxic effect. Metallic poisons, such as lead, are removed rapidly from the circulation, stored in the bones, and then slowly mobilized and excreted over an extended period of time. Mechanisms for eliminating toxic substances include the bile, upper intestinal secretions, and excretion through the kidneys and sweat glands. The liver has a special ability to detoxify some classes of organic poisons by splitting them into harmless products for excretion.

Problems of overabundance or deficiency in nutritional elements are minimized by the wide tolerance of the body with respect to daily intake and to its ability to adapt metabolically to deficiency. Excess caloric intake is stored in the form of body fat which can be mobilized in time of caloric restriction, often with a beneficial effect on the silhouette of the host. The bones serve as depots for calcium and other minerals which can be mobilized when intake is inadequate. Particularly interesting is the decrease in nitrogen utilization when the dietary source of nitrogen (protein) is inadequate.

Defenses against living parasites   A variety of defense mechanisms confront the living agent that has penetrated the protective envelope of the body. Extracellular parasites such as bacteria commonly stimulate the development of inflammation at the site of invasion. This inflammation represents the body's effort to wall off and destroy the invaders. A fine retaining network of fibrin is deposited and numerous phagocytic cells congregate at the scene and attempt to engulf and digest the parasites. Escaping parasites are transported via lymph channels to the regional lymph nodes (filterlike organs) where they run a gauntlet of sinusoidal passages lined by still other phagocytic cells. If these regional barriers fail to hold and the parasites gain access to the bloodstream, a final battery of large phagocyte-filled filters (bone marrow, spleen, and liver) awaits them. Meanwhile (as will be discussed in more detail in a later section), the infection will have stimulated the formation of specific antibody which will combine with any persisting parasites and render them more vulnerable to phagocytosis and digestion. The initial presence of such antibody because of a previous infection would, of course, have prevented or greatly limited the invasion of the host. Viruses, because of their small size and usual intracellular position, are less easily localized. Also, although viruses are highly vulnerable to antibody during the stage of invasion in which they are still extracellular, they are little affected once they have gained entrance into cells. Fortunately, viruses still are vulnerable to the inhibitory action of interferon, a protein of low molecular weight elaborated by virus-infected cells.

5-4   Age, Sex, Ethnic Group or Race, and Family

In this and the following sections of this chapter we will be considering host characteristics of widely differing natures but which relate to disease occurrence in one or more of three basic ways: by determining degree of exposure, differences in susceptibility, or the likelihood of specific immunity. Age, sex, and ethnic group or race are characteristics of such great importance that determination of their relation to disease occurrence is the usual first step in the epidemiologic description of a disease.

Age   Poliomyelitis and measles well illustrate how age influences the occurrence of infectious diseases. In both instances infection and disease occur predominantly among young children who are selected because of their lack of immunity and high risk of exposure. Older persons are very likely to be immune because of infection during childhood and, unless they are parents of small children, they have little opportunity for contact with infected persons. Younger children, on the other hand, have ample opportunity for such contact, since they and their playmates represent the age segment of the population in which most infections occur. The predominance of immunes among older persons often masks the relation of age to susceptibility. For most infectious agents, both the proportion of infections in nonimmune persons that are clinically overt and the severity of the resulting disease increase directly with age. This age factor is most evident when outbreaks occur in populations which, because of their isolation, have been free of infection for many years and so are largely nonimmune. The Faroe Islands experience with measles in 1846 is shown in Table 5-1. Although attack rates were high in all age groups,

TABLE 5-1
Measles on the Faroe Islands in 1846. Attack rates and case fatality by age

AGE (YEARS)	POPULATION	NUMBER ATTACKED	ATTACK RATE (PER CENT)	NUMBER OF DEATHS	CASE FATALITY (PER CENT)
<1	198	154	77.8	44	28.6
1–9	1440	1117	77.7	3	0.3
10–19	1525	1183	77.6	2	0.2
20–29	1470	1140	77.6	4	0.3
30–39	842	653	77.6	10	1.5
40–59	1519	1178	77.6	46	3.9
60–79	752	583	77.5	46	7.9
80+	118	92	78.0	15	16.3
Total	7864	6100	77.6	170	2.8

Source: Peter L. Panum. Observations Made During the Epidemic of Measles on the Faroe Islands in the Year 1846. New York: Delta Omega Society, 1940, p. 82. Notes by the editor (Dr. J. A. Doull) and translators (Ada Hatcher and Joseph Dimont).

case fatality varied significantly, being highest under one year and then rising steadily for those over age thirty. The 1949 outbreak of poliomyelitis among Hudson Bay Eskimos (Table 5-2) revealed an attack rate for overt disease rising with age up to twenty years in an almost totally infected population and a low case fatality under age ten (3).

Sex Variations in disease occurrence between the sexes often reflect differences in exposure which relate to differences in play habits among children and in occupations during adulthood. Typical, for example, is the increased risk of intra-household exposure that is built into the role of mother or older sister who nurses an ill family member. Differences in susceptibility intrinsically owing to sex are less readily documented. Below age twenty poliovirus infections are equally frequent in both sexes, but

TABLE 5-2

Poliomyelitis among Eskimos in Chesterfield Inlet, Hudson Bay, in 1949. Attack rates and case fatality by age

AGE (YEARS)	POPULATION	NUMBER OF CASES	ATTACK RATE (PER CENT)	NUMBER OF DEATHS	CASE FATALITY (PER CENT)
0–4	53	2	4	0	
5–9	56	13	23	1	7.7
10–14	33	8	25	3	37.5
15–19	26	11	42	3	27.2
20–29	30	6	20	0	0
30–49	52	12	23	4	33.3
50+	25	5	20	3	60.0
Total	275	57		14	

Source: A. F. W. Peart. An outbreak of poliomyelitis in Canadian Eskimos in wintertime. Epidemiological features. *Canad. J. Public Health* **40**: 410, 1949 (Oct.).

the frequency of paralytic disease in boys has for years been 1.3 times that in girls. Although a sex-linked difference in susceptibility cannot be excluded, boys and girls commonly differ in the frequency with which they engage in strenuous physical activities which are known to predispose to paralytic disease. Above age twenty, paralytic poliomyelitis is more common among women than among men. Two possible explanations are: (1) mothers of young children are at greater risk of intrahousehold exposure than are fathers; (2) women have the added risk of pregnancy which predisposes to paralytic disease when infection occurs.

Ethnic group   Ethnic or racial groups often differ in disease experience. Frequently, this can be attributed to differences in exposure or the frequency of immunity determined by environmental factors which in the United States are often closely correlated with ethnic background. However, members of an ethnic group share many genetically determined traits which, in addition to obvious physical characteristics, may include increased susceptibility or resistance to specific disease agents. This concept is easy to understand, but demonstration that differences in disease experience are genetically determined is very difficult, since the effect of all relevant environmental factors must be taken into account. That genetic differences could result from natural selection is reasonable for diseases that are highly lethal before the years of reproduction. A very controversial example is the possibly greater resistance to tuberculosis of Caucasians than of Negroes. Caucasian experience with the tubercle bacillus presumably began in prehistoric times, whereas the first contact of Negroes with tuberculosis was little more than three hundred years ago. Epidemic typhus also may provide an illustration. In population groups in which it is truly epidemic, a high proportion of infections result in disease and case fatality rises sharply with age. However, among the Andean Indian population of South America, who apparently have lived with typhus since the Spanish invasion, infection is endemic and only one in twenty-five or thirty infections results in recognized disease (4). The question here is whether the host has become resistant or the agent less pathogenic.

Family   If ethnic groups may differ from one another with respect to genetically determined susceptibilities to disease, so may individuals within ethnic groups. Indeed, it has long been accepted that hereditary factors may contribute to the occurrence of disease. Demonstration of their contribution, however, again requires taking adequate account of the many environmental influences that affect families as groups, for example, common exposure to infectious agents, diet, education, and socioeconomic status. In a major study of a possible genetic contribution to paralytic poliomyelitis, a geneticist began with all patients who experienced disease in one year and determined that, in the five preceding years, their close relatives had experienced significantly more disease than had the community at large (5). This geneticist unfortunately ignored the fact that the close relatives generally shared the same characteristics of socioeconomic status and personal hygiene that had contributed to the original selection of the index patients from the general community population (6). Better conceived was the classic study of Kallman and Reisner (7) who focused on twins as index cases of tuberculosis and clearly showed the operation of a genetic factor. This study is described in more detail in Chapter 9. For presumably noninfectious diseases such as breast cancer and coronary heart disease, a larger well-controlled and more convincing body of evidence suggests that predisposition to the disease in question is genetically transmitted.

5-5   General Health Status of Host

Another constellation of "built-in" factors influencing host reaction to disease agents are those which describe the general health status of the host. These include aspects of the physiologic state, the nutritional status, the presence of intercurrent disease, and stress.

Physiologic state   Puberty, with its accompanying periods of rapid growth and change in endocrine balance, appears to contribute to the occurrence of such divergent diseases as acne and tuberculosis. Pregnancy also enhances the risk of tuberculosis, clearly predisposes to infection of the urinary bladder, and may well exacerbate various pre-existing pathologic conditions.

Nutritional status   Nutritional status is described in relation to many specific requirements and the consequences of specific deficiencies differ in surprising ways. Gross malnutrition associated with low intake of nitrogen results in definite impairment of immune responses and a corresponding increase in susceptibility to bacterial diseases. However, when we turn to viruses and rickettsia, which depend for their replication on the intracellular metabolic pathways of the host, generalizations about the effects of deficiencies are not possible. In controlled laboratory experiments some specific deficiencies have been shown to increase susceptibility and others have been shown to increase resistance. Although there is little valid documentation in man, there are suggestive fragments of evidence. For example, inmates of concentration camps in Germany during World War II were grossly malnourished and heavily louse-infested at the end of the war and epidemic typhus was common among them. However, the disease occurring was relatively benign. Nonetheless, as the camps were liberated by the advancing allied troops, the inmates scattered over the countryside and spread their infection to the well-nourished German civilian population who responded with disease of classical severity (8).

Intercurrent or pre-existing disease   Although it is known that infection with one virus may, by an interfering effect, induce temporary resistance to a second virus, the operation of the interference phenomenon probably exerts little influence on natural occurrence of disease (9). More commonly, one disease state paves the way for a second one. The most common example is the frequent occurrence of bacterial bronchopneumonia (the "old man's friend") as a terminal event in persons dying with a chronic noninfectious disease. Also well known are the peculiar susceptibility of diabetics to many bacterial infections and the tendency for measles and pertussis to activate pre-existing but quiescent infection with the tubercle bacillus. Finally, otherwise benign respiratory viral infections may pave the way for severe bacterial disease, a phenomenon best documented by the relation between influenza virus infection and the development of bacterial pneumonias (10).

Stress   The term "general health status" also embraces a number of less tangible factors. In addition to psychic state or mental attitude, which was discussed in relation to disease agents, stress induced by a variety of means is commonly believed to contribute substantially to disease occurrence. The possible results of stress are most readily illustrated with disease agents such as the polioviruses or the tubercle bacillus, infection with which infrequently develops into "characteristic" disease. The tendency for active tuberculosis to develop during puberty, during young adulthood in females, and during older adulthood in males may be explained in part by stress engendered, respectively, by the rapid growth which characterizes puberty, by the phenomenon of pregnancy and the caring for small children during young female adulthood, or by strenuous or increasingly responsible occupations of the older males. Similarly, chilling, physical exertion, inoculations with irritant materials, and pregnancy are included among the stress factors which help determine which few individuals out of each thousand infected with polioviruses will develop paralytic disease. As described by Dr. Hans Selye, stressful stimuli of quite divergent types, including fears or emotions, strenuous physical exertion, traumatic injury, or unusual exposure to heat or cold may all express themselves through a common pituitary-adrenocortical hormonal path (11).

5-6 Immunity and Immunologic Response in the Individual

"Immunity" means freedom or exemption from some penalty. Biologically, the penalty is infection (and possible disease) because of a living agent. The immune state may be an inborn characteristic of a vertebrate species. Examples are the resistance of man to many pathogens of lower animals, for example, the viruses of canine distemper and canine infectious hepatitis, or the resistance of lower animals to pathogens of man, for example, that of canine species to influenza virus. This species-determined, inherent resistance is called natural immunity and is not our present concern. Rather, we shall discuss immunity to pathogens, chiefly those of man, acquired either naturally (as by infection) or artificially (as by vaccination).

Forms of immunologic response In man and other vertebrates immunologic response is triggered by the presence in the host of antigens. These may be invading living organisms or large molecular protein or polysaccharide substances (commonly derived from such organisms) which the host recognizes as non-self or foreign. The usual ability of the host to discriminate between self and non-self substances is of critical importance since, when host tissues become the targets of the immune response, "auto-immune" diseases result. In this latter category are such serious entities as systemic lupus erythematosus, multiple sclerosis, rheumatic fever, and chronic glomerulonephritis.

Occasionally, the host mistakenly identifies truly foreign antigens as self, especially if they are present during fetal or (for lower vertebrates) early postnatal life before the immunologic apparatus is fully functional. The resulting failure of immunologic response is called *immunologic tolerance*. How to achieve a state of selective tolerance is a major current problem in surgery where technically feasible tissue and organ transplants (grafts) will fail to be accepted by the recipient host (will be immunologically rejected) unless tolerance can be established. Tolerance to infectious agents apparently is uncommon but, when it occurs, may permit serial congenital transmission of infection. This has been documented for the virus of lymphocytic choriomeningitis in mice which, if infected congenitally, harbor the virus for life* and transmit it congenitally to their progeny. Similar congenital transmission in man is suspected to occur with the virus of serum hepatitis.

Immunologic response has two principal results. One is the development of a state of hypersensitivity. This state is characterized by rapid and excessive reaction to further contact with the inciting antigen. The second is the production of protective antibodies (chemically, molecules of several types of gamma globulin) which have the ability to combine specifically with the inciting antigen and which are found in blood serum, tissue fluids, and mucous secretions.

Hypersensitivity   Hypersensitivity is nearly always harmful to the host and is a potential cause of disease. Some hypersensitivities (the immediate type) depend on the presence of antibody (called reagin). Combination of antigen with this antibody forms a complex which provokes the reaction. The most common forms of immediate hypersensitivity are the numerous allergies to pollens, house dust, or other airborne allergens which cause hayfever; to many food items, for example, strawberries or seafoods; and to certain drugs. Most serious are the potentially lethal anaphylactic reactions provoked by injections of serum from lower animals, drug, or vaccine in a person sensitive to some component of the substance injected. In persons not previously sensitive, injection of large doses of serum from horses or other animals containing rabies antibody or tetanus antitoxin often stimulates development of hypersensitivity before all of the foreign serum has been eliminated. Reaction of the persisting foreign serum with the newly formed antibody results in disease called "serum sickness."

Hypersensitivity of the delayed type, typified by skin sensitivity to tuberculin, is believed to be mediated by small lymphocytes which possess a specific ability to attack the inciting antigen. Such cell-mediated hypersensitivity plays major roles in the pathogenesis of chronic infectious diseases such as tuberculosis and of the "auto-immune" diseases and in the immunologic rejection of skin grafts and organ transplants. It also is essential to the production in mice of acute disease resulting from lymphocytic choriomeningitis virus (only the tolerant mouse escapes such disease) and may well be involved in the pathogenesis of some viral diseases in man. Interestingly, antiserum to lymphocytes (anti-lymphocytic serum or ALS) temporarily depresses delayed hypersensitivity and may be the key to achieving the selective tolerance needed to avoid rejection of surgical transplants.

---

*Congenitally infected mice remain healthy for most of their lives. However, it is now recognized that such infection does result in slowly developing kidney disease (12).

Protective antibodies Specific immunity to infection and disease caused by microorganisms usually is mediated by antibody. The immune host is characterized by the presence of antibody in his blood serum, tissue fluids and, in many cases, mucous secretions. His immunity is classified according to the origin of the antibody. If he produced the antibody himself, the immunity is called active. If it was produced by another host, it is called passive. As illustrated below, immunity of either type may be acquired by natural means (naturally acquired) or with human intervention (artificially acquired).

The possession of antibody most often signifies the *naturally acquired active immunity* that results from previous infection. Also common is the *naturally acquired passive immunity* to many agents possessed by newborn infants who acquired it from their mothers, chiefly by transplacental passage of maternal antibodies into the fetal circulation. These passively acquired antibodies disappear with a half-life of about twenty-five days, i.e., the level (or titer) of antibody in the infant serum declines by half every twenty-five days. How long they persist, therefore, depends on the level present at birth, as seen for poliovirus antibodies in Figure 5-1. However, nearly all maternally derived antibodies disappear by six months of age (13). *Artificially acquired active immunity* is that stimulated by administration of vaccines (or toxoids) prepared from cultures of important microbial pathogens. Technically, "vaccine" describes preparations containing all or some portion of the agent particle, whereas "toxoid" refers to those containing only a modified (detoxified) bacterially-produced toxin. Important vaccines are those against smallpox, poliomyelitis, yellow fever, typhus, typhoid, and influenza. To protect against diphtheria and tetanus, toxoids are employed. *Artificially acquired passive immunity* also exists. This is most frequently conferred through use of gamma globulin, the antibody-containing fraction of pooled adult human plasma, in the short-term prophylaxis of measles and infectious hepatitis. The antibody so conveyed has a half-life of twelve to fourteen days and the resulting immunity persists for no more than four or five weeks. Antibody produced in lower vertebrates (usually horses) is also used to provide temporary protection against suspected exposure to tetanus or rabies. As pointed out in the discussion of hypersensitivity, the use of such preparations is associated with significant risk of serum sickness or, in already sensitized persons, of anaphylactic reactions.

As a final note, let us examine the consequences of immunity to the individual. The key point is that immunity is a relative term. At its maximum, it renders the individual completely refractory to infection and disease. This presumably would be the case with respect to measles during the first few years after infection. At the other extreme, the occurrence of infection may not be impeded and disease not fully prevented (although usually it will be beneficially modified). This situation may result when immunity wanes following vaccination, as has been observed for smallpox, whooping cough, and diphtheria.

5-7   Immunity and Immunization in the Group

Herd immunity   The individual inevitably is part of a group, and it is of interest to consider the phenomenon of resistance and susceptibility in the group as a whole. Regardless of the agent or its source, the proportion of susceptibles in a population is an important factor influencing the occurrence of disease. This is especially important for agents which pass from one individual to another. If the proportion of immunes is too great, the agent cannot penetrate and spread. This relationship applies to both human and vertebrate populations and has been zoonotically

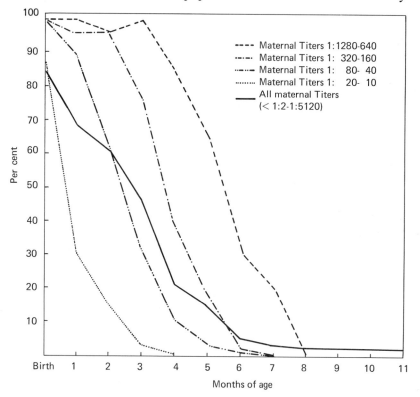

FIG. 5-1 Percentage of infants of given age with neutralizing antibody of titer 1:10 or greater against poliovirus according to maternal titer against the homologous virus type. (Henry M. Gelfand *et al.* Studies on the development of natural immunity to poliomyelitis in Louisiana. V. Passive transfer of polio-antibody from mother to fetus, and natural decline and disappearance of antibody in the infant. *J. Immunol.* **85**:46–55, 1960.)

christened "herd immunity." From the standpoint of controlling specific diseases such as measles in man or rabies in dogs, it would be desirable to know just what proportion of the population must be immune to make spread of infection highly improbable. This proportion will vary with the infectiousness of the infected host, the length of time during which he is infectious, and the density and degree of mixing of the population. Although estimates are available for some disease agents, e.g., 70 to 80 per cent immune for measles, precise information does not exist. Work with mathematical models of epidemics, however, suggests that in no case must the proportion immune approach 100 per cent before spread halts.

Immunity resulting from natural infection   For immunity resulting from natural infection to influence disease occurrence, the disease agent must be frequently encountered and must give rise to durable and effective immunity. With most zoonotic agents, including those of Rocky Mountain spotted fever, tularemia, and St. Louis encephalitis, too few people become infected for the resulting immunity to reduce disease incidence significantly. A sharp contrast is provided by the widely prevalent agents of measles, chickenpox, and poliomyelitis which provoke durable, possibly lifelong immunity. Disease caused by these ubiquitous agents occurs chiefly in children, because few adults are nonimmune. No similar age pattern is evident for diseases such as influenza or the common cold caused by agents which are equally ubiquitous but give rise to only short-lived immunity.

Immunity induced by vaccination   Use of vaccines to induce active immunity represents an effort to obtain for the vaccinated person the same benefits that would result from natural infection, but without the risk of disease. To the extent that the resulting immunity reduces the vaccinee's ability to serve as a link in the chain of transmission, vaccine-induced immunity also contributes to herd immunity. How vaccines may differ in this contribution can be illustrated by comparing inactivated (Salk) and attenuated live virus (Sabin) vaccines against poliomyelitis. Both types of vaccine are highly protective against disease. However, infection with the Sabin vaccine strains of poliovirus resembles natural infection in that it greatly increases the resistance of the alimentary tract to reinfection, whereas immunity resulting from the Salk vaccine exerts little such effect. This is illustrated by comparing the occurrence of infections following intra-household exposure in persons immune because of previous natural infection with that in persons immunized with Salk vaccine, as shown in Table 5-3 (14). Vaccination which protects against infection as well as disease will, if widely used, restrict the spread of natural infection and so serve to protect even those who remain unimmunized. Although the Sabin live poliovirus vaccine offers this promise, it must be noted that in Sweden use of a highly potent inactivated vaccine also has effectively restricted spread of wild polioviruses. Another example of a disease similarly susceptible to restriction by vaccination is smallpox which, largely

typhoid bacilli, brucella organisms, streptococci, and before rigorous inspection of dairy herds was introduced, tubercle bacilli of bovine origin.

A more modern problem is the great variety of substances not naturally present in food. These include not only additives such as synthetic flavoring materials and chemicals intended to preserve color or the freshness of bread, but also many unnatural residual substances. These latter derive from synthetic hormones and other growth-promoting chemicals included in poultry and livestock feed or from insecticides used to insure bigger and better fruits and vegetables. The presence of such additives or residues in foods, even though only in trace amounts, is of concern because the long-term effects on man of continuing exposure are unknown.

Disposal of human excreta   Lack of concern for places where human feces are deposited characterizes the populations of less-developed areas and the young children and poorly educated segments of populations of more advanced areas. Feces freshly deposited near human habitations attract filth flies which become active vehicles for disseminating enteric infectious agents. Such casual defecation, together with failure to wear shoes, contributes to the extensive prevalence of hookworm in many parts of the world. In India there is a compulsion, with cultural basis, for feces to be deposited in or near running water. This fact, coupled with lack of knowledge or concern about water contamination, helps explain the endemicity of many important enteric infections in that country. In the Orient and some other parts of the world, human night soil is regarded (quite properly) as a valuable source of organic nitrogen and used (quite improperly) for purposes of fertilization. This practice leads to direct contamination of crops such as strawberries or lettuce, which usually are consumed raw and uncleansed. For this reason, persons traveling to areas of uncertain hygiene are warned to avoid food that has not been cooked or peeled. Diseases transmitted by night soil contamination include typhoid, dysentery, amoebiasis, infectious hepatitis, and poliomyellis.

Problems concerning disposal of feces still persist in highly developed countries. In Scandinavia extensive outbreaks of hepatitis have been traced to shellfish which were harvested from waters over which "sanitary" privies had been constructed. Oysters and clams harvested from sewage-polluted waters have been responsible for similar outbreaks in the United States. Although rapidly being replaced by the septic tank and tile drain field, the rural outdoor privy still exists in the United States and is a hazard when inadequately protected against flies or when improperly located with respect to wells.

Personal hygiene   Personal hygiene varies widely between cultures and between individuals within cultures. As one example, infestation with body lice is directly related to infrequent bathing and laundering of clothes. This may be a result of poverty, because of which soap and changes of clothing are in short supply, or of climate, as in the Andes, where the water available for bathing and laundering averages a chilly 5°C. Bathing also has a direct relation to some bacterial and fungal infections of the skin. Washing of hands is chiefly important to minimize their role in the indirect transmission of fecal contamination. Although this is most obviously important for food handlers, it is also important for small children who frequently put much-handled toys and objects into their mouths, a mechanism contributing to the ready spread of polio and other enteroviruses in the young-child population. In some cultures in which washing of hands may be ignored, the concept of "hand contamination" is honored by the custom of reserving one hand for feeding oneself and the other for cleaning after defecation (without benefit of toilet tissue).

The control of respiratory secretions includes the use of disposable tissues for nasal secretions, the avoidance of uncovered coughing, refraining from indiscriminate spitting, and not talking directly into the face of another person (such intimate conversation characterizes some cultures). Oral hygiene, meaning proper care of the teeth and the gums, is principally important to the individual himself and may minimize or prevent the development of chronic foci of infection, as well as insure the long retention of teeth. The care of skin infections is important to both self and other persons. Bacterial (chiefly staphylococcal) and fungal infections frequently spread from one part of the body to another and the lesions are potential sources of infections for other persons. Of special importance are lesions on the hands of food handlers which frequently have been responsible for outbreaks of staphylococcal food poisoning.

Use of appropriately protective clothing is another important element of personal hygiene. Not only do we require protection against strong sunlight or excessive cold, but properly designed clothing protects against such arthropod vectors as mites, ticks and mosquitoes, and the wearing of shoes prevents the acquisition of hookworm infestations.

Forms of personal contact   The types of contact we have with our fellows may influence contact-transmitted diseases. Different methods of greeting such as handshaking, the impulsive kiss, the Latin *abrazo*, or the Eskimo rubbing of noses are dictated by social custom. The Oriental custom of greeting (the *wai*, or shaking hands with oneself) has much to recommend it insofar as health is concerned. Also, sound health reasons support the modern mother who protects her young infant from indiscriminate kissing by affectionate friends and relatives. Occurrence of the several venereal diseases is related to cultural and individual habits with respect to sexual intercourse, including degree of promiscuity and use of prophylactic devices. Finally, in nearly all cultures and societies the play habits of young children result in highly intimate interpersonal contact which greatly facilitates the spread of disease agents of many types, including the mites which cause scabies, the streptococci which cause impetigo, numerous respiratory viruses, polioviruses, and even pinworms.

Household hygiene   Familial health depends greatly on the environmental sanitation or hygiene of the individual household. Many aspects of household hygiene relate to the culture. Sleeping *en famille* in a single bed, as is usual among Andean Indians and other impoverished groups, greatly facilitates intra-household spread of contact-transmitted agents and body lice. Groups also vary in respect to the sharing of houses with livestock, the provision of windows for light and ventilation, and customs relating to domestic animal pets, including both the types of pets and the intimacy of contact with them. On a more individual basis are measures taken to protect against rodents, roaches, filth flies, and mosquitoes and the general maintenance of cleanliness throughout the house and in relation to food handling.

Occupation   The risk of acquiring many diseases is directly related to occupation. Although this factor will be considered further in relation to the environment, some examples of disease hazards related to occupation may be mentioned now. These include the development of bone cancers among workers who applied radium paint to watch dials and hands, the high rate of leukemia in physicians and others exposed to X-ray apparatus, and the occurrence of lead poisoning in battery workers and painters. Less well known, perhaps, are the high frequencies of urinary bladder cancers in aniline dye workers, of lung cancer in miners of radioactive ores, and of silicosis and tuberculosis in miners exposed to dusts with high silica content. Often overlooked are the hazards related to the "healthy, rural" life of the farmer. These include increased risks of skin cancer as a result of exposure to the sun, of serious accidents associated with the use of powerful and complex machinery, and of such zoonotic diseases as Rocky Mountain spotted fever resulting from contact with arthropod vectors. Finally, we most often forget the hazards of the housewife who spends most of her time in the home. Although commonly regarded as citadels of safety, homes typically abound in such built-in accident hazards as the loose carpeting on the stairway, the carelessly disposed child's roller skates, or the improperly grounded electrical appliance. The housewife also is exposed to infectious disease agents imported by the small children in her charge or inadvertently present in food she prepares and test-tastes prior to adequate cooking.

Recreation   Although recreation in general is healthy, our recreational habits do result in increased disease hazards. Travel in itself, particularly by automobile, has a significant accident risk, whereas that to foreign areas may result in unusual exposures to a variety of infectious agents, particularly if the travel is to less well-developed parts. Even the "healthy outdoor life" as typified by hunting, fishing, and camping trips or the Sunday family picnic results in disruption of our usual personal hygiene and brings us into contact with many unfriendly aspects of nature, ranging from poison ivy to the arthropod vectors of serious diseases.

Other aspects of behavior   Many other aspects of individual and group behavior also may influence disease occurrence. Important among these is the utilization of medical care. Conscientious acceptance of a well-planned program of immunizations is but one aspect of health care. Calling the physician early when infectious illness occurs may lessen the chances of serious, possibly permanent sequellae such as may follow untreated streptococcal infections. It also may minimize spread of the infectious agent, either because specific treatment shortens the period of patient infectivity (e.g., streptococcal infection treated with penicillin) or because specific precautions are advised to protect other family members.

Certain individual traits such as accident proneness (still something of a controversial concept) and overindulgence in or addiction to tobacco, alcohol, or drugs engender disease in their own right (e.g., cigarette smoking and lung cancer), enhance susceptibility to infections (e.g., alcoholism and pneumococcal pneumonia), or afford unusual pathways for infection (e.g., drug addicts who share common instruments for administering heroin intravenously, with the resulting transmission of viral hepatitis). Educational level and individual intelligence relate to the knowledge of specific disease hazards and how they may be avoided. Finally, individual temperament largely determines whether we ignore or act upon the health information available to us. With the approaching solar eclipse of 1963 a widespread publicity campaign sought to warn people of the hazards to eyesight of trying to view the eclipse directly. In one notable instance, an educated adult male in Indiana listened to the publicity but still could not resist inspecting the eclipse directly for a period of ten seconds, an act which resulted in 30 per cent reduction in his visual acuity.

5-9   Summary

Many factors relating to the human host contribute to disease occurrence. Some are inherent and others are acquired. The latter include aspects of human behavior dictated by habits and customs.

Infection provides a model for agent–host interaction. Possible immediate results form a gradient of response from inapparent to overt to severe or lethal. The last outcome is unsatisfactory to parasites that depend on man for species survival (and, of course, to man). Longer-term outcomes may include persisting defect or deformity, progressive chronic disease, persistence of the agent with shedding (carrier state) or without, and post-infection resistance of variable degree and duration.

Host defences are both structural and functional, the specific mechanisms depending on the nature of the disease agent. The skin and mucous membranes form a protective envelope against microbial, chemical, and some physical agents. Evasive action and quick elimination of agents depend on the special senses and various reflexes. Microbial agents are confronted with local inflammatory response, regional and systemic filters, and the immune response.

Biologic factors indirectly influencing disease occurrence include age, sex, genetic constitution (racial and familial), and aspects (physiologic, nutritional, stress, and pre-existing or intercurrent disease) of the general health of the host. They are important as they relate to susceptibility to the effects of the agent, to the risk of exposure, or to the probability of specific immunity.

Immunologic response usually is triggered only by non-self or foreign antigens. Responses directed against self antigens cause autoimmune diseases. Failure of response to foreign antigens (tolerance) is a possible factor in serial congenital transmission of infections. Response includes both hypersensitivity (immediate or delayed, and in either case harmful) and antibody-mediated protective immunity.

The individual host, specifically immune to a microbial agent, possesses protective antibody because: (1) he made it himself (active immunity) after natural infection (naturally acquired) or vaccination (artificially acquired); or (2) he acquired it ready-made (passive immunity) by placental transfer from his mother (naturally acquired) or by inoculation of antiserum or gamma globulin (artificially acquired). Passive immunity is of very short duration. Protection conferred by specific immunity is relative and may range from minimal to absolute.

Immunity also influences disease occurrence in the population. Disease resulting from highly prevalent agents which cause effective and durable immunity occurs chiefly in young children, because most older people are naturally immune (and less exposed). For several diseases effective vaccines exist, the systematic use of which also limits disease occurrence. Active immunity, naturally acquired or vaccine induced, also may render the individual host unable to serve as a source of infection. If a sufficient proportion of the host population is so immune, spread of the agent is restricted and "herd immunity" has been achieved.

Disease occurrence also is influenced by human behavior as governed by habits and customs. Important aspects, chiefly affecting exposure to disease agents, include practices regarding water use, food and milk, waste disposal, hand washing, other aspects of personal hygiene, social customs, occupation, recreation, use of medical care, and abuse of tobacco, alcohol, or drugs. These factors are closely related to the environmental realm.

GLOSSARY

Anaphylaxis (anaphylactic reactions) Manifestation of immediate hypersensitivity in which antigen-antibody complex stimulates spasm of smooth muscle (of blood vessels or bronchioles); unless counteracted by adrenalin, acute anaphylaxis can cause death.

Attack rate   Number of persons attacked with a specific disease per 100 or 1000 at risk, i.e., in the population groups specified.

Auto-immune disease   Disease caused by immunologic response to a host's own tissue antigen.

Case fatality rate   Number of deaths per 100 cases of a disease.

Half-life   Applied to states of declining activity, e.g., radioactivity of isotopes or passively acquired antibody; time required for level of activity to be reduced by 50 per cent.

Herd immunity   Resistance of a group to invasion and spread of an infectious agent, based on the immunity of a high proportion of individual members of the group.

Immunity—natural   Species-determined inherent resistance to a disease agent, e.g., resistance of man to virus of canine distemper.

Immunity—acquired   Immunity acquired by host to a natural pathogen for the host, e.g., immunity to measles acquired by man.

Immunity—active   Immunity developed in response to stimulus by an antigen (infecting agent or vaccine) and usually characterized by presence of antibody produced by the host himself.

Immunity—passive   That immunity conferred by antibody produced in another host and acquired naturally by an infant from its mother or artificially by administration of an antibody-containing preparation (antiserum or gamma globulin).

Immunologic tolerance   State of selective inability to respond immunologically to a specific antigen.

Inflammation (inflammatory process)   Normal tissue response to cellular injury or presence in the tissue of foreign material, characterized by dilation of small blood vessels (capillaries) and mobilization of defense cells (blood and tissue leucocytes and phagocytes).

Interference phenomenon   State of temporary resistance to infections with other viruses induced by an existing virus infection; mediated in part by interferon.

Interferon   Low-molecular-weight protein produced by cells infected with viruses which has the property of blocking viral infection of new cells and suppressing viral multiplication in cells already infected; active against a wide range of viruses.

Lymphocyte   One of the types of white blood cells; a small round cell which plays a role in immune response, especially in delayed hypersensitivity.

Phagocyte (phagocytosis)   Cell which engulfs and, hopefully, destroys foreign particles or microorganisms by digestion (the activity of phagocytic cells).

Serum sickness A manifestation of delayed hypersensitivity to long-persisting antiserum of nonhuman origin, e.g., diphtheria or tetanus antotoxin or rabies antiserum produced in horses; typically begins ten to twelve days after inoculation and may be very crippling.

Subclinical (silent, inapparent) infection Infection resulting in no clinically evident disease.

Toxoid A preparation containing detoxified toxin; employed to induce specific active resistance to the toxin, e.g., of diphtheria or tetanus bacilli.

Vaccine A preparation containing whole microorganisms (killed or living) or a fraction of the organisms possessing the immunizing antigen; employed to induce specific active immunity.

REFERENCES

1. Panum, Peter L. Observations Made During the Epidemic of Measles on the Faroe Islands in the Year 1846. New York: Delta Omega Society, 1940.
2. Soper, George A. Typhoid Mary. *Milit. Surg.* **45**:1–15, 1919.
3. Peart, A. F. W. An outbreak of poliomyelitis in Canadian Eskimos in wintertime. Epidemiological features. *Canad. J. Public Health* **40**:405–417, 1949 (Oct.).
4. Montoya, Juan A., Jordan, Martha E., Kvamme, Liev, Quiros, Carlos, and Fox, J. P. A survey of sero-immunity against epidemic typhus among certain population groups in Peru. *Amer. J. Hyg.* **62**:255–269, 1955 (Nov.).
5. Reedy, John J. Recessive inheritance of susceptibility to poliomyelitis in fifty pedigrees. *J. Hered.* **48**:37–44, 1957 (Jan.-Feb.).
6. Gelfand, Henry M. Inheritance of susceptibility to poliomyelitis. (Letter to the editor). *New Eng. J. Med.* **258**:964–965, 1958.
7. Kallman, F. J. and Reisner, D. Twin studies on the significance of genetic factors in tuberculosis. *Amer. Rev. Tuberc.* **47**:549–574, 1943.
8. Gordon, John E. Louse-Borne Typhus Fever in the European Theater of Operations, U.S. Army, 1945, in *Rickettsial Diseases of Man.* Malcolm H. Soule, org. Washington, D.C.: American Association for the Advancement of Science, 1948, pp. 16–27.
9. Fox, John P. Interference Phenomenon Observed in the Field, in *Recent Progress in Microbiology*, VIII. Toronto: University of Toronto Press, 1963, pp. 445–453.
10. Stuart-Harris, C. H. *Influenza and Other Virus Infections of the Respiratory Tract.* Baltimore: Williams and Wilkins, 1965, pp. 28–46.
11. Selye, Hans. *The Physiology and Pathology of Exposure to Stress.* Montreal: Acta Inc., 1950.

12. Oldstone, Michael B. A., and Dixon, Frank J. Pathogenesis of chronic disease associated with persistent lymphocytic choriomeningitis viral infection. 1. Relationship of antibody production to disease in neonatally infected mice. *J. Exp. Med.* **129**:483–505, 1969.

13. Gelfand, Henry M., Fox, John P., LeBlanc, Dorothy R., and Elveback, Lila. Studies on the development of natural immunity to poliomyelitis in Louisiana. V. Passive transfer of polioantibody from mother to fetus, and natural decline and disappearance of antibody in the infant. *J. Immun.* **85**:46–55, 1960 (July).

14. Fox, John P., Gelfand, Henry M., Le Blanc, Dorothy R., Rowan, Dighton F. The influence of natural and artificially induced immunity on alimentary infections with polioviruses. *Amer. J. Public Health* **48**:1181–1192, 1958.

6

Environmental Factors in Causation of Disease

Environment is all inclusive, embracing the entire ambient external to the individual human host and so includes not only the agent, but also the host's fellow man. For descriptive convenience we recognize three broad environmental areas: the physical, or inanimate, which includes geologic, geographic, and climatic or meteorologic features; the animate, or biological, which comprises all of the flora and fauna, including pathogenic parasites and many other disease agents; and the socio-economic, which includes, among other things, man's relation to his fellow man.

In the analysis of causation of disease, the contribution of environmental factors is difficult to evaluate for four principal reasons. The first is the multiplicity of such factors. Second, environmental factors typically operate concurrently and in an interrelated manner. Together, these two features greatly complicate the task of identifying the factors which most influence disease occurrence and of measuring their individual contributions. Third, many environmental factors contribute by very indirect, sometimes almost circular paths. In such instances, the situation resembles the legendary horseshoe nail, the loss of which led sequentially to the loss of the horse-shoe, the horse, the rider, and—ultimately—the battle. Finally, some environmental factors have the potential to act on the agent, on the host, and on the agent–host relationship. Sunlight is one factor which possesses this triple-barrelled potential. For an agent such as the tubercle bacillus, ultraviolet radiation from the sun may be lethal. For man, sunlight helps him synthesize vitamin D, is a source of bodily warmth, and is also an agent of disease (sunburn). Excessive sunlight may disturb the equilibrium between a latently infecting virus, herpes simplex, and its human host, leading to the occurrence of fever blisters. The following discussion represents an effort to simplify what necessarily is a complex relationship.

Before proceeding, one general truth must be recognized. Man does not accept the unfavorable aspects of environment without attempting to modify them. Hence, man's capacity to cope with his environment is an important factor which indirectly influences the occurrence of disease. This capacity varies with the degree of social organization and level of civilization. For single individuals or family groups, clearing small areas for cultivation and erecting primitive shelters may represent man's maximum capacity. In modern urban populations, in contrast, man's cooperative efforts provide every amenity, from abundant and potable water springing forth at the turn of a spigot to dwellings that ensure a year-round interior climate adjusted to man's tastes and needs. Unfortunately, the achievement of such victories over the environment has been accompanied by the evolution of new adverse environmental influences (high population density, air and water pollution, and so on) which we will consider in later sections of this chapter.

6-1 Physical Environment

Geography and geographic epidemiology As here employed, geography relates to position on and physical aspects of the earth's surface. The geographic distribution of diseases and the implications of such distributions to the nature of the causative agents and their transmission and reservoir mechanisms constitute the field of geographic epidemiology or medical geography as defined by Dr. Jacques May (1). One might note, as examples of the importance of medical geography, the divergent distributions of diseases caused by similar agents. Murine typhus, caused by *Rickettsia typhi* and transmitted by rat fleas, occurs widely in the tropic and subtropical lowlands whereas epidemic typhus, caused by *R. prowazekii* and transmitted by the human body louse, is restricted to temperate zones and high altitudes in the subtropics. Equally great differences are observed for two worm parasites of man: pinworms occur throughout the world, whereas hookworms are encountered only in the tropics and subtropics.

Frequently, the geographic distributions of disease are described in much more specific terms. Sandfly fever, for example, is said to occur "in parts of the European and African littoral of the Mediterranean, Asia Minor, the Russian shores of the Black Sea, Pakistan and northwest and central India" (2). From such specificity, one might infer that geographic factors act chiefly to determine disease spread. Thus, distance alone and such geographic features as mountains and rivers act as natural barriers or aids to human travel and so to disease spread. Such influences are far less important in the United States now than they were fifty or a hundred years ago, but they are still of substantial importance in developing countries.

The more important role of geography, and to Dr. May the more intriguing, is indirect: geography acts as a determinant of other aspects of the environment, beginning with climate. Basically determined by latitude, longitude, altitude, and relation to nearby mountain ranges and bodies of water, climate, in turn, determines the biologic environment and many aspects of human activity. Warm climate, by favoring abundance of rat fleas and development of hookworm eggs into invasive larvae, helps define the distribution of murine typhus and hookworm disease. Cool weather encourages the wearing of many clothes, a condition which (together with infrequent laundering) favors the human body louse and so helps determine the distribution of epidemic typhus. Pinworms, on the other hand, are little affected by climate, because their entire life cycle is within the human host. Climatic influence on flora and fauna is particularly important to the occurrence of all arthropod-transmitted zoonotic diseases, including such rickettsial diseases as murine typhus, Rocky Mountain spotted fever, and scrub typhus and the many arbovirus diseases (yellow fever, Japanese B encephalitis, St. Louis encephalitis, and so on).

Geography also influences the socioeconomic environment. The natural paths of overland travel, the natural waterways, and natural harbors, by facilitating or impeding transportation, help determine where populations will concentrate and the types of industry they will develop. The city of New Orleans, for example, developed at a convenient transfer point between an arm of the Gulf of Mexico, known as Lake Ponchartrain, and the Mississippi River about 100 tortuous and, for sailing ships, hard-to-navigate miles above its true mouth. As will be evident when we consider climatologic factors, geography also influences socioeconomic environment more indirectly, but no less importantly, by its influence on climate.

Geologic factors   Improbable as it may seem at first glance, geologic structures and formations contribute significantly to health status. Relating to their physical character (ranging from clay to nearly pure sand), soil types vary greatly in ability to hold and purify water. Depending on their content of organic matter and essential minerals, soils also differ in capacity to support vegetation which, in turn, relates to the types and abundance of animal life. Thus, soil helps determine the nature and availability of food for man and lower vertebrates, is an important determinant of the type and the importance of agriculture, and is a major factor influencing the total biologic environment. Soil also is an aspect of environment that man can greatly influence. This is clearly seen when we compare primitive land use (clearing and cultivation until soil exhaustion forces a move to a fresh tract) with modern practices of soil management (irrigation, soil enrichment, crop rotation, and protection against erosion). Even more dramatic is the salvage of vast areas of arid and barren lands in New Mexico, Arizona, and the Imperial Valley of California in the United States and, more recently, in Israel and the Egyptian Sahara.

Geologic formations determine water supply and fuel and mineral deposits. Water supply is a factor limiting population size and, together with fuel and mineral deposits, also influences the location, the type, and the extent of industrial development. Thus, the location of major steel mills near Chicago, Cleveland, and Pittsburgh was determined by the locations of deposits of iron ore, coal, and limestone and the availability of waterways to bring these essential ingredients together most economically. The importance of such developments to the socioeconomic pattern seems self-evident. However, man's influence with respect to geologic formations is largely developmental. He cannot add to the natural fuel and mineral deposits, although he can conserve them. Similarly, men can conserve and improve the use of water supplies by means of dams, irrigation, and forestation projects. However, despite major efforts, rainmaking has not yet become a respectable profession nor have economical means for large-scale demineralization of sea water been developed.

Climate   As noted in an earlier chapter, climate has long figured prominently in efforts to explain disease occurrence. The original belief in supernatural origins of disease was replaced by the concept of epidemic constitutions. This concept, initiated by Hippocrates and still retained by Sir Thomas Sydenham, invoked atmospheric changes, depending on season and year, which were believed to determine the nature of prevailing epidemics of disease. Until the time of Louis Pasteur, many diseases were attributed to such vague atmospheric qualities as miasmas and fetid air.

We must begin our discussion of modern views of the effects of climate on disease with some definitions. Climatologic factors include solar effects such as visible light and ultraviolet irradiation, temperature, precipitation (rain or snow) or the lack thereof, barometric pressure, winds, and even lightning. The term *climate* describes the typical pattern of weather conditions throughout the year in a specified region. Thus, Minnesota and New England have cool, temperate zone climates, whereas Louisiana and Florida are warm and subtropical. *Season* refers to the usual conditions of weather during certain parts of the year which follow a regular predictable annual cycle. *Weather* is something predicted with notorious unreliability on a day-to-day basis, as a consequence of which umbrellas and raincoats are consistently at the wrong end of the path between home and office. Climatologic factors influence disease occurrence directly by their effects on disease agents and the host and indirectly by their important influence on the biologic and socioeconomic environments.

Let us look first at the influence of climatologic factors on disease agents. Such factors as temperature, humidity, and radiation of both visible and invisible nature are directly important in the survival of microbial agents in the free state and in the life cycles and reservoir mechanisms of many microbes and higher parasites. Undue warmth, excessive irradiation, and uncontrolled drying are likely to be lethal to agents such as the tubercle bacillus or the virus of poliomyelitis. Critical phases of the life cycle of other microbial parasites are highly dependent on temperature and humidity. The development and hatching of hookworm larvae from ova deposited in the soil depend not only on the suitability of the soil but also on reasonable humidity and a relatively warm temperature. The multiplication of malarial parasites and of yellow fever virus in their mosquito vectors and, indeed, the breeding and activity of the vectors themselves are favored by warm temperatures.

Climate also may exert a significant effect on the host. In the most direct sense, unduly low barometric pressure at high altitudes or excessively high pressure in the depths of the sea; extremes of heat, cold, or sunlight; and the all-powerful bolt of lightning are in themselves physical agents of disease. In addition, Mills (3) argues that man's general well being is adversely influenced by the effect of warm climates on body heat economy. In warmer, tropical climates difficulty in dissipating internally generated heat results in depression of body functions, lowering of vitality, and a predisposition to infection. In temperate climates, the facility of heat loss is presumed to stimulate vitality and quicken bodily function. In this light, the desirability of substantial resettlement of man in tropical areas, deriving from the pressure of population increase, makes it urgent to resolve the problem of man's physiologic adaptation to warmer temperatures.

Morbidity and mortality from many diseases vary with season and short-term weather changes for reasons still poorly understood. Notably, respiratory diseases are most frequent in the colder months. Possible explanations include increased congregation of people indoors, which would facilitate transmission, or increased susceptibility to disease owing to fluctuations in either temperature or humidity or, more directly, to chilling. Interestingly, efforts to demonstrate an effect of chilling on the occurrence of colds (subjects wrapped in wet sheets and exposed to a fan) were successful only when attempted with women in the middle of their menstrual cycle (4). Even less well understood are the spring peaks seen in the incidence of diabetes and heart disease and summer peaks in deaths from leukemia. Short-term changes, appropriately, have been associated with short-term effects. Many years ago Peterson (5) noted that brief peaks in daily death rates coincided with the passage of cold fronts, presumably reflecting the inability of near moribund persons to withstand such weather-induced stress. Of greater significance to basic health, sudden atmospheric inversions also are associated with sharp rises in daily deaths, presumably because of the related increase in concentration of air pollutants (6). The need for man to adapt to abrupt changes in climate is rapidly growing with his ever-increasing mobility and use of high-speed jet air transport. The dimensions of the continental United States, for example, are roughly two and a half hours north–south by five hours east–west when expressed in jet air travel time.

Season and climate also effect health indirectly by influencing human habits and customs. As was pointed out in the previous chapter, these operate to increase or decrease exposure to particular etiologic factors. Aspects of behavior most influenced by climate or season are clothing, recreation, occupation, and intimacy of social contact. The amount of clothing we wear varies inversely with temperatures. During summer months our clothing may give little protection against insect bites, sunburn, exposure to irritating vegetation, or even, among small children who play intimately together, exposure to fecal contamination. These also are the months when vector-borne diseases tend to occur and when, in years gone by, typhoid and dysentery were most prevalent. Recreation is particularly dependent on season. Camping, picnicking, hiking, and swimming (often in potentially polluted streams) are typical activities which reflect the summer urge for the great outdoors. Winter recreation is less predictable, because some of us risk our lives on snowy ski slopes, whereas others flee to warmer regions such as Florida or the Caribbean. Occupations other than those related to agriculture are little influenced by climate directly, but may vary with season. In addition to agricultural activities, many service jobs related to recreation are seasonally determined in temperate zone climates. Also, there is significant seasonal variation in the type and intimacy of social contact in temperate zones. The tendency to congregate indoors during winter greatly assists in the spread of respiratory infections. In summer, the outdoor play of scantily clad children facilitates spread of skin infections and fecally excreted agents such as polioviruses. Finally, in the springtime a young man's fancy, presumably reciprocated by a young woman's fancy, may lead to particular intimacy of social contact.

Superabundance or undue lack of rainfall also may influence human health. Drought brings crop failure and resulting famine, and leads to concentration of microbial contaminants in that water still available. Excess rainfall leads to floods which may threaten human life directly, wash out newly planted crops, and cause serious contamination of surface water supplies. In the period immediately after floods, the safety of drinking water should be insured by chlorination or boiling.

Finally, in the familiar circular pattern, climate operates still more indirectly by its influence on both the biologic and socioeconomic environments. The relation of these sectors of environment to disease will be elaborated in detail shortly. However, it should be evident that climate affects the biologic environment in at least two important ways. First, temperature and humidity help determine the abundance and particular species of the flora and fauna. Second, season determines the stage of development of the flora and in many instances the developmental cycles and abundance of the fauna. These biologic factors are of great importance to reservoirs and mechanisms of transmission of microbial agents and to food supplies for man.

Through its influence on the biologic environment, climate helps determine the type and importance of agriculture and so becomes a partial determinant of the socioeconomic environment. Climate also may influence the level of civilization on a teleologic basis. It helps determine the availability of naturally occurring food (e.g., bananas and coconuts) and the inversely related need for cultivated crops, and it also determines need for and type of shelter. The typical temperate zone winter, indeed, may provide a special incentive to work simply to ensure survival during this harsh season.

In more advanced civilizations, man has proved reasonably capable of coping with the adverse aspects of climate. He can control temperature and humidity within doors or within automobiles and, for out-of-doors, he can select minimally or highly protective clothing. His improving ability to predict the immediately coming weather enables him to avoid major weather hazards such as hurricanes. Finally, there is hope that the profession of rainmaker may yet earn respectability.

6-2   Biologic Environment

The biologic environment includes all living things—plant, animal, or indeterminate—and, particularly important for health in man, includes the pathogenic parasites. It influences human health, favorably or unfavorably, in many direct and indirect ways.

The quality and quantity of human nutrition depend directly on plant and animal life. To the extent that total quantity or specific nutritive elements are seriously lacking, the components of man's food supply may be in themselves agents of disease. We have also seen how nutrition may act to alter human susceptibility to disease agents. Man's ability to exploit the biologic environment for food, of course, is related to his level of civilization. In his most primitive state he utilizes only naturally occurring plants, fish, and game. As recently as the time of the first New World settlements, the early settlers were heavily dependent on foods native to the new area and might well have starved without the guidance of friendly natives. Currently, despite great technologic advances in agriculture that have resulted in incredible surpluses of food in the United States, the constantly rising population of the world puts in serious question the future adequacy of man's food supply on a worldwide basis.

Numerous noxious agents come from the biologic environment. Most numerous are those substances referred to as allergens. Plant pollens, organic house dust, feathers, and the "dandruff" from the skin of many animals provoke severe hay fever; plant juices from various forms of poison ivy and sumac induce a severe vesicular dermatitis; and foods as different as strawberries and seafood may cause marked hives or urticaria. Highly toxic substances occur in potentially lethal, inedible mushrooms and cyanide-containing raw mandioca root of Latin America, in certain poisonous shellfish and, at unpredictable times, in several normally edible species of fish found in tropical waters. Finally, a number of substances of plant origin have specific therapeutic or pain-relieving effects in appropriate dose, but are toxic in overdose. These include extracts of cinchona tree bark (quinine, used for treating malaria), of foxglove leaves (the powerful heart stimulant, digitalis), and of the Oriental poppy (opium and its various derivatives, which include the most effective pain relievers known). In addition to their toxic potential, opium derivatives have the added hazard of causing addiction.

Various forms of animal life participate in the transmission and reservoir mechanisms of infectious disease agents. For some agents, including those of malaria, epidemic typhus, and dengue, man is the only vertebrate involved but transmission is by arthropod vectors. For other diseases, referred to as zoonoses, the basic reservoir involves only subhuman vertebrates. Some of these, including scrub typhus, murine typhus, and Rocky Mountain spotted fever (all caused by rickettsiae), tularemia and plague (caused by bacteria), and yellow fever, St. Louis encephalitis, and Russian Spring Summer encephalitis (all caused by viruses), require an arthropod vector for their transmission. However, many zoonotic disease agents require no insect vector to reach man. These include bacteria such as the salmonellae, the viruses of cowpox, rabies, and psittacosis, and animal parasites such as canine hookworm (the cause of "creeping eruption").

Plant and animal life also influence the health of man in many less direct and often interrelated ways. Plant life, for example, provides food and shelter for many arthropod and animal species. The nature and abundance of plant life and its seasonal stage of development determine how much wild life and which species are present. Herbivorous species thrive best in grassy plains, whereas some birds commonly are attracted by fruits and berries in their proper seasons. Arthropods often breed in tree holes and plant axils which collect water, and utilize plant foliage for shelter from predatory animal life and as a resting place in a suitable microclimate. For arthropods with a taste for blood, lower vertebrates constitute both the usual food source and potential sources of infection for vector species.

Human health is affected still more indirectly by the biologic environment through its influence on man's habits and customs, the type and relative importance of agriculture in his economy and his actual occupation. The availability of fish and game or other wildlife determines the popularity of fishing and hunting or birdwatching, whereas a superabundance of biting insects may cause people to desist from camping and picnicking. The importance of major crops such as coffee, sugar, wheat, and cotton to the economy of areas or countries is obvious.

The biologic environment has been particularly susceptible to modification by man. Indeed, change inevitably begins when man first plants his foot on virgin soil. Semihistorically, and to oversimplify the case, man's first step has been to clear the forests to provide land for cultivation and wood for shelter and fuel. His second step is cultivation itself, including determination of the crops to be introduced. Concomitantly, his hunting activities deplete and drive away game and other vertebrate species; these are replaced in time as domestic animal stocks are developed. Manipulation of biologic environment has not always contributed to the ultimate welfare of man. For various reasons, for example, to provide wild game, to combat local pests, or because of their beauty, animal and plant species have been introduced into regions distant from their normal habitat and lacking biologic control mechanisms such as natural predator species. As unforeseen consequences of such transplantation, European rabbits became serious threats to Australian crops, Indian mongooses became pests in Puerto Rico, and the water hyacinth has clogged inland navigation channels from Texas to Florida. In many parts of the world, including the United States, destruction of forests over large areas has decreased their capacity for retaining water and the resulting lowering of the water table has threatened the water supply. The drought-afflicted regions of northern India illustrate the extreme end result of this process. Deforestation, coupled with overgrazing or breaking up the sod for cultivation of grain, also has led to major soil erosion and, in periods of reduced rainfall, to the creation of huge dustbowl areas in the United States. The consequences of man's war against insects, particularly those of agricultural importance, cannot yet be fully evaluated. There is little doubt that the extensive use of chemical pesticides has played a major role in increasing the agricultural output of the United States. However, the fear has been dramatically articulated by Rachel Carson (7) that man and nature may seriously suffer from the gradual accumulation of the relatively stable and highly toxic chemicals now so widely employed. Their presence, even in trace amounts, in animal and vegetable foods constitutes the most direct threat to man. The foregoing examples suggest that, in future efforts to modify his biologic environment, man must weigh the long-term effects against the immediate advantages far more carefully than he has in the past.

6-3   Socioeconomic Environment

The sector of environment most difficult to define depends on population density and distribution; on the availability of natural resources; on the economic level achieved; on the stage of social, political, cultural and scientific development; and, of critical importance, on man's relation to his fellow man. Almost without exception, socioeconomic factors influence man's health by indirect and often highly circuitous means. Further, because they characteristically act concurrently and are so closely interrelated, evaluation of the contribution of individual socioeconomic factors may be extremely difficult.

Prior to the industrial revolution, the most important environmental influences on disease occurrence were considered to be climatic. Beginning in the middle of the eighteenth century in England and somewhat later in France and Germany, the shift to a predominantly industrial economy gave vastly increased importance to the socioeconomic environment. This was recognized in France by 1828 when Villerme (8) showed that morbidity and mortality rates were functions of the living conditions of different classes in the population and concluded that "not primarily climatic, but to a large extent social factors are the basic element in the causation of disease." In 1848 the German pathologist Rudolf Virchow (9) wrote that the health of the people was a matter of direct social concern. Recognizing the important effect of social and economic conditions on health and disease, Virchow stressed the need for reliable statistics so that the causal relations between these factors and disease could be scientifically investigated.

Population distribution   The overall density of population not only determines whether available food supplies and natural resources are adequate, but also relates to the ease of dissemination of infectious agents and so to the occurrence of both disease and immunity. Very simply, increasing density of population favors the spread of infectious agents to man, whether from human or nonhuman sources and whether by direct or indirect means. In relatively dense (and large) populations infections with ubiquitous agents such as measles virus tend to occur in early childhood and the agents persist because sufficient numbers of new susceptibles continue to enter the population by birth. In less densely populated areas such agents cannot persist and are reintroduced after unpredictable intervals, with the result that "childhood" diseases may be long delayed. This accounts for the very frequent occurrence of measles and other childhood diseases among military recruits from rural areas. Population density varies tremendously from one country to another and between different parts of the same country. Estimates as of the early 1960s, expressed as people per square mile, give such figures as 1130 in Java, 793 in England and Wales, 215 in France, 52 in the United States, and 3 in Australia.* Within the United States in 1960 illustrative figures are 0.4 for Alaska (the lowest), 11.5 for Arizona, 129 for Illinois, 655 for Massachusetts, and 12,525 for the District of Columbia (the highest).

The relative distribution of population between urban and rural areas is important with respect to several factors. Particularly great are differences in the biologic environment. In cities the most abundant vertebrate species may well be man and both vegetation and the arthropod fauna are limited in variety and abundance. Exposure to insects, various animals, and poisonous vegetation tends to be more frequent in rural areas, although stray dogs and domestic rats may be abundant in city slums. An obvious point of major difference, population density, has been discussed. Related to this are the more complex social structure and greater degree of political organization that characterize the denser populations of cities. Urban aggregation of people facilitates cooperative efforts to insure safe milk and water supplies, to dispose safely of sewage and waste, and to provide for the preservation, storage, and distribution of food. In contrast, for the rural resident satisfactory sanitation becomes a much more personal problem. The lives of urban and rural residents also may differ in aspects of human behavior and other conditions of living. Outdoor living, a more closely knit family life, and fewer distracting influences characterize rural living, whereas city life at its best is much more subject to tensions and pressures deriving from occupation and from the intimacy of social contact. In urban slums such pressures are magnified by overcrowding, lack of employment, and poverty. It is also obvious that urban and rural areas will differ greatly in types of industry and occupation which are characterized by their own special hazards to health.

In many parts of the United States, differentiation between urban and rural is becoming progressively more difficult. The Eastern seaboard from Washington to Boston has become a nearly unbroken metropolitan strip containing several focal concentrations of population and industry or business. Each urban area is surrounded by a wide and expanding zone of densely settled suburbia whose inhabitants, dwelling in semirural environments, commute daily to the city to work. Unfortunately, in such large metropolitan areas development of cooperative efforts to cope with the many adverse aspects of environment is impeded by an archaic political structure characterized by a patchwork of overlapping county, township, and town or city governments. In the field of education some of these political barriers have been overcome, at least in more rural regions, by the consolidation of school districts to permit construction of modern centralized schools. This pooling of educational resources brings large

*Sources: Demographic Yearbook, United Nations, 1962; Statistical Abstract of the United States, 1961.

numbers of rural children into close proximity each school day. Thus, at least at the school age, the degree of isolation of the rural inhabitant is substantially decreased. The influence of these changes on the time-honored urban and rural disease patterns remains to be evaluated, but one might speculate that the differences will become progressively less distinct.

The basic unit of population distribution is the household. Whether in urban or rural areas, belonging to a household carries the same basic implications to health. Intrafamilial contacts are both prolonged and intimate. Also, the degree of intrahousehold exposure increases with crowding or density (commonly expressed as persons per room). Children are particularly affected. Prolongation of contact is most important for chronic infectious diseases such as tuberculosis or leprosy. The latter disease probably requires just such prolonged and intimate contact for its persistence, because removal from a leprous household protects infants from future development of disease. Crowding is most important for acute infections and favors early exposure of children to pathogens. This may actually be beneficial when, as with measles or polioviruses, the consequences are least likely to be serious when infection is acquired in early childhood. However, very early exposure is not desirable when, as with whooping cough, infancy is the time of greatest susceptibility.

Evaluating the contribution of household crowding to disease occurrence requires the same caution needed in similar evaluations of other environmental factors and, indeed, provides a relatively simple illustration of the basic problem. In addition to crowding, several other readily identifiable factors also operate on a household basis. Members of a family are genetically related, eat the same food, are exposed to the same local physical and biologic environment (including insect and animal pests), have the same economic status, and are governed by the same religious, cultural, ethnic, and educational influences. The contribution of household crowding to increased disease in families can be evaluated only when allowance has been made for the contributions of these other influences.

Social and political structure   A stable and highly developed society should achieve many health advantages through its capacity for cooperative action. This is most directly illustrated in the provision of agencies, facilities, and services for the prevention and the care of disease. Official and voluntary public health agencies traditionally have played the major role in prevention. They provide numerous specific services (e.g., prenatal clinics, food and milk inspection, chlorination of water) and implement many programs (e.g., control of air pollution, mass immunizations against polio and measles) related to current important disease problems. These agencies also have a major responsibility for recognizing new problems and securing effective action for their control. Thus, the United States Public Health Service has officially recognized that smoking of cigarettes constitutes a serious health hazard and is now attempting to secure appropriate action to minimize its influence. Medical care facilities of high quality and medical personnel of high competence are most available in highly developed societies. However, governmental action appears essential to providing good medical care for all segments of the population, for example, the National Health Service in Great Britain and Medicare, Medicaid, and the Regional Heart, Cancer, and Stroke program in the United States.

A well-educated population and educational institutions of high quality also are important characteristics of the highly developed society. Education relates closely to personal health practices, which are based on understanding how diseases are spread and what should be done individually to avoid disease hazards and to control spread. The degree of literacy of the population is a major determinant of the methods employed in and the effectiveness of mass programs for specific health education. Such programs are essential to attacking problems of worldwide importance, for example, family planning, malaria control, and cigarette smoking.

The process of acquiring education in itself has special connotations. Schools commonly play a major function in child health programs. Children are examined in school or at the request of the school for physical defects and, more recently, for mental or emotional problems so that early corrective measures can be applied. In addition, school programs motivate important immunizations and make provision in their curricula for specific health education. Schools also serve to bring children together under circumstances which facilitate the airborne spread of agents of respiratory and childhood diseases. This latter influence is counterbalanced only for the few diseases such as diphtheria and, very recently, measles for which specific immunization procedures are included in the school immunization program.

The relation of social and political structure to man's capacity to combat the adverse aspects of his environment has been pointed out already, with emphasis on various aspects of environmental sanitation. Other phases of the fight against the physical and biologic environment include measures for flood control, campaigns to control such allergens as ragweed, control of mosquito and rodent pests, weather forecasting, and exploration of ways to control weather (e.g., inducing rain and snuffing out hurricanes). Ascent to the highly developed state, however, has led to the creation of new and potentially serious environmental hazards. These include the pollution of air with possible carcinogens, toxic pesticides, and even radioactive fallout.

The state of a poorly developed society is essentially the obverse of that just described. The most important lack is cooperative endeavor for environmental sanitation. As a result, vector-borne diseases such as malaria and diseases of insanitation such as cholera and typhoid are widely prevalent. Because of the overpopulation common to these societies, such contact-transmitted diseases as smallpox and measles are abundant. The latter, because of the frequent severe malnutrition and high prevalence of intercurrent infections among infants, does not appear in its familiar benign character, but is associated with unbelievably high case fatality rates, in some instances up to 25 per cent (10). Even when, as in the metropolitan centers, sanitation programs and facilities for good medical care and immunization exist, they are unavailable to the majority of the population because of lack of communication and inadequate transportation.

Even the most highly developed society is vulnerable to catastrophic social upheavals related to war or revolution. Such upheavals disrupt cooperative health efforts and greatly disturb individual morale. The population returns abruptly to a state of primitive insanitation which opens the door to new activity of diseases long under control such as typhoid, tuberculosis, or, as in Naples in 1943, epidemic typhus. War also is associated with forced migrations of large numbers of people, both organized as in the movement of troops and totally disorganized as in the flight of civilian populations. The possible consequences are several. First, there may be important changes in herd immunity. In particular, the proportion of persons susceptible to local disease agents may increase sharply, as when American and British troops were exposed to scrub typhus in the Far East during World War II. Second, the migrating population may bear disease agents to the populations they join, such as smallpox, typhus, or various venereal diseases. Finally, general susceptibility to infectious disease may be increased because of famine and exposure following the breakdown of transport and communication and the resulting exhaustion of supplies of food, clothing, and shelter.

Economic development   Although bank balances and other indices of wealth are relatively tangible, the influence of economic factors on health is often difficult to delineate. One may start with economic status itself. The close correlation of poverty and disease is obvious, but it sometimes is hard to decide which is the cause and which is the effect. Assuming that low economic status contributes to disease occurrence, we have the problem of tracing its mode of action. Economic status determines the abundance and quality of clothing, the type of housing, the degree of household crowding, the adequacy of nutrition, the availability of medical care, the level of education; unfortunately, it is also inversely related to family size. Through these and other subordinate factors, economic status becomes tremendously important to human health.

The key to economic status is occupation, which, however, relates to disease occurrence in still other ways. Occupation is an aspect of host behavior and its relation to specific disease hazards was discussed in the preceding chapter. Association of occupation with disease also results from the relation between certain occupations and population groups defined by ethnic or racial origin. Such relations are illustrated by the predominantly Jewish immigrant composition of garment workers on the Lower East Side of Manhattan in the first part of this century; by the typically Slavic composition of steel workers in Pittsburgh, Gary, and South Chicago; and by the typical Negro sharecropper in the southern United States. Obviously, the over- and underabundance of diseases that appear to parallel certain occupations may sometimes be determined by behavioral and genetic factors deriving from ethnic or racial associations.

We come finally to economic structure, the contrasting forms of which are typified by the industrial and the agrarian states. Since the industrial revolution there has been a gradual but constant shift of population from rural to urban residence and similarly gradual development of a high level of social and political structure. In the United States the southeastern section is only now undergoing this shift. The pace of this development normally has been sufficiently gradual that development of the facilities and services necessary to urban populations, from sanitation to educational institutions, has kept pace. The net effect, despite the adverse environmental influences introduced with industrialization, has been a substantial gain in human health. However, when this shift occurs too rapidly, serious health problems arise. During World War II the massive industrial mobilization in the United States, including the creation of whole new industries, led to large and rapid migrations of population from basically rural areas to newly developing or expanding urban centers. The migrating populations were greeted initially with inadequate sanitary, educational, and other facilities and brought with them large numbers of persons susceptible to those infectious agents common in urban centers. Sharp increases in venereal diseases were often observed, presumably reflecting the lonesomeness of single individuals (or temporarily separated married workers) in strange communities. Fortunately, adequate social resources were mobilized fairly rapidly and the problem was not of long duration.

The agrarian state is basically characterized by a relatively primitive social structure and a high proportion of the population in rural circumstances. Although the major agrarian countries in the second half of the twentieth century are no longer characterized by sparse populations, the rural populations still are substantially less dense than the urban. Within these populations, furthermore, there is relatively little development of cooperative endeavor to improve the sanitary environment or to combat other adverse environmental influences. In effect, the situation resembles that already described in relation to the society with poorly developed social structure.

6-4 Summary

Environment is all inclusive and embraces the entire ambient external to the individual human host. Environmental factors, hence, are potentially very numerous and typically operate concurrently and in a strongly interrelated manner. In practice this situation complicates the task of identifying and measuring the influence of the most important factors. For purposes of discussion, we divide the environment arbitrarily into three broad areas: physical, biologic, and socioeconomic.

Environmental factors can influence disease occurrence quite directly by acting on the agent or on the host or by influencing the agent–host relationship. They also, perhaps more frequently, act indirectly. Man typically strives to combat the adverse aspects of environment and his ability to succeed is closely related to his social and economic development.

Important aspects of the physical environment are geographic, geologic, or climatologic in nature. Geographic location influences disease occurrence because of its relation to natural barriers to or avenues for human travel and because of its influence on climate. Climate, in terms of solar effects, precipitation, and temperature, affects man directly and also determines the biologic environment in part. Geologic aspects include soil type (important to plant life and agriculture) and basic formations which determine water availability and deposits of minerals and fuel, all of which—together with place and climate—act to determine socioeconomic development.

The biologic environment embraces all living things and their products. It includes disease agents (allergens, poisons, microbial pathogens), the vertebrate and invertebrate species essential to the transmission and reservoir mechanisms of living parasites, and the nutritional necessities for human life. Type of economy, occupation, and recreational habits vary with the biologic environment which, in turn, is highly susceptible to change by man.

Man's relation to his fellow man is central to socioeconomic development, which further depends on density and distribution of population, availability of natural resources, type and level of the economy, stage of social and political organization, and cultural and scientific development. Population density relates to adequacy of food and natural resources, to spread of disease agents, and, in some part, to social structure and potential for cooperative action in combating the environment. The basic unit of population distribution is the family or household. Urban and rural populations differ in density, in exposure to biologic environment, in degree of social organization, and in type of economy—agrarian or industrial.

Industrialization, urbanization, and a stable and highly developed social and political structure tend to evolve in parallel. At the price, still uncounted, of new adverse features of the environment such as air pollution, these trends have important positive implications for health. These include provision for environmental sanitation, preventive medical services, curative medical services, and facilities for education. Poorly developed, typically agrarian societies are correspondingly deficient. Economic status and health are strongly correlated, presumably by way of the adequacy of food, clothing, housing, education, occupation, and medical care.

GLOSSARY

Arbovirus(es)   A class of virus(es) transmitted by arthropods (contracted from *ar*thropod-*bo*rne *viruses*).

Larva (hookworm)   Developmental stage of the hookworm as it leaves the ovum, characterized by its ability to infect by penetrating the skin.

Life cycle   Term usually employed for multicellular forms of animal life that produce eggs or ova; refers to the usual developmental sequence from the ovum to the adult capable of producing more ova.

Rickettsia(e)   Microbial agent(s) appearing like small bacteria and multiplying by simple fission, but only within a living host cell.

REFERENCES

1. May, Jacques M. *The Ecology of Human Disease*. Studies in Medical Geography, No. 1. New York: MD Publications, Inc., 1958.
2. Fox, John P. Sandfly Fever, in *Cecil-Loeb Textbook of Medicine*, 12th ed. Philadelphia: W. B. Saunders Co., 1967, p. 89.
3. Mills, Clarence A. *Climate Makes the Man*. London: Gollancz Press, 1944, p. 11.
4. Andrewes, Christopher H. The complex epidemiology of respiratory virus infections. *Science* **146**:1274–1277, 1964.
5. Peterson, William F. *Man, Weather and Sun*. Springfield: Charles C. Thomas, 1947.
6. McCarroll, James, and Bradley, William. Excess mortality as an indicator of health effects of air pollution. *Amer. J. Public Health* **56**:1933–1942, 1966.
7. Carson, Rachel. *Silent Spring*. Boston: Houghton Mifflin, 1962.
8. Shryock, Richard H. *The Development of Modern Medicine*. New York: Alfred A. Knopf, 1947, p. 225.
9. Ackerknecht, E. H. *Rudolph Virchow. Doctor, Statesman, Anthropologist*. Madison: University of Wisconsin Press, 1953, pp. 122–137.
10. Morley, D., Woodland, Margaret, and Martin, W. J. Measles in Nigerian children. A study of the disease in West Africa, and its manifestations in England and other countries during different epochs. *J. Hyg. (Camb.)* **61**:115–134, 1963.

7

Vital Statistics

The stage upon which the epidemiologist focuses his attention is a city, state, nation, continent, or the entire world. The principal actors are the human inhabitants, supported by (or exposed to) the animal and plant life. The stage set includes the entire environment. The plot of the drama is the development of disease or the maintenance of health. The epidemiologist plays various roles, from that of director (in experimental studies), to that of an interested but noninterfering member of the audience (in observational studies), or even that of librarian (in maintenance or study of records of vital events).

The human inhabitants come in many shapes, sizes, and colors, and although they are highly differentiated and individually highly unpredictable, they do fall into recognizable groups by residence, age, race, sex, social customs, and so on.

7-1 Census

Content and methods For centuries (beginning as early as B.C. 3800 in Babylonia) nations have undertaken to enumerate the populations for reasons beginning with military service and taxation and evolving today to include a complex set of information concerning each individual to serve governmental, economic, social, and medical purposes.

In the United States the decennial census was established in 1790, enumerating some four million persons along the Eastern seaboard, and has continued in unbroken sequence to the determination in 1960 of many characteristics of some 180 million persons in the fifty states and territories. As the census coverage grew, so also did the amount of information collected concerning each individual. The 1960 census of population and housing called for place of residence, age, sex, race or color, occupation,

111

national origin, marital status, education, income, and relationship to head of household, in addition to information on the dwelling place.

Censuses in other countries range from the absence of collection of information on a national scale to decennial enumerations closely resembling those of the United States in completeness and content. One interesting difference is that several European countries conduct their censuses by distribution of census forms to the householders, who fill them out unassisted, whereas in the United States trained enumerators have been used to complete the forms during direct interview (prior to 1960) or at least to collect and review the forms with the householders who completed them (in 1960). In the United States in 1970, according to current plans (1), census information for households in certain metropolitan areas will be obtained insofar as possible by return of mailed questionnaires. In these areas enumerators will visit only those households from which incompletely filled out forms or no forms at all are received. It is hoped that this change will not result in loss of accuracy and completeness.

Some definitions   Certain important terms used to describe characteristics of populations require definition. The use of the word *race* in publications of the Bureau of the Census conforms to that commonly accepted by the general public; it does not attempt to define biological stock, and some of the categories refer to national origin. The designation "nonwhite" includes Negroes (92 per cent of the total), American Indians, Japanese, Chinese, Filipinos, Koreans, Hawaiians, Asian Indians, Malayans, Eskimos, and Aleuts. Mexicans are included as white, unless they are Indians.

Inhabitants are classed by place of residence as *urban* or *rural* under definitions which have been changed periodically to recognize more realistically population concentrations with densities approaching those in cities but developing outside of municipal corporate limits. As defined in 1960, urban populations included, in addition to incorporated or other communities with 2,500 or more inhabitants, the densely settled fringe surrounding large cities and other areas in which population density was at least 1,500 per square mile. In 1960, 69.9 per cent of the United States population were classed as urban and the rest as rural. However, the rural population is further subdivided into rural farm and rural nonfarm, a classification useful to both economists and epidemiologists.

Tabulation of census returns   The information collected in the decennial census, including numbers of inhabitants and their distribution by age, sex, race, marital status, income, education, occupation, and other recorded characteristics, is published in varying detail for the country as a whole, and by state, county, places with 1,000 or more inhabitants, and several types of special statistical areas. Similar information is available on request (2) for various lesser civil divisions and individual census tracts and, for 1970, numerous special tabulations will be provided on request (and at cost), including block face data for areas defined by the user.

The most important of the special statistical areas are the Standard Metropolitan Statistical Areas (SMSA). These have been defined following county boundaries, with certain exceptions in New England, about cities with populations of at least 50,000. In 1960, 113,000,000 persons resided in the 212 then defined SMSAs, each of which was made up of one or more counties containing a major central city and its surrounding metropolitan area. By 1967 there were 231 SMSAs with a total population of 119,000,000 (3). Two larger Standard Consolidated Areas have been formed to recognize the special importance of the metropolitan complex around two of the largest cities in the United States, New York and Chicago. The census also defines urbanized areas about cities of 50,000 or more, the boundaries of which follow streets or streams clearly demarcating densely settled areas rather than the boundaries of political units. Such urbanized areas are usually smaller and more homogeneously urban than SMSAs and, as they are not limited by county lines, are not always fully contained in an SMSA. Finally, to meet a rather special need, states have been subdivided into state economic areas and larger economic subregions.

For statistical purposes, census tracts have been formed in certain cities and most SMSAs. These are small areas, initially averaging 4,000 inhabitants but now much larger, the boundaries of which are established jointly by local committees and the Bureau of the Census to achieve some homogeneity of such population characteristics as economic status and living conditions. In 1960, census tracts were formed in 2 cities and 178 SMSAs, of which 136 were completely tracted. The detailed information available for census tracts is of great value in the design of sampling surveys of metropolitan areas.

Errors in the United States census   Omissions in enumeration in the 1960 census have been estimated at 3.0 per cent and erroneous inclusions (counting persons more than once) at 1.3 per cent for a net underenumeration of approximately 1.7 per cent (4). The underenumeration is largest for nonwhites, single working adults, and at the extremes of age. Infants, apparently not yet thought of as "people," are often omitted from the report to the enumerator. Underenumeration in 1960 for those less than five years of age, has been estimated to range from 1.4 per cent for white females to 7.9 per cent for nonwhite males and 2.6 per cent overall. The underenumeration error, as well as the heaping at certain ages, has been decreasing. In 1890, 27.4 per cent of the population fell into ages ending in zero and five, whereas in 1960 only 20.2 per cent fell in this class. Spiegelman's very useful textbook (4) devotes an entire chapter to a discussion of errors of coverage, response, records, compiling, and processing.

Epidemiologic usefulness of census data   The publications of the Bureau of the Census provide us with quantitative population information against which we can measure the frequency of vital events as rates, such as the number of births or deaths per 1,000 population per year or the annual number of deaths from cancer per 100,000 males in the age group 30–39. The fact that the population composition is constantly changing results in changes in overall disease incidence and death rates. In interpreting time trends in such rates it is necessary to know and take into account the many ways in which the population composition has changed. For example, we know that the United States population is becoming larger, older, better educated, richer, more urban, and more mobile. Only one in two United States citizens occupied the same residence in 1960 as in 1955, and one in every twelve had moved into a different state during this period. Levels of medical care are improving, the ratio of the number of females to the number of males is increasing, more married women are working, and the proportion of employed persons who are in white collar jobs is increasing. The center of the United States population is still moving westward. The association of these and other population variables with diseases is discussed in detail in Chapters 9, 10 and 11.

Intercensal population estimates   In the ten-year intervals between regular censuses substantial changes occur in the size and distribution of the population and, for many purposes, it is necessary to estimate population size in intercensal years. In 1954 there were 109,445 deaths among residents in California. The death rate involves the population as of July 1, 1954. Calculation of this rate, in 1955, required estimation of the population prior to the 1960 census. The census bureau publishes such estimates, but for our example here we will illustrate a simple method based on linear extrapolation from the 1940 and 1950 census figures. This method, as illustrated below, is adequate for most purposes in epidemiology and is useful for small communities for which no estimates are published.

POSTCENSAL ESTIMATE

Population April 1, 1950	10,586,000
Population April 1, 1940	6,907,000
10-year gain	3,679,000
1-year gain	367,900
4-year gain	1,471,600
3-months gain	91,975

July 1 population of 1954 $= 10,586,000 + 1,471,600$
$+ 91,975 = 12,149,575$

After the 1960 census figures became available, linear interpolation between the 1950 and 1960 figures gave a better approximation, since it took into account the new rate of growth in the 1950s instead of relying on the rate from the 1940s.

INTERCENSAL ESTIMATE

Population April 1, 1960   15,717,000
Population April 1, 1950   10,586,000
   10-year gain   5,131,000
   1-year gain   513,100
   4-year gain   2,052,400
   3-months gain   128,275
July 1 population of 1954 $= 10,586,000 + 2,052,400$
                          $+ 128,275 = 12,766,675$

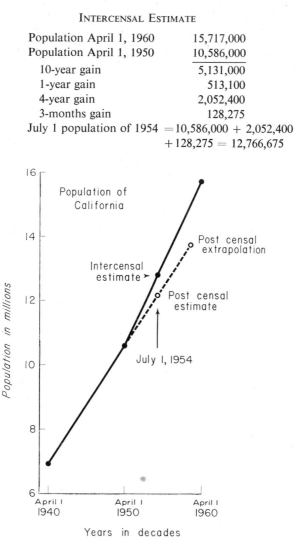

FIG. 7-1 Postcensal and intercensal population estimates, California, July 1, 1954.

The postcensal and intercensal methods are shown graphically in Figure 7-1. The postcensal estimate published by the census bureau for 1954 was 12,500,000 (5). The death rates of California residents as estimated by using the three population estimates were:

DEATHS PER 1,000 POPULATION

Postcensal linear extrapolation   9.0
Intercensal linear interpolation   8.6
Census bureau estimate (postcensal)   8.8

Although linear interpolation between census figures is usually adequate for use in vital statistics for the country as a whole, the problems are much more complex when information is desired for smaller areas or when information by age is needed. Intercensal and postcensal information is published by the Bureau of the Census and by a number of other agencies. The Census Bureau estimates involve the use of births and elementary school registration figures in addition to census data.

7-2   Registration of Vital Events

The basic events recorded by vital statistics are births, deaths, marriages, and divorces. Morbidity is also usually included, but is mentioned separately because the mechanisms of obtaining information are quite different and the completeness and reliability of the information obtained are far less than those for the first four items. In the early days of the census in the United States, attempts were made to obtain information concerning births and deaths that had occurred in the last year. The results were incomplete and involved errors in statements of cause of death. In the United States today, state laws call for the registration of births, deaths, marriages, and divorces as these events occur. These events are recorded with the local registrar and are transmitted to the state office where they are kept on file and are copied for the National Center for Health Statistics.*

The birth certificate   The birth certificate shown in Figure 7-2 is one the National Center for Health Statistics (NCHS) has recommended as a model for use by all states. It is to be noted that the state registration laws are not identical, and the NCHS is not in a position to do more than make recommendations to the states. The Birth Registration Area (with the requirement that 90 per cent of all births be registered) was not completed for the entire United States until the admission of Texas in 1933. Currently all states conform to the recommended model law (6). Several states (and New York City) use a birth certificate which includes all the information called for by the model and, in addition, much valuable information concerning complications of pregnancy and congenital malformations. Some state birth certificates still call for a statement of legitimacy, and New York City has in recent years moved the statement of legitimacy and of race from the face of the certificate to the confidential section which is not included in the copy issued to the individual. Currently, the completeness of birth registration is estimated to be between 98 and 99 per cent. Estimates differ among the states and are, in general, related

*Formerly the National Office of Vital Statistics.

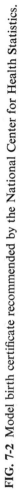

FIG. 7-2 Model birth certificate recommended by the National Center for Health Statistics.

117

to the percentages of births that occur in hospitals. Underreporting for the white population is estimated to be less than 1 per cent, whereas among nonwhites it is approximately 3 per cent (7).

The fetal death certificate   One other difference in state laws is in the definition of a fetal death or stillbirth. Some health jurisdictions (including New York City) require the use of a fetal death certificate for all products of conception, whereas others require its use only in cases in which gestation has reached the twentieth week. The certificate shown in Figure 7-3 is the NCHS model.

The death certificate   The Death Registration Area for the entire United States was also completed with the admission of Texas in 1933. The model death certificate of the NCHS (Figure 7-4) calls for place of residence, place of occurrence, age, sex, race, national origin, cause of death, and contributing causes. It is recommended that, in filling out the death certificate, physicians use guidelines contained in a pamphlet published by the United States Public Health Service (6). Cause of death must be regarded as a somewhat arbitrary concept, since in all of the routine publications each death is assigned to one and only one cause, by use of the International Classification of Diseases which has been subject to periodic revision (about every ten years).* Until 1949 the difficulties stemming from the listing of a number of contributing causes were resolved by the Manual of Joint Causes of Death (MJCD).† The MJCD established a heirarchy of precedence and in early days the rules were set up in order to give precedence to the infectious diseases. Over the years the rules were changed periodically and definitions such as that of "death from diabetes" or of "death from syphilis" were changed. In studies of the secular trend of death rates from specific causes it is necessary to study these changes and make appropriate corrections.

In 1949 major changes were introduced by the international conference into the 6th revision of the International Classification of Diseases and the use of the MJCD was stopped. Judgment as to the *underlying cause* or *the disease or condition directly leading to death* was left largely to the physician. To facilitate comparison of 1949 and subsequent data with pre-1949 data, the National Office of Vital Statistics drew a 10 per cent sample of 1949 and 1950 deaths in the United States and assigned them to cause in accordance with the new (6th) and the old (5th) revisions. From this a comparability ratio was derived (deaths assigned to a specific cause under 6th revision as a proportion of the deaths assigned to same cause under 5th revision). Some examples are

---

*The Eighth Revision of the International Classification of Diseases was adopted in Geneva in July 1965. See Vital and Health Statistics, Series 4, Number 6, NCHS, Report of the U.S. delegation to the international conference for the Eighth Revision of the International Classification of Diseases, Geneva, Switzerland, July 6–12, 1965.

†Fourth Edition, 1939, based on the Proceedings of the International Commission at Paris, 1938, and issued by the Bureau of the Census.

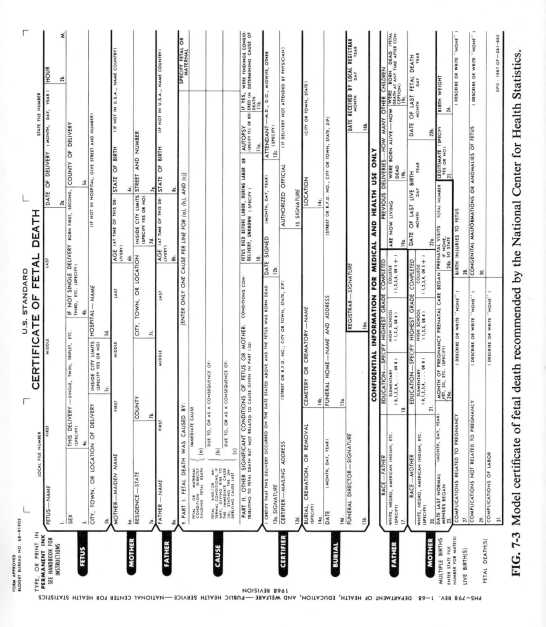

FIG. 7-3 Model certificate of fetal death recommended by the National Center for Health Statistics.

119

FORM APPROVED
BUDGET BUREAU NO. 68–R1901

(PHYSICIAN, MEDICAL EXAMINER OR CORONER)

U.S. STANDARD

CERTIFICATE OF DEATH

U.S. GOVERNMENT PRINTING OFFICE: 1967 OF–241-659

TYPE, OR PRINT IN **PERMANENT INK**
SEE HANDBOOK FOR INSTRUCTIONS

LOCAL FILE NUMBER | STATE FILE NUMBER

DECEASED

DECEASED—NAME FIRST MIDDLE LAST 1. | SEX 2. | DATE OF DEATH (MONTH, DAY, YEAR) 3.

RACE WHITE, NEGRO, AMERICAN INDIAN, ETC. (SPECIFY) 4. | AGE—LAST BIRTHDAY (YEARS) 5a. | UNDER 1 YEAR MOS. DAYS 5b. | UNDER 1 DAY HOURS MIN. 5c. | DATE OF BIRTH (MONTH, DAY, YEAR) 6. | COUNTY OF DEATH 7a.

CITY, TOWN, OR LOCATION OF DEATH 7b. | INSIDE CITY LIMITS (SPECIFY YES OR NO) 7c. | HOSPITAL OR OTHER INSTITUTION—NAME (IF NOT IN EITHER, GIVE STREET AND NUMBER) 7d.

STATE OF BIRTH (IF NOT IN U.S.A., NAME COUNTRY) 8. | CITIZEN OF WHAT COUNTRY 9. | MARRIED, NEVER MARRIED, WIDOWED, DIVORCED (SPECIFY) 10. | SURVIVING SPOUSE (IF WIFE, GIVE MAIDEN NAME) 11.

SOCIAL SECURITY NUMBER 12. | USUAL OCCUPATION (GIVE KIND OF WORK DONE DURING MOST OF WORKING LIFE, EVEN IF RETIRED) 13a. | KIND OF BUSINESS OR INDUSTRY 13b.

USUAL RESIDENCE WHERE DECEASED LIVED. IF DEATH OCCURRED IN INSTITUTION, GIVE RESIDENCE BEFORE ADMISSION. →

RESIDENCE—STATE 14a. | COUNTY 14b. | CITY, TOWN, OR LOCATION 14c. | INSIDE CITY LIMITS (SPECIFY YES OR NO) 14d. | STREET AND NUMBER 14e.

PARENTS

FATHER—NAME FIRST MIDDLE LAST 15. | MOTHER—MAIDEN NAME FIRST MIDDLE LAST 16.

INFORMANT—NAME 17a. | MAILING ADDRESS (STREET OR R.F.D. NO., CITY OR TOWN, STATE, ZIP) 17b.

CAUSE

PART I. DEATH WAS CAUSED BY: [ENTER ONLY ONE CAUSE PER LINE FOR (a), (b), AND (c)] | APPROXIMATE INTERVAL BETWEEN ONSET AND DEATH

18. IMMEDIATE CAUSE

(a)

DUE TO, OR AS A CONSEQUENCE OF:

CONDITIONS, IF ANY, WHICH GAVE RISE TO IMMEDIATE CAUSE (a), STATING THE UNDERLYING CAUSE LAST

(b)

DUE TO, OR AS A CONSEQUENCE OF:

(c)

PART II. OTHER SIGNIFICANT CONDITIONS: CONDITIONS CONTRIBUTING TO DEATH BUT NOT RELATED TO CAUSE GIVEN IN PART I (a) | AUTOPSY (YES OR NO) 19a. | IF YES WERE FINDINGS CONSIDERED IN DETERMINING CAUSE OF DEATH 19b.

ACCIDENT, SUICIDE, HOMICIDE, OR UNDETERMINED (SPECIFY) 20a. | DATE OF INJURY (MONTH, DAY, YEAR) 20b. | HOUR 20c. M. | HOW INJURY OCCURRED (ENTER NATURE OF INJURY IN PART I OR PART II, ITEM 18) 20d.

INJURY AT WORK (SPECIFY YES OR NO) 20e. | PLACE OF INJURY AT HOME, FARM, STREET, FACTORY, OFFICE BLDG., ETC. (SPECIFY) 20f. | LOCATION (STREET OR R.F.D. NO., CITY OR TOWN, STATE) 20g.

CERTIFIER

CERTIFICATION—PHYSICIAN: I ATTENDED THE DECEASED FROM 21a. MONTH DAY YEAR TO MONTH DAY YEAR 21b. | AND LAST SAW HIM/HER ALIVE ON MONTH DAY YEAR 21c. | I DID/DID NOT VIEW THE BODY AFTER DEATH. 21d. | DEATH OCCURRED (HOUR) 21e. M. AT THE PLACE, ON THE DATE, AND, TO THE BEST OF MY KNOWLEDGE, DUE TO THE CAUSE(S) STATED.

CERTIFICATION—MEDICAL EXAMINER OR CORONER: ON THE BASIS OF THE EXAMINATION OF THE BODY AND/OR THE INVESTIGATION, IN MY OPINION, DEATH OCCURRED ON THE DATE AND DUE TO THE CAUSE(S) STATED. 22a. HOUR OF DEATH M. | THE DECEDENT WAS PRONOUNCED DEAD MONTH DAY YEAR HOUR 22b. M.

CERTIFIER—NAME (TYPE OR PRINT) 23a. | SIGNATURE DEGREE OR TITLE 23b. | DATE SIGNED (MONTH, DAY, YEAR) 23c.

MAILING ADDRESS—CERTIFIER STREET OR R.F.D. NO. CITY OR TOWN STATE ZIP 23d.

BURIAL

BURIAL, CREMATION, REMOVAL (SPECIFY) 24a. | CEMETERY OR CREMATORY—NAME 24b. | LOCATION CITY OR TOWN STATE 24c.

DATE (MONTH, DAY, YEAR) 24d. | FUNERAL HOME—NAME AND ADDRESS (STREET OR R.F.D. NO., CITY OR TOWN, STATE, ZIP) 25a.

FUNERAL DIRECTOR—SIGNATURE 25b. | REGISTRAR—SIGNATURE 26a. | DATE RECEIVED BY LOCAL REGISTRAR 26b.

PHS–797–1 REV. 1–68 DEPARTMENT OF HEALTH, EDUCATION, AND WELFARE—PUBLIC HEALTH SERVICE—NATIONAL CENTER FOR HEALTH STATISTICS
1968 REVISION

FIG. 7-4 Model death certificate recommended by the National Center for Health Statistics.

CAUSE OF DEATH	RATIO
Diabetes	0.57
Syphilis	0.74
Malignant neoplasms	1.01
Arteriosclerotic and other degenerative heart disease	1.10

In New York City a similar double assignment was maintained for the first eight months of 1949. By the 5th revision there were 2,367 deaths assigned to diabetes; of these, only 1,038 were so assigned by the 6th revision. The new distribution of the 1,329 deaths dropped from diabetes was as follows:

CAUSE OF DEATH	PER CENT
Arteriosclerotic heart disease	54
Hypertensive disease	18
Cerebrovascular lesions	14
Other causes	14

In recent years classification of deaths with respect to multiple causes has been receiving growing attention (8). With the use of electronic computers it is becoming more feasible to utilize for epidemiologic purposes all of the information on the cause-of-death portion of the death certificate. The necessary coding of the information contained in the certificates, however, does require occasional questioning of the physician when it appears that the general concept of the underlying cause has been misinterpreted. Also, although uses of the classification of deaths by cause are numerous and important in many ways to research in the health sciences, many problems remain in development of a satisfactory scheme of classification of deaths in terms of multiple causes (9).

7-3   Morbidity Statistics

Notifiable disease statistics   Within the United States laws requiring the reporting of cases of specified infectious diseases (*notifiable diseases*) differ from state to state. The National Communicable Disease Center of the United States Public Health Service publishes the accumulated state reports in the "Morbidity and Mortality Weekly Reports," both for the diseases reported by all states and for those which are reported by only a few. The completeness of reporting is satisfactory for the few more serious diseases such as smallpox and very poor for others such as measles, which is believed to have averaged below 15 per cent of the total cases

prior to the advent of the highly effective Enders vaccine. One may antici-
pate that reporting of measles will become progressively more complete
as use of the vaccine is extended in efforts to eradicate the disease.

Chronic disease morbidity (except for tuberculosis) usually is not included and the only data on the occurrence of such diseases available on
an official registration basis are the mortality statistics. Semiofficial and
incomplete data for selected chronic diseases exist in the many state
tumor registries or are collected by voluntary health agencies oriented
to such specific diseases as multiple sclerosis or cystic fibrosis. For diseases
which are highly lethal after a short course, such as lung cancer, the
number of deaths may be taken as an indication of the number of cases
occurring during the year. However, the personal and national losses
resulting from the crippling effect of nonfatal diseases must be estimated
by other methods which involve large and expensive undertakings.

The foregoing paragraphs apply particularly to the United States. In
many less developed countries the situation is even less satisfactory, as
will be discussed in Chapter 10. However, in other developed countries
where much or most of the medical care is provided by the governments,
the available morbidity information is far more complete than that in
the United States. England, with its National Health Service, is a notable
example.

Special studies of population subgroups   Incidence and prevalence rates
are expressed as relative frequencies in which the base or denominator is
the population from which the cases come. The usefulness of data available
from clinics and hospitals on the number of cases diagnosed or hospitalized
is limited, unless it is possible to define the population served by the
institutions. As an example, the Mayo Clinic and the Olmsted County
Medical Group provide medical care for approximately 95 per cent of
the residents of Rochester, Minnesota. Thus, the medical records available
from these two sources would make it possible to identify most cases,
both mild and severe, coming to medical attention, and would provide
more accurate estimates of incidence or prevalence than are usually
obtainable.

More typically, defined (or easily definable) populations make use of
many sources of medical care. In smaller communities and in rural areas,
the numbers of physicians and hospitals available may be small and can
be canvassed with reasonable facility. In such situations, however, important specialized facilities, for example, a heart-lung machine or powerful X-ray therapy equipment may not be available and physicians with
equally specialized training also may be lacking. The result is that patients
with diseases requiring such services are cared for elsewhere. In large
metropolitan areas, such special needs ordinarily can be met, but collection of complete health information becomes impractical because of
the very large numbers of physicians and hospitals.

Until 1956, when the National Health Survey was instituted (see a following section), the occurrence of disease in specific subgroups of the population, such as the armed services, schools, employee and insured groups, and populations receiving prepaid medical care have provided a major part of morbidity information, and special studies in such populations continue to yield epidemiologic information of great value. As an example, a number of important studies dealing with such diverse problems as congenital malformations (10) and coronary heart disease (11) have come from the Health Insurance Plan of Greater New York (HIP). As a detailed example of how such records can be exploited, 4,210 children under the age of nine were vaccinated with the Sabin live poliovirus vaccine, type 1, at two of the HIP medical groups during a weekend in May 1962. There was interest in whether or not immunizing infection with the vaccine virus would, by operation of the interference phenomenon, reduce the frequency of disease caused by other viruses during a period following vaccination. The information that could be extracted from existing medical records concerned visits to the HIP physicians for reasons which were later classified as possibly viral, nonviral, or routine, for all the vaccinated and unvaccinated children whose families were enrolled. In terms of number of visits for possibly viral reasons before and after vaccination, it was not possible to detect the action of interference (12).

With the increasing coverage of comprehensive medical care plans, their importance as sources of morbidity data should increase. They are potential sources for studies of a prospective nature as well as for retrospective studies of records.

Surveys   Estimation of disease frequency in a community by house-to-house interview of the entire population, or more frequently of a random sample of households, is, overall, the most powerful method of obtaining morbidity information. The most valuable information, of course, comes from surveys based on medical examinations. However, because of expense and difficulties in obtaining cooperation, these have been relatively limited in scope. An example of the power of the medical examination method is the Framingham study of heart disease in which approximately 4,500 persons in Framingham, Massachusetts have been kept under surveillance for heart disease for nearly twenty years with repeated medical examinations (13). This study is discussed further in Chapter 12 as an example of continuing surveillance.

The National Health Survey   As recently as 1956, morbidity data for the United States were grossly inadequate. Need for a great deal of unavailable information existed in national, state, local, and voluntary health agencies as a basis for planning, evaluation, disease control, and research. Similarly, information was needed by institutions concerned with medical care, rehabilitation, manpower resources, and medical insurance, and by drug and appliance manufacturers.

In 1956, years of planning for continuing surveillance of morbidity in the nation bore fruit. With the advantage of new methods of survey design, and information from previous surveys such as the Hagerstown, Eastern Health District Studies and British, Canadian, Danish, and United States 1935–36 national surveys, a national undertaking was begun in the United States when Congress established the National Health Survey (NHS) on a continuing basis under the Public Health Service. *The Origin, Program and Operation of the U.S. National Health Survey* (14) describes the "program to produce statistics on disease, injury, impairment, disability, and related topics on a uniform basis for the Nation." The data of the NHS are based on approximately 40,000 interviews per year, selected in such a way that each week's interviews provide a probability sample of the fifty states and the District of Columbia. The complex design of the survey involves highly stratified multistage sampling. The importance of the resulting data, reported in certain series of issues of *Vital and Health Statistics*, published by the National Center for Health Statistics (NCHS), cannot be overstated. A recent issue (15) outlines the content of all the reports of the NCHS as indicated in the following:

Outline of Report Series for Vital and Health Statistics

Series 1.   PROGRAMS AND COLLECTION PROCEDURES. Reports which describe the general programs of the National Center for Health Statistics and its offices and divisions, data collection methods used, definitions, and other material necessary for understanding the data.

Series 2.   DATA EVALUATION AND METHODS RESEARCH. Studies of new statistical methodology, including: experimental tests of new survey methods, studies of vital statistics collection methods, new analytical techniques, objective evaluations of reliability of collected data, contributions to statistical theory.

Series 3.   ANALYTICAL STUDIES. Reports presenting analytical or interpretive studies based on vital and health statistics, carrying the analysis further than the expository types of reports in the other series.

Series 4.   DOCUMENTS AND COMMITTEE REPORTS. Final reports of major committees concerned with vital and health statistics, and documents such as recommended model vital registration laws and revised birth and death certificates.

Series 10.   DATA FROM THE HEALTH INTERVIEW SURVEY. Statistics on illness, accidental injuries, disability, use of hospital, medical, dental, and other services, and other health-related topics, based on data collected in a continuing national household interview survey.

Series 11.   DATA FROM THE HEALTH EXAMINATION SURVEY. Data from direct examination, testing, and measurement of national samples of the population provide the basis for two types of reports: (1) estimates of the medically defined prevalence of specific diseases in the United States and distributions of the population with respect to physical, physiological, and psychological characteristics; and (2) analysis of relationships among the various measurements without reference to an explicit finite universe of persons.

Series 12. DATA FROM THE INSTITUTIONAL POPULATION SURVEYS. Statistics relating to the health characteristics of persons in institutions, and on medical, nursing and personal care received, based on national samples of establishments providing these services and samples of the residents or patients.

Series 13. DATA FROM THE HOSPITAL DISCHARGE SURVEY. Statistics relating to discharged patients in short-stay hospitals, based on a sample of patient records in a national sample of hospitals.

Series 20–22. DATA FROM THE NATIONAL VITAL STATISTICS SYSTEM.

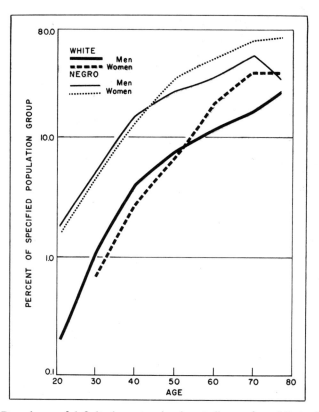

FIG. 7-5 Prevalence of definite hypertensive heart disease for white and Negro adults, by age and sex. (Published by the National Center for Health Statistics, Series 11, No. 6.)

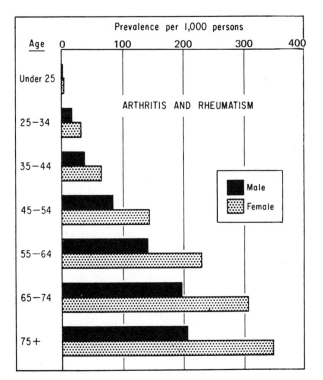

Prevalence per 1,000 persons

ARTHRITIS AND RHEUMATISM

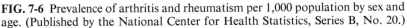

FIG. 7-6 Prevalence of arthritis and rheumatism per 1,000 population by sex and age. (Published by the National Center for Health Statistics, Series B, No. 20.)

Not only do the data of the NCHS (including that of the NHS) provide basic information of descriptive epidemiology in its incidence and prevalence rates* for the population by subgroups, but it also gives information on exposure to environmental and personal risk factors, such as smoking, which is most valuable in the study of the etiology of various diseases. The methodology studies constitute a further contribution of major importance in epidemiology. These include not only the Series 2 reports on evaluations of and advances in sampling and survey techniques but, from the Division of Health Examination Statistics, the Series 11 reports on the evaluation of diagnostic testing procedures.

The accompanying figures illustrate the types of morbidity information collected by the NHS. Figure 7-5 shows the prevalence by age of hypertensive heart disease, with higher rates in Negroes than whites, and higher rates for women in the older age groups. Figure 7-6 shows the prevalence of arthritis and rheumatism by age groups, and also shows higher rates

---

*The NHS is basically a single-visit survey in which information on illness occurrence during the previous two weeks, as well as at the time of interview, is obtained. See Series A-1, A-2 of Health Statistics from the U.S. National Health Survey.

in women for all age groups. Figure 7-7 shows the seasonal pattern for several types of illness, in particular the large waves of respiratory illnesses in the winter and early spring. Injuries also show a marked seasonal pattern, with peak incidence in late summer. Only the digestive conditions fail to show a consistent seasonal pattern.

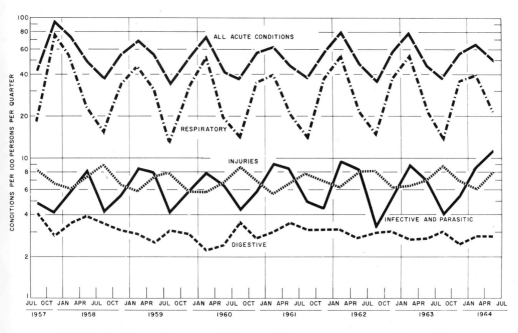

FIG. 7-7 Incidence of acute conditions per 100 persons per quarter, by condition group. (Published by the National Center for Health Statistics, Series 10, No. 15.)

7-4　Conventional Rates of Vital Statistics

Births and deaths　The *birth rate* for a given community for a calendar year is defined as the ratio of the number of live births occurring to the residents of that community during the calendar year to the population at midyear, and the results are quoted as live births per 1,000 population per year, or

$$\text{birth rate} = \frac{\text{number of live births during the calendar year}}{\text{population at midyear}} \times 1{,}000$$

As shown in the following examples (16), birth rates may differ greatly between different parts of the United States. In El Paso, Texas in 1960 there were 13,098 births to residents and an estimated population of 277,128 on July 1, 1960. The birth rate was thus 41.7 births per 1,000 population. In the SMSA of Atlantic City, New Jersey, with a midyear population of 160,880, there were 3,072 live births during 1960; the birth rate was 19.1 births per 1,000 population. It is to be noted that 36 per cent of the population of El Paso is in the age group 20–45, whereas in Atlantic City, this group accounts for only 29 per cent of the population.

A number of measures other than the birth rate have been used as measures of fertility of the population. Alternative measures restrict the denominator to the female population, either total, that part in certain age groups, or married women of appropriate ages. One of the most frequently used in this country is the *fertility ratio*, defined as

$$\frac{\text{number of children under 5 years of age}}{\text{number of women in the 15–49 age group}} \times 1,000$$

In the United States this ratio has increased since 1940. In 1960 it was 488, a level at which the population would eventually increase by two thirds in each generation. A fertility ratio of 291 would have been adequate for maintenance of the population size (17).

The crude death rate for a given community is, like the birth rate, usually computed on a residence basis and is quoted as deaths per 1,000 population per year.

$$\text{crude death rate} = \frac{\text{deaths among residents during a calendar year}}{\text{population at midyear}} \times 1,000$$

To illustrate the important difference between death rates by occurrence and by residence we need only to look at any city which serves as a medical center for the surrounding area, particularly cities with medical schools, clinics, and hospitals to which difficult cases are referred by physicians in a fairly large surrounding area. Olmsted County, Minnesota (which includes Rochester, with its Mayo Clinic and Graduate School of Medicine) may be used as an example. In 1960 1,397 deaths occurred in the county. Of these 412 were among county residents. An additional 48 deaths among county residents occurred outside the county. These counts lead to a death rate by occurrence (21.3) which is three times as large as the death rate among residents (7.0).

Specific death rates   Death rates for specific subgroups of the population are, in general, more meaningful than the crude death rate. Death rates may be specific in the sense that they refer to some subgroup of the population defined in terms of race, age, and sex, or they may refer to the entire population but be specific for some single cause of death. As a first step the relationship of the crude rate to the *color (or race)* specific rates*

---

*Although the census data provide information as to race in the more specific sense, it is customary for summary purposes to divide the population into white and nonwhite. Rates for the corresponding segments of the population, hence, usually are referred to as *color specific*.

will be considered, using the data for Georgia and Wisconsin shown in Table 7-1.

TABLE 7-1

Relationship of color-specific death rates to crude death rates in two states, 1960

STATE	COLOR-SPECIFIC DEATH RATES*		PROPORTION OF POPULATION		CRUDE DEATH RATE
	W	NW	W	NW	
Georgia	8.0	11.4	.714	.286	9.0
Wisconsin	9.8	6.5	.976	.024	9.7

*Deaths per 1,000 population.
Source: Vital Statistics of the United States, 1960; United States Census of Population, 1960.

The crude rates are weighted averages of the color-specific rates,

for Georgia: $.714 \times 8.0 + .286 \times 11.4 = 9.0$
for Wisconsin: $.976 \times 9.8 + .024 \times 6.5 = 9.7$

Note that in the Wisconsin crude rate, 98 per cent of the total weight goes to the death rate for whites, whereas in the Georgia crude rate only 71 per cent of the weight is so allocated.

Because death rates vary significantly with sex, it often is important to calculate *sex specific* death rates. This ratio is of special interest in study of specific diseases. As one example, we may look at deaths in 1960 assigned to coronary heart disease (CHD) in New York City and in the United States, the respective *cause specific* death rates being 185.0 and 160.1 per 100,000 population per year. The corresponding *sex and cause specific* rates were:

for New York City: 260.6 (males) and 115.8 (females)
for the United States: 218.4 (males) and 103.6 (females)

Thus, in both populations, male rates were more than twice those for females. Fortunately, although usual populations are not evenly distributed by sex (the usual pattern being a progressively increasing excess of females with age), important differences in distribution by sex occur only between relatively special types of populations such as occupational groups, prisons, schools, and so on. Hence, despite the usual strong relation between sex and death rates, it is not usually necessary to take account of differences in distribution by sex when comparing death rates in different populations.

Age-specific rates   The age-specific rates are defined in the same terms as the crude rate, except that both the numerator and denominator are confined to a particular age group. For example, the death rate for persons under the age of ten years is

$$\frac{\text{number of deaths of persons aged 0–9 in a calendar year}}{\text{population of persons aged 0–9 at midyear}} \times 1{,}000$$

The age distribution and the age-specific death rates for the United States in 1965 are shown graphically in Figure 7-8. The crude death rate, if plotted, would appear as a horizontal straight line summarizing all of the age-specific rates. It is important to understand the nature of this summary. The crude rate is a weighted average of the age-specific rates in which the weight (relative importance) of the age-specific rate for any age group is given directly by the proportion of the population in that age group. This is discussed in more detail below.

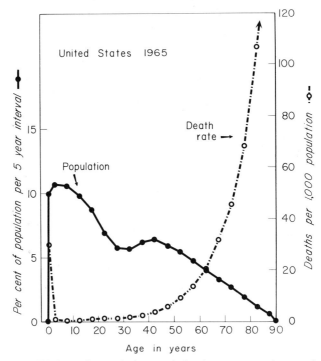

FIG. 7-8 Distribution of population and death rates per thousand, by age, United States, 1965.

It can be seen from the definitions that the crude rate has as its numerator the sum of all the numerators of the age-specific rates (i.e., the total number of deaths at all ages) and for its denominator the sum of all of the denominators of the specific rates (i.e., the total population). The

most easily understood expression for the relationship of the crude rate
to the specific rates is the weighted average

> crude rate = sum of [(age specific rate) × (proportion of
> population in age group)]

or

$$R = \Sigma\left(\frac{P_i}{P}\right)R_i$$

where P = total population; P_i and R_i respectively, are the populations
and the death rates for successive age groups i into which the total population is divided. Note that each age-specific rate is weighted (or multiplied)
by the proportion of the total population to which it applies.

It is important to recognize that the crude death rate summarizes not
only the age-specific rates, R_i, which measure the force of mortality, but
also the particular age characteristics of the population of the community

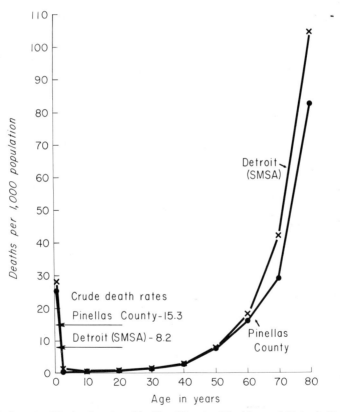

FIG. 7-9 Age-specific death rates, Pinellas County, Florida, and Detroit Standard Metropolitan Statistical Area, 1960.

under consideration. We find that in the Standard Metropolitan Statistical Area of Detroit the crude rate gives 15.7 per cent of the total weight to the death rate for age groups over sixty, whereas in Pinellas County, Florida, the crude rate gives these rates 38.7 per cent of the total weight. The respective crude rates were 8.2 and 15.3 deaths per 1,000 population in 1960. If we are interested in the rate at which persons of various ages are dying in the two cities it is necessary to look at the age-specific rates (later we will also take into account differences in race and sex). Figure 7-9 shows the age-specific rates for the two communities graphically. The only satisfactory comparison of the occurrence of death is made in terms of age-specific rates.

It is apparent that the crude rates of the two cities cannot be compared. The crude rates have two disadvantages. The first and most important is that they oversummarize the complex patterns of rates. The pattern of changes of the death rates with age shown in the graph cannot be expressed in terms of any single number, and any attempt to do so will result in serious loss of information. The second disadvantage of the crude rate is the lack of comparability for two communities (or a single community in different years) which have different age composition and hence different weighting systems for the age-specific rates.

As another example of the importance of a population's age distribution in determining the size of the crude rate, it is interesting to note that in 1960 the crude death rate in Vermont was 11.3, and in Alaska was 5.5 deaths per 1,000 population. Inspection of the age-specific rates is immediately suggested and would prove rewarding.

The crude death rates of South Dakota in 1940 and 1960 serve as an example of the importance of changes in the age composition of the population over time. As seen in Figure 7-10 the 1960 age-specific rates are uniformly lower than those in 1940, and yet the crude rate has risen from 8.9 to 9.7. Inspection of the census figures reveals that the percentage of population over fifty-five years of age rose during this period from 15 per cent to 19 per cent. The following section deals with a method of correcting for difference in age distribution which, for the South Dakota rates, leads to corrected rates of 8.6 in 1940 and 7.1 in 1960 (age-adjusted by the direct method to the 1940 United States age distribution).

7-5   Adjusted Rates

It was noted earlier in discussion of the data of Table 7-1 that the crude rates for Georgia and Wisconsin involve giving 98 per cent of the total weight to the death rate for whites in Wisconsin, whereas the corresponding figure for Georgia was only 71 per cent. *Adjustment for color* involves summarizing the two sets of color-specific rates by using the *same weights*.

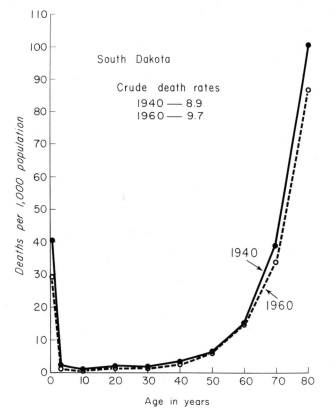

FIG. 7-10 Age-specific death rates, South Dakota, 1940 and 1960.

If those weights are obtained from the color distribution of the United States, 1960 population, in which 11.4 per cent were nonwhite, the color-adjusted rates are

$$\text{Georgia:} \quad .886 \times 8.0 + .114 \times 11.4 = 8.4$$
$$\text{Wisconsin:} \quad .886 \times 9.8 + .114 \times \ 6.5 = 9.4$$

Different choices of standard populations will give different results, as illustrated in Table 7-2. How the choice of standard population influences the adjusted rates is discussed in detail in a following paragraph.

Adjustment for color, without adjustment also for age, is not very useful in this case. From the color-specific rates themselves we see that the death rate for whites in Wisconsin is much higher than that for whites in Georgia. How much of this difference is because the Wisconsin white population is older than the white population of Georgia? Similarly, the rates suggest that the nonwhite population of Wisconsin is younger than that of Georgia. These questions will be left for the reader to investigate by seeking out the census volumes and the Vital Statistics publications

TABLE 7-2

Color-adjusted death rates per 1,000 population for two
states in 1960 using different standard populations

STANDARD POPULATION	COLOR-ADJUSTED RATES	
	GEORGIA	WISCONSIN
United States	8.4	9.4
Georgia	9.0	8.1
Wisconsin	8.9	9.7

Source: Vital Statistics of the United States, 1960; United
States Census of Population, 1960.

of the National Center for Health Statistics. In a following section another
example will be used to illustrate age and age–color adjustment.

Adjustment is a method of correcting for the second and less serious
of the disadvantages of the crude rate, that is, for unequal weights. The
first and most important disadvantage, oversimplification, is one the
crude and adjusted rates have in common. The two crude rates are replaced by two other single numbers that are the result of using the same
weighting system in summarizing the two sets of subgroup (e.g., age, race,
or sex) specific rates. Just what this weighting system is is not very important; the real purpose is to correct for the differences (in this case,
distributions of the populations by age) in Detroit and Pinellas County.
For comparison of two communities within the United States, it is common practice to use the weights from the last census for the entire United
States population, in which case the 1960 United States population is
said to be the *standard population.*

Table 7-3 gives the proportion of the total United States 1960 population in each age, sex, and color group. Table 7-4 gives the basic vital
statistics and census data for the Standard Metropolitan Statistical Area
of Detroit and for Pinellas County, Florida. Table 7-5 is set up for the
adjustment procedure that will give us rates for these two communities
which are comparable in the sense that any difference in the resulting
adjustment must be caused by something other than differences in age
distribution.

The age adjusted rates are then given by:

Detroit: $.023 \times 25.4 + .090 \times .8 + \ldots + .031 \times 106.1 = 9.7$
Pinellas: $.023 \times 28.2 + .090 \times 1.4 + \ldots + .031 \times 82.5 = 8.2$

This adjustment procedure corrects for differences in the age distribution of the population, but not for differences in the color distribution.

TABLE 7-3

Percentage distribution, 1960 population of the United States, by age, sex, and color

AGE GROUP (YEARS)	WHITE			NONWHITE			ALL		
	MALE	FEMALE	TOTAL	MALE	FEMALE	TOTAL	MALE	FEMALE	TOTAL
<5	4.9	4.7	9.6	.9	.8	1.7	5.8	5.5	11.3
5–14	8.8	8.5	17.3	1.3	1.3	2.6	10.1	9.8	19.9
15–24	5.8	6.0	11.8	.8	.8	1.6	6.6	6.8	13.4
25–34	5.5	5.7	11.2	.7	.8	1.5	6.2	6.5	12.7
35–44	5.9	6.1	12.0	.7	.7	1.4	6.6	6.8	13.4
45–54	5.1	5.2	10.3	.5	.6	1.1	5.6	5.8	11.4
55–64	3.8	4.1	7.9	.4	.4	.8	4.2	4.5	8.7
65–74	2.7	2.9	5.6	.2	.3	.5	2.9	3.2	6.1
75+	1.2	1.7	2.9	.1	.1	.2	1.3	1.8	3.1
Total	43.7	44.9	88.6	5.6	5.8	11.4	49.3	50.7	100.0

Source: United States Census of Population, 1960.

TABLE 7-4

Age distribution of population and deaths, Detroit SMSA and Pinellas County, Florida, 1960

AGE (YEARS)	DETROIT SMSA		PINELLAS COUNTY, FLORIDA	
	DEATHS	POPULATION (IN THOUSANDS)	DEATHS	POPULATION (IN THOUSANDS)
<1	2,316	91.2	160	5.7
1–4	304	376.3	30	22.2
5–14	262	768.7	30	51.9
15–24	406	443.2	26	32.6
25–34	696	506.8	47	33.9
35–44	1,585	555.0	124	41.6
45–54	3,387	429.8	320	41.7
55–64	5,802	322.0	829	52.0
65–74	8,225	196.1	1,901	65.8
75+	7,764	73.2	2,259	27.4
Total	30,747	3,762.2	5,726	374.8

Source: Vital Statistics of the United States, 1960; United States Census of Population, 1960.

TABLE 7-5

Table for computation of age-adjusted death rates with the United States 1960 population as standard

AGE (YEARS)	PROPORTION OF U.S. 1960 POPULATION IN AGE GROUP	AGE-SPECIFIC DEATH RATES PER 1,000 POPULATION	
		DETROIT SMSA	PINELLAS COUNTY, FLORIDA
<1	.023	25.4	28.2
1–4	.090	.8	1.4
5–14	.199	.3	.6
15–24	.134	.9	.8
25–34	.127	1.4	1.4
35–44	.134	2.9	3.0
45–54	.114	7.9	7.7
55–64	.087	18.0	15.9
65–74	.061	41.9	28.9
75+	.031	106.1	82.5
Crude death rates		8.2	15.3
Age-adjusted death rates		9.7	8.2

Source: Vital Statistics of the United States, 1960; United States Census of Population, 1960.

Table 7-6 is set up to demonstrate the method of simultaneous adjustment for age and color. Since each population has been divided into twice as many subgroups, there are twice as many multiplications and additions involved. However, the basic method is exactly the same: Each subgroup-specific rate is multiplied by the proportion of the standard population which falls into that subgroup and the sum of the products over all subgroups gives the adjusted rate.

It is to be noted that the differences between the age distributions could be corrected for by use of weights derived from the age distribution of any community such as Chicago, New Orleans, or either of the two communities under discussion. Some textbooks give illustrations in which the standard population is taken to be the pooled populations of the two communities to be compared. This is, of course, just as reasonable as any that could be chosen, but it does involve a little additional calculation that is hard to justify. It should be noted carefully, however, that if a different standard population were used, the two adjusted rates would have different values, their ratio would be different, and the difference between them would change and conceivably be of different sign. In short, one of the major weaknesses of the adjustment procedure lies in its lack

TABLE 7-6

Table for computation of age- and color-adjusted death rates with the U.S. 1960 population as standard

AGE (YEARS)	PROPORTION OF U.S. 1960 POPULATION IN SUBGROUP		AGE- AND COLOR-SPECIFIC DEATH RATES PER 1,000 POPULATION			
			DETROIT SMSA		PINELLAS COUNTY	
	White	*Nonwhite*	*White*	*Nonwhite*	*White*	*Nonwhite*
<1	.0195	.0034	22.154	41.555	21.455	54.640
1–4	.0773	.0131	0.759	1.044	1.335	1.433
5–14	.1713	.0265	0.333	0.381	0.601	0.430
15–24	.1175	.0164	0.860	1.230	0.800	0.791
25–34	.1123	.0149	1.105	2.773	1.104	3.064
35–44	.1202	.0141	2.497	4.810	2.658	5.979
45–54	.1031	.0112	7.185	12.112	6.897	16.514
55–64	.0790	.0078	17.110	24.695	15.063	36.654
65–74	.0565	.0048	41.333	47.751	28.317	63.419
75	.0289	.0022	108.819	75.793	82.946	57.447
Age- and color-adjusted rates			9.664		8.321	

Source: Vital Statistics of the United States, 1960; United States Census of Population, 1960.

of uniqueness, or in the influence which the choice of a standard population exerts on the outcome of the desired comparisons. This has been illustrated already in relation to color-specific death rates in Wisconsin and Georgia (cf. Table 7-2). As an additional illustration of the loss of information involved in bringing the standard population into the comparison of the age-specific rates, consider a situation in which community A has higher rates from birth to age thirty and community B has higher rates from age thirty on. It is easy to see that, by choice of a very young population as standard, we can arrive at the conclusion that the adjusted rate is higher for community A, whereas by choice of an old population we can arrive at exactly the opposite conclusion. In fact, with one choice of the standard population, the age-adjusted rates will be equal. The point is that, in view of the vastly different age patterns of death rates in this case, which indicate some very real difference in environment or medical care practice, we do not want to compare summary rates at all. A further general point is that no adjustment for age or other characteristic should be undertaken until the age- or other subgroup-specific rates have been studied carefully.

The standardized mortality ratio   It is often desirable to compare the mortality experience (either total or from a selected cause) of a designated group (occupational or other) with that of the total population. One could, of course, compute the age-sex-adjusted rate for the studied group (using the general population as standard) and compare it directly with the general population rate. An alternate method expresses the extent to which the observed number of deaths in the group exceeds (or falls below) the number expected on the basis of applying the age-sex-specific rates of the general population to the corresponding age-sex subgroups of the group under study. The ratio of the number of deaths observed to the number expected, expressed in per cent, is the standardized mortality ratio (SMR).

As an example, we can compare the 1960 mortality experience of the population of Pinellas County, Florida (shown in Table 7-4) with that of the United States as a whole. Observed deaths numbered 5,726. Table 7-7 provides the information needed to compute the number of deaths expected if the 1960 United States age-specific death rates were applied. Summing the products $27.0 \times 5.7 \ldots 106.1 \times 27.4$ gives 7,058 as the number of deaths expected. The SMR is calculated as $5726/7058 \times 100$ or, 81 per cent, i.e., the observed deaths were only 81 per cent of those expected under United States rates. It may be noted that in this and other

TABLE 7-7

Table for the computation of the standardized mortality ratio for Pinellas County, Florida in 1960

AGE (YEARS)	U.S. 1960 DEATH RATES (PER 1,000 POP.)	PINELLAS COUNTY 1960 POPULATION (IN 1,000's)	PINELLAS COUNTY DEATHS	
			OBSERVED	EXPECTED
<1	27.0	5.7	160	154
1–4	1.1	22.2	30	24
5–14	.5	51.9	30	26
15–24	1.1	32.6	26	36
25–34	1.5	33.9	47	51
35–44	3.0	41.6	124	125
45–54	7.6	41.7	320	317
55–64	17.4	52.0	829	905
65–74	38.2	65.8	1,901	2,513
75+	106.1	27.4	2,259	2,907
All	9.5	374.8	5,726	7,058

Source: Vital Statistics of the United States, 1960; United States Census of Population, 1960.

examples involving communities with the usual distribution of populations by sex, it is not necessary to take account of sex-specific rates in computing the SMR. It should also be evident that computing the SMR is a special form of adjusting for differences in the distributions of the studied population and of the general population with respect to age and (when necessary for groups with unusual distributions) to sex.

7-6   Cause-Specific Death Rates

Death rates for any specific disease, such as tuberculosis, may be given for the entire population or for any age, race, or sex subgroup. *Cause-specific death rates* are computed as:

$$\frac{\text{deaths assigned to the disease among the specified population in a given year}}{\text{total specified population as of July 1 of the given year}} \times 100,000$$

and so are expressed as deaths per 100,000 population per year. Data for deaths resulting from respiratory tuberculosis in the New York City SMSA, 1959–1961, illustrate the application of cause-specific death rates to populations defined by sex and color (18). Cause-, sex-, and color-specific rates per 100,000 population per year were:

	MALE	FEMALE
White	31.6	7.9
Nonwhite	103.7	38.3

It must be noted that the foregoing sex- and color-specific rates cannot be compared until adjustment has been made for differences in the age distributions of the respective sex–race populations. Using the combined 1960 population of all 212 SMSAs as standard, the resulting age-, sex-, and color-specific death rates per 100,000 population per year were:

	MALE	FEMALE
White	9.3	2.2
Nonwhite	43.7	15.5

One could, of course, compare directly cause-, sex-, and color-specific death rates for corresponding age groups (i.e., rates in which both numerators and denominators are from the same age groups and, hence, are age-specific) as shown here for respiratory tuberculosis for the New York City SMSA:

	MALES 45–54 YEARS	FEMALES 45–54 YEARS
White	16	4
Nonwhite	81	19

Indeed, for many diseases such as tuberculosis the age pattern of deaths for each sex is quite distinctive and we may prefer comparing successive age-specific rates for one sex with those for the other to comparing age-adjusted summary rates. The data in Table 7-8 for deaths from respiratory tuberculosis in the New York City SMSA permit such a comparison between sexes for both whites and nonwhites. This table reveals the important fact (lost in the summary rate) that the difference between sexes is not important until after age 45 among whites and age 35 among nonwhites.

TABLE 7-8

Death rates for respiratory tuberculosis per 100,000 population in the New York City SMSA, 1959–1961, by age, sex, and race

AGE (YEARS)	WHITE		NONWHITE	
	MALE	FEMALE	MALE	FEMALE
0–4	0	0	1	3
5–14	0	0	0	0
15–24	0	1	4	4
25–34	2	1	21	17
35–44	5	4	56	24
45–54	16	4	81	19
55–64	28	4	106	18
65–74	41	6	103	28
75–84	56	10	126	24
85+	58	21	110	61
All	31.6	7.9	103.7	38.3

Source: Duffy, Edward A. and Carroll, Robert E. *United States Metropolitan Mortality*, 1959–1961, PHS Publication No. 999-AP-39, U.S. Public Health Service, National Center for Air Pollution Control, 1967.

7-7   Other Rates Used for Mortality from Specific Causes

The proportional mortality* rate (PMR)   The 1958 PMR for tuberculosis in Puerto Rico equals

*Use of the adjective *death* is reserved for rates in which the denominator is a population number; when the denominator is something other than a population (e.g., all deaths, all cases, or all live births) a different adjective, *mortality* or *fatality*, is used.

$$\frac{\text{deaths assigned to tuberculosis in Puerto Rico residents in 1958}}{\text{total deaths among Puerto Rico residents in 1958}} \times 100 = \frac{667}{16{,}074} = 4.1\%$$

This is a simple statement of the proportion of all deaths which were assigned to the cause tuberculosis. Since the denominator is deaths among persons of both sexes and all ages and races, proportional mortality rates will in general need adjustment, just as crude death rates do.

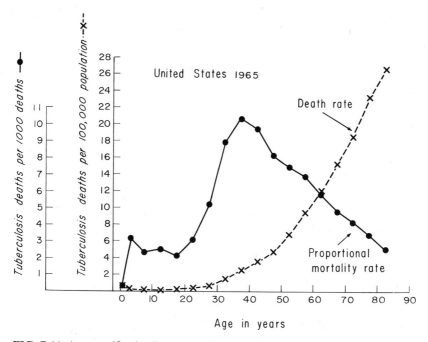

FIG. 7-11 Age-specific death rates and proportional mortality rates for tuberculosis, United States, 1965.

Figure 7-11 shows the 1965 United States PMR for tuberculosis and the death rate (for all causes) by age. To understand the entirely different slope of these age patterns, we note that

$$\text{PMR} = \frac{\text{tuberculosis death rates}}{\text{tuberculosis death rates} + \text{death rates for all other causes}} \times 100$$

and that the PMR decreases in older age groups in response to an increase in deaths from *other* causes (such as heart disease and cancer) which is much more rapid than the increase in deaths from tuberculosis.

The case fatality rate   The case fatality rate for smallpox is defined as

$$\frac{\text{the number of deaths assigned to smallpox in a specified period of time}}{\text{the number of cases occurring in the same period of time}} \times 100$$

The period of time may cover a particular local outbreak or may cover many years of experience with an endemic disease. The purpose is to measure a property of the disease (related to virulence) and to provide a basis for prognosis. The case fatality rate is used mostly for acute infectious diseases such as paralytic poliomyelitis and diphtheria. Its usefulness for chronic diseases (even when, as with tuberculosis, they are infectious) is limited, because the period from onset to fatal outcome is typically long and very variable. The number of deaths in a given period of time will have little relation to the number of cases occurring in that period and the outcome of all current new cases may not be known until many years have passed.

Mortality rates based on live births   The infant mortality rate (IMR) for the residents of any specified community is defined as:

$$\frac{\text{the number of deaths in a calendar year among persons aged less than one year}}{\text{the number of live births during that calendar year}} \times 1000$$

For the State of Washington in 1960, the IMR was 23.4 infant deaths per 1,000 live births. For Australia in 1961 the corresponding figure was 19.5. The importance of the IMR arises from the fact that the denominator of the death rate for persons under one year of age is very difficult to determine even in a census year. Experience indicates that when an adult is asked to list all of the persons who were living in the house on April 1, a month-old infant is frequently forgotten and the infant population is underenumerated. It is to be noted that the IMR as defined above cannot be considered an exact measure of "risk," because some of the infant deaths in a calendar year are from births of the previous year and some of the deaths under the age of one year among the births of the calendar year will occur in the following year. If the birth rate remains relatively constant this is not an important factor, but in years of sudden change (such as the war years) the result can be misleading. The NCHS adjusts for this effect by using corrections for changes in the birth rate.

Although the infant mortality rate involves deaths in the first year of age, changes in the rates and in the predominant causes of death within this single year are so striking that for many purposes we must look at a shorter period after birth. Figure 7-12 shows the marked skewing of infant deaths toward the time of birth and suggests that a rate reflecting

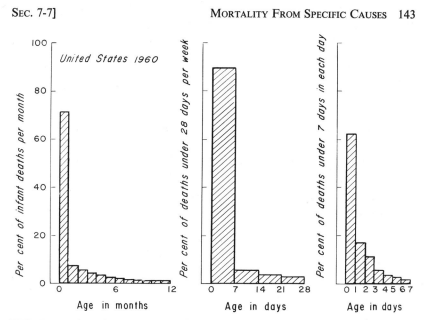

FIG. 7-12 Infant deaths by age, United States, 1960.

deaths in the first month of life would be useful. The *neonatal mortality rate* is defined as

$$\frac{\text{number of deaths in a calendar year among infants under 28 days of age}}{\text{number of live births in that calendar year}} \times 1,000$$

In 1960 the rate in the state of Washington was 1,126 deaths under 28 days × 1,000/65,278 live births, or 16.2 deaths per 1,000 live births.

Figure 7-12 also suggests that, for some purposes, the first month of life is too long a period as, perhaps, even the first week may be. To assist in the study of reproductive loss, the *fetal death ratio* (*FDR*) was defined as a measure of risk in the late stages of gestation:

$$FDR = \frac{\text{the number of fetal deaths after 28 weeks or more gestation}}{\text{the number of live births in the calendar year}} \times 1,000$$

The high proportion of infant deaths in the first day of life suggests the continuing operation after birth of factors contributing to late fetal deaths. For the study of reproductive loss the distinction between a child who dies within hours or minutes after birth and one dying shortly before birth (i.e., stillborn) is not important. To provide a measure of risk based on deaths in both periods the *perinatal mortality rate* (*PerMR*) is introduced:

$$\text{PerMR} = \frac{\text{the number of deaths of infants under 7 days of age and fetuses over 28 weeks' gestation*}}{\text{the number of live births plus fetal deaths in a calendar year}} \times 1,000$$

When the rate of decrease of the United States infant mortality rate slowed sharply after 1950 (and in New York City increased from 24.8 to 27.3 infant deaths per 1,000 live births), it was suggested that improvements in medical practice had resulted in bringing to live birth and early death what had previously been late fetal deaths. This hypothesis was explored in New York City by comparing the trends from 1940 to 1962 in the IMR, FDR, and PerMR (see Table 7-9). Between 1940 and 1950

TABLE 7-9

Trends in infant mortality and perinatal deaths in New York City

Rate*	1940	1950	1962
IMR	34.9	24.8	27.3
FDR	25.3	15.4	13.6
PerMR	44.7	31.3	31.1

*See text for definitions of the three rates.
Source: New York City Department of Health: Summary of Vital Statistics, 1962, The City of New York.

dramatic relative decreases of approximately 30, 40, and 30 per cent are noted in the IMR, FDR, and PerMR, respectively. However, in the next twelve years, the infant mortality rate increased by 8 per cent, the FDR decreased by 10 per cent, and the PerMR did not change. The decline in the FDR was perhaps sufficient to have caused a small increase in the IMR. However, the failure of the IMR to continue its dramatic drop (another 30 per cent relative decrease would have brought it to 17.5) apparently cannot be fully explained, as suggested above, on the basis of increased success in bringing nonviable progeny to live birth.

Changes in the infant mortality rate by age and cause   The infant mortality rate in the United States decreased rapidly until 1950 when the annual rate of decrease in the rate changed from 4.3 per cent to 2 per cent. The 1960 IMR was about one third of the 1920 rate. Decline in deaths due to infectious diseases accounted for most of the decrease up to 1950 and

*The definition of the perinatal period as extending from the twenty-eighth week of gestation to the seventh day of life was endorsed by the International Conference for the Eighth Revision of the International Classification of Diseases.

for some thereafter. For example, during the period between 1950 and 1965 the IMR for "certain diseases of early infancy" (chiefly noninfectious) decreased by 14 per cent, while in the same period the rates for dysentery and whooping cough decreased by 84 per cent and 95 per cent respectively.

The shifts in the proportional mortality by cause away from common infectious agents has been accompanied by a shift in the age distribution of infant deaths. Thus, 52 per cent of all infant deaths in 1920–1924 were of infants under one month of age; in 1965 this figure had risen to 72 per cent. The rate at which this shift took place is indicated in Figure 7-13 which shows the trends of the infant mortality and neonatal mortality rates 1920–1965.

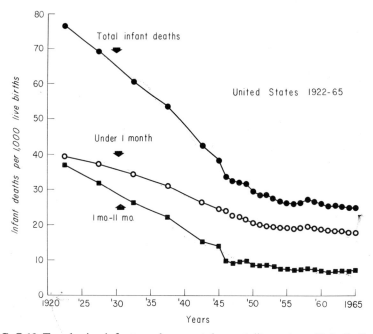

FIG. 7-13 Trends in infant and neonatal mortality rates, United States, 1922–1965.

Figure 7-14 shows the seasonal variations in neonatal mortality and postneonatal mortality (ages 1–11 months) in Norway in the five-year period, 1955–1959. The sharp seasonality of the postneonatal rates and relative lack of seasonal influence on neonatal rates provides further evidence for the operation of quite different causes of death during and after the first month of life. The predominance of infectious causes after the neonatal period largely explains the observed seasonality. Although the causes of neonatal deaths are now being intensively studied, their lack

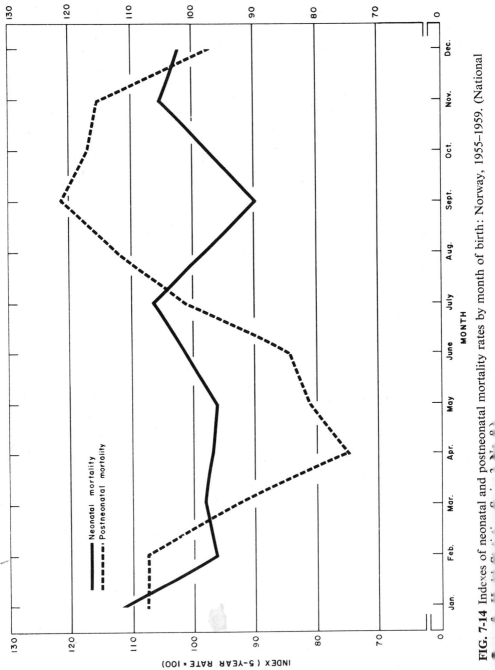

FIG. 7-14 Indexes of neonatal and postneonatal mortality rates by month of birth: Norway, 1955–1959. (National

146

of seasonality suggests that common infectious causes play no more than a minor role.

⌐The maternal mortality rate (MMR) is defined traditionally as:

$$\frac{\text{number of deaths assigned to puerperal causes in a calendar year}}{\text{number of live births in that calendar year}} \times 1{,}000$$

Because of the decline in the MMR in the United States (by decade from 1920 to 1960: 6.9 to .37 maternal deaths per 1,000 live births) it is customary now to quote the 1960 MMR as 37.1 maternal deaths per 100,000 live births. In some countries the base of 1,000 live births is still convenient. The risk of death resulting from pregnancy is not measurable in any way that is sufficiently accurate to be useful. Because many pregnancies terminate as spontaneous abortions before they are recognized (and an unknown number are terminated by induced abortion, both legal and illegal), the true number of pregnancies is not known and no legislation requiring the registration of pregnancy is likely to improve the situation to the point where a good measure of risk can be evaluated. Thus, the MMR is not a measure of risk (good or poor) and should not be criticized because it is not. It is instead an excellent measure of the cost in maternal deaths assigned to puerperal causes per live births.

7-8   Morbidity Rates

In considering the impact on our society of a chronic disease such as tuberculosis, we are concerned with two aspects of disease occurrence, prevalence and incidence. In each case the rates are quoted per 1,000 population if convenient, although other powers of 10 may be used for particular diseases (e.g., per 100 for very common diseases or per 10,000 or 100,000 for uncommon diseases). *The prevalence rate* is defined as

$$\frac{\text{number of known cases at a given point in time}}{\text{population at that time}} \times 100,\ 1{,}000,\ 10{,}000,\ \text{or } 100{,}000$$

It measures the magnitude of the disease problem at a stated point in time. The prevalence rate is particularly useful as an indicator of needs for medical and social care to cope with the current cases (and, if the patients are bread winners, their families). It is useful only for diseases of long duration (months or years), commonly referred to as chronic diseases. *The incidence rate* is defined as

$$\frac{\text{number of newly reported cases in a defined period, often a calendar year}}{\text{population at midperiod}} \times 100,\ 1{,}000,\ 10{,}000,\ \text{or } 100{,}000$$

It measures the rate at which new cases are occurring in the population. It is particularly important as an indicator of the need for preventive measures and is potentially useful for both acute and chronic diseases.

Information on morbidity is not as readily available, nor is what we do have nearly as reliable or complete as are data for natality and mortality. The reasons for this were discussed in the section on morbidity statistics. However, to further illustrate the problem we can look at a case of tuberculosis which, to be included in the numerator of either the prevalence or incidence rates, must first be diagnosed and then be reported. The first step requires that the patient see a doctor or have an X ray as part of a mass screening public health program. The second step requires the cooperation of the physician in reporting the case to the local health department. Finally, because only active cases of tuberculosis are of interest in prevalence studies, some mechanism must exist for removing cases from the roster. The proportion of tuberculosis cases known to the local health authorities differs widely among communities, even within the United States.

For chronic diseases such as tuberculosis both the prevalence rate and the incidence rate carry important information. Prevalence measures the need for treatment and hospital beds and the economic loss to the community. Incidence serves as a measure for evaluating control programs (if any) and has implications for the future problems of medical care.

Ideally, the incidence rate would be based on prospective surveillance of the population of an entire community under conditions of medical care which would result in early diagnosis of all cases. This situation is approximated in the population of Olmsted County, Minnesota, where the overwhelming majority of persons receive their medical care from either the Mayo Clinic or the Olmsted County Medical Group. The combined medical records of these two institutions make possible studies of incidence and prevalence of diseases requiring medical care which are based on exceptionally good case ascertainment. One example is a study of the trend of leukemia over a thirty-year period, 1935–1964 (19). This study was undertaken in an effort to understand the increase in the United States annual death rate for leukemia which rose from 2.3 per 100,000 population in 1930 to 7.5 in 1963. Because of the exceptional quality and coverage of medical care in Olmsted County throughout the period of the study, it was felt that no change had occurred in the probability that a case of leukemia would be recognized and recorded as such. Examination of the age-adjusted rates in this study revealed no increase in leukemia incidence, a finding which led the authors to suggest that changing patterns of medical care in the rest of the United States may have been responsible for the national increase. Unfortunately, the ideal situation in Olmsted County has few counterparts elsewhere in the country. Hence, both prevalence and incidence rates are usually subject to the same errors and lack of completeness that characterize morbidity data in general.

The secondary attack rate (SAR) is a measure of the occurrence of a contagious disease among known (or presumed) susceptible persons following exposure to a primary case. The SAR is defined as:

$$\frac{\text{number of contacts developing disease within the maximum incubation period}}{\text{total number of "susceptible" exposed persons (contacts)}} \times 100$$

It represents an attempt to measure the spread of infection following contact and, as such, provides an indication of the infectivity of the causative agent. Typically, it is applied to relatively closed groups, households or classrooms, where contact can be safely presumed for all members. The first case occurring in such a group is called the primary case (two or more cases occurring on the same day or within an interval less than the shortest incubation period are called co-primary cases). Subsequent cases occurring within the maximum incubation period are called secondary cases. Cases occurring after a longer interval are excluded as representing tertiary spread or deriving from sources outside the group. Given information concerning a number of households containing primary cases, the numerator of the SAR is the total number of secondary cases as defined above and the denominator is the total number of exposed "susceptible" members of the affected households. (Note that the primary cases are excluded from both numerator and denominator.) The limitation to "susceptibles" is feasible only for such diseases as measles or chickenpox which lead to long-enduring immunity and which are sufficiently characteristic clinically that history can be used as the basis for classification. When, as with common respiratory diseases or influenza, susceptibles cannot be reliably identified, the SAR is based on all exposed family members and still remains a useful tool.

The SAR, as illustrated above, is limited in application to infectious disease in which the primary or index case is infective for only a short period of time (measured in days). When the index person is infective over a long period of time, as in tuberculosis, duration of exposure is an important factor in determining the extent of spread. To take this into account, exposure units are defined (person-week, month, or year) and the measure of spread (equivalent of the SAR in concept) is *the number of cases per number of person-weeks (months or years) of exposure* × 100. This rate has the additional advantage that the experience of persons with exposures of differing duration can be summarized conveniently. Thus, two persons exposed for six months plus four persons exposed for eighteen months provide seven person-years of exposure ($2 \times \frac{1}{2}$ + $4 \times \frac{3}{2}$ years).

7-9   Life Tables

In the section on age adjustment of rates we discussed methods of summarizing the age-specific death rates of a given community in a given year. It was pointed out that the age-adjusted rate shares with the crude rate the weakness that it is a single number and cannot summarize adequately the pattern of variation in the age-specific rates.

The life table is also a summary of the age-specific rates of a given calendar year. It offers a number of different summaries, of which two will be discussed here. Each of these is a function of age, as is shown in Figure 7-15. The mathematical calculations required for these functions, to be found in textbooks on actuarial methods, are quite complex.* The interpretations, however, are fairly simple, provided one fact is kept in mind: Both of the summaries refer to an imaginary population born into the set of age-specific rates operating during the specified calendar year and living their entire lives under that set of rates. In reality, a child born in 1960 will be subject at age ten to the death rate for ten-year-olds (DR_{10-11}) of 1970 and at age thirty to the DR_{30-31} of 1990, and so will reap the advantages of medical advances as they occur. The 1960 life table, on the other hand, summarizes the mortality experience of a completely fictitious cohort upon which is imposed in each year of age the death rate for that age as it was in 1960.

The survivorship function, 1_x   The survivorship function is a statement of the number of persons, out of 100,000 live births, who would survive

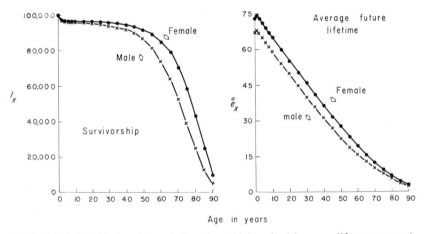

FIG. 7-15 Life table functions: 1_x (survivorship) and e_x^0 (average life expectancy), United States white population, 1960.

*There is a whole range of approximate methods, some quite simple, which are adequate for epidemiologic use.

to age x under the age-specific rates for the specified year. The value of 1_{40}, for example, is determined by the cumulative operation of the specific death rates for all ages below forty.

The average future lifetime, or expectation of life function, e_x^o The expectation of life function is a statement of the average number of years of life remaining to those persons who survive to age x. The value of e_{40}^o is determined by the sequential application of the age-specific death rates for each year of age after forty. The value of e_0^o is referred to as the expectation of life at birth. It should be noted that e_0^o for 1960 cannot be interpreted as the average of the deaths occurring in 1960, because these deaths come from the 1960 population, the age distribution of which was determined by the changing age-specific rates of the preceding century. The value of e_0^o for United States males born in 1960 was 66.6, whereas the average age of United States males dying in 1960 was 60.7. The sharp increase in the e_x^o function (and the parallel drop in the 1_x function) between birth and age one year are reflections of the high death rate in infancy, much of which is accounted for by neonatal deaths of infants born alive but with life-threatening defects.

Some implications of life tables The occurrence of death is commonly accepted as the ultimate in poor health. Hence, the crude death rate is commonly (and incorrectly) taken as a rough measure of the health status of a population. As we have seen in preceding sections, the age composition of a population exerts great influence on the death rate and, if we wish to make valid comparisons based on deaths, we must use age-adjusted rates. The life table offers still another way of comparing the mortality experience of populations and, in a rough way, their general health status.

Within a country, one may wish to compare the experience of different segments of the population. In Figure 7-15 the experiences of United States males and females are compared with respect to survival (1_x) and life expectation (e_x^o) by age, based on age- and sex-specific death rates in 1960. Both bases of comparison reveal the superior survival rate of females. One may also wish to examine the mortality experience at different periods as a basis for visualizing progress in promoting health. Because John Graunt is credited with developing the first life table, it is particularly interesting to compare early British experience, represented by Graunt's life table for London in 1662, with more modern experience, as in Table 7-10, using survival to specified ages as the basis for comparison. Although tremendous changes in survival occurred between 1662 and 1901–1910, it is encouraging to note that the proportions of people reaching older ages continued to increase significantly, at least up to 1955.

Comparisons between countries are commonly based on expectation of life at birth or at other specified ages. Table 7-11 presents the latest readily available data for selected countries by sex and illustrates a number

TABLE 7-10
Survival to specified age in Britain, 1662–1955

		ENGLAND AND WALES‡		
LONDON, 1662*			NO. SURVIVING	
AGE	NO. SURVIVING†	AGE	1901–10	1930–32	1955
0	100	0	100	100	100
6	64	5	81	91	97
16	40	15	79	89	97
26	25	20	77	88	96
36	16	30	74	86	95
46	10	40	69	82	94
56	6	50	62	77	90
66	3	60	51	67	81
76	1	70	34	48	63
86	0				

*Wilcox, W. F., ed. *Natural and Political Observations made upon the Bills of Mortality by John Graunt* (a reprint of the first edition, 1662). Baltimore, Johns Hopkins Press, 1937.

†Number of persons who would survive to the exact age specified out of 100 born alive and subject to mortality conditions of the period specified.

‡*Demographic Yearbook*, 1957, 9th ed. New York, United Nations, 1957.

of points of interest. One is the fact that the greater life expectancy of females is a presumably universal phenomenon (only among Asiatics in South Africa and the population of Guatemala were females at a slight disadvantage, presumably reflecting some aspect of the respective cultural patterns). Second, in countries with lower life expectancy at birth (South African Colored and Asiatics, Chile, Guatemala, and India), life expectancy at age five exceeded that at birth (an indication of the toll taken by high infant mortality rates and major infectious diseases in early childhood). Finally, of special interest to United States citizens, the United States female fares as well as females in any other country, whereas, among the countries listed, the United States male ranks fourth in life expectancy at any age shown and is approached (age thirty) or outranked (age fifty) by males in India. The obvious moral is that there is still room for improvement in the health of United States males.

7-10   Graphical Methods for Secular Trends

Death rates from tuberculosis and typhoid fever have dropped sharply since 1900. Panel A of Figure 7-16 shows the death rate as a function of

TABLE 7-11

Expectation of life at specified ages by sex, for selected countries at times indicated

COUNTRY		YEAR	MALES, AGE IN YEARS				FEMALES, AGE IN YEARS			
			0	5	30	50	0	5	30	50
United States		1961	67.0	64.3	40.7	23.1	73.6	70.5	46.3	28.0
United Kingdom		1961	68.0	65.0	41.0	22.6	73.8	70.4	46.0	27.4
Israel		1961	70.5	67.7	43.8	25.0	73.6	70.5	46.2	27.4
Sweden		1960	71.2	67.9	43.9	25.5	74.9	71.2	46.8	28.0
South Africa	Colored	1950–52	44.8	52.2	32.3	19.0	47.8	55.1	36.2	22.1
	Asiatic	1950–52	55.8	57.6	34.5	18.3	54.8	55.6	34.2	18.4
	White	1950–52	64.6	62.8	39.6	22.4	70.1	67.8	44.1	26.3
Chile		1952	49.8	55.6	34.8	20.4	53.9	59.9	39.3	23.6
Guatemala		1949–51	43.8	51.3	33.9	20.5	43.5	50.4	33.4	20.4
Japan		1960	65.4	63.3	40.1	22.4	70.3	67.9	44.2	26.1
Taiwan		1959–60	61.3	61.2	38.1	21.0	65.6	65.7	42.4	24.8
India		1957–58	45.2	55.8	40.3	23.3	46.6	57.6	43.1	27.2

Source: *Demographic Yearbook, 1962*, 14th issue. New York, United Nations, 1962.

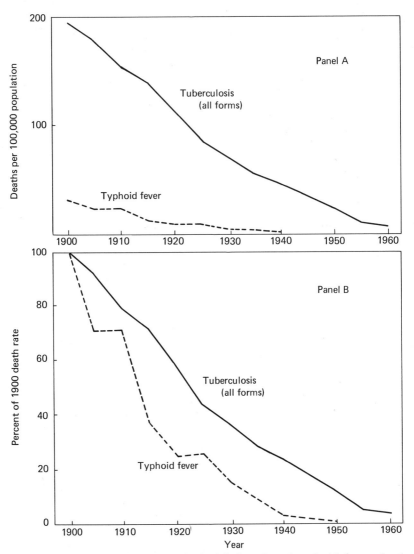

FIG. 7-16 Death rates for tuberculosis (all forms) and typhoid fever, death registration states 1900–1930 and the United States 1940–1960, plotted on an arithmetic scale. (Vital Statistics of the U.S. 1960, Vol. II Mortality, Part A, Table 1K, pp. 1–24.)

time. Tuberculosis, which accounted for 11.3 per cent of all deaths in 1900, with a rate of 194 per 100,000 population, accounted for less than 1 per cent of all deaths in 1960, with a death rate of 6 deaths per 100,000 population. Typhoid fever, with 31.3 deaths per 100,000 population in 1900, fell to 0.01 deaths per 100,000 population in 1960. In panel B the relative rates of decrease for the two diseases are shown by expressing each rate as a percentage of the 1900 rate for the same disease. On this scale we see that up to 1920 the percentage decrease in typhoid fever as a cause of death was greater than that for tuberculosis.

Figure 7-17 illustrates a second method of depicting the relative rates of decrease. The graph is made on four-cycle "arith-log" paper in which the horizontal scale is arithmetic and the vertical scale is logarithmic. On arith-log paper, equal slopes denote equal relative rates of decrease, and an exponential function, $y = A.10^{bx}$ (or e^{ax+b}) becomes a straight line. In later chapters graphs are presented in which death rates by age have been plotted on arith-log paper. The reader is cautioned that this distorts the shapes of the curves and exaggerates changes at the low levels between the ages of one and forty. This can be seen by a comparison of Figures 7-18 and 7-19 which show the United States 1960 death rates plotted by age on an arithmetic and a logarithmic scale, respectively.

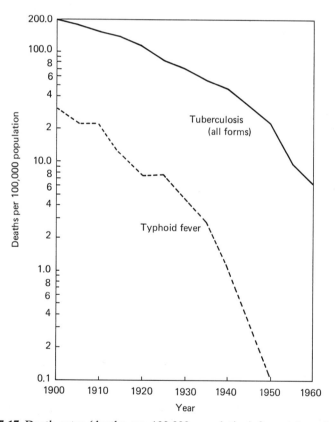

FIG. 7-17 Death rates (deaths per 100,000 population) from tuberculosis and typhoid fever, United States death registration area 1900–1930 and United States 1940–1960, plotted on a logarithmic scale. (Vital Statistics of the U.S. 1960, Vol. II, Mortality, Part A, Table 1K, pp. 1–24.)

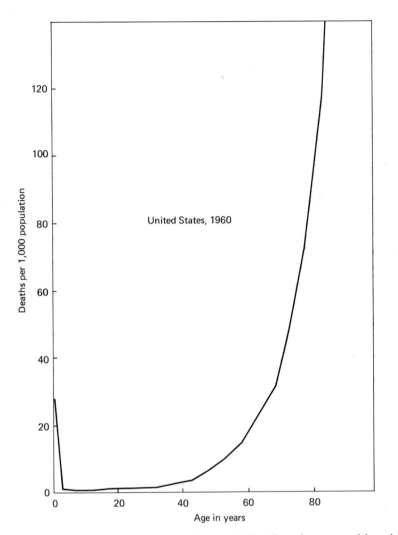

FIG. 7-18 Death rates of the United States, 1960, plotted on an arithmetic scale. (Vital Statistics of the U.S. 1960, Vol. II, Part A, Table 1D, pp. 1–21.)

7-11 Summary

The phrase "vital statistics" is usually used to cover the body of knowledge contained in the routinely collected and published data concerning the structure of population of the nation and the events of births, deaths, marriages, divorces, and cases of certain diseases that occur in that population. In addition, the phrase covers the branch of knowledge concerning the inherent errors in such data and methods of summarizing, graphing, and interpreting the data.

Vital statistics frequently provides background for the descriptive epidemiologic study of a disease, that is, its geographical pattern of occurrence as well as the patterns by age, sex, occupation, religion, ethnic background, and so on. The broad national pattern of disease occurrence contained in the publications of the National Center for Health Statistics provides baseline information against which the current experience of a specialized group may be assessed.

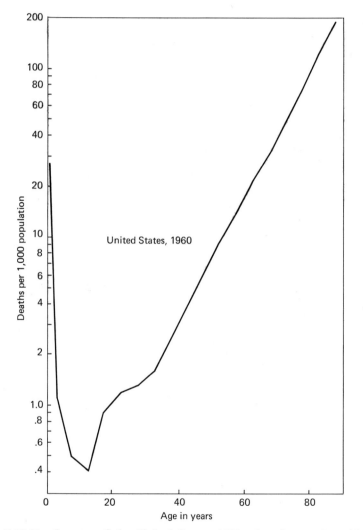

FIG. 7-19 Death rates of the United States, 1960, plotted on a logarithmic scale. (Vital Statistics of the U.S. 1960, Vol. II, Part A, Table 1D, pp. 1–21.)

Familiarity with the publications that contain the data of vital statistics, and with the methods appropriate to their use, is a fundamental and important tool in epidemiology.

GLOSSARY

Adjustment of rates   A method of correcting for noncomparability with respect to age, race, sex, and so on (see text).

Census data   The data of the decennial national census (and of special censuses) of population and housing, the special population censuses, the special census of agriculture, labor, and so on.

Life table   A method of summarizing the age-specific death rates of a single calendar year (see text).

Registration data   Data derived from certificates of vital events: births, deaths, marriages, divorces; and notifiable diseases.

Standardized mortality ratio   The ratio of the number of deaths observed in the study group to the number of deaths "expected" in the study group under the set of rates for the control population.

Vital Statistics   The body of knowledge encompassing the study of the census and registration data.

REFERENCES

1. Self-Enumeration as a Method for the 1960 Census of Housing. Working Paper No. 24. Washington, D.C.: U.S. Department of Commerce, Bureau of the Census.
2. Directory of Federal Statistics for Local Areas. Bureau of the Census (USGPO, S O D).
3. Standard Metropolitan Statistical Areas—1967. Executive Office of the President, Bureau of the Budget (USGPO, 0-257-095).
4. Spiegelman, Mortimer, *Introduction to Demography*, rev. ed. Cambridge, Mass.: Harvard University Press, 1968.
5. Current Population Reports, Series P-25, No. 165. Washington, D.C.: U.S. Department of Commerce, Bureau of the Census, November 4, 1957.
6. Physicians' Handbook on Medical Certification: Death, Fetal Death, Birth. Public Health Service Publication No. 593 B, Washington, D.C.: National Center for Health Statistics, 1967.
7. Vital Statistics of the U.S., Vol. 1, 1965, Natality. Washington, D.C.: U.S. Department of Health, Education, and Welfare, Public Health Service.
8. Procedures for Coding Multiple Causes of Deaths Occurring in 1955, in Vital Statistics Instruction Manual. Washington, D.C.: U.S.

Department of Health, Education, and Welfare, National Vital Statistics Division, April 1962.

9. Weiner, L., Bellows, M., McAvoy, G., and Cohen, E. Use of multiple causes in the classification of deaths from cardiovascular-renal disease. *Amer. J. Public Health*, **45**(4):492–501, 1955.

10. Shapiro, S., Ross, L. J., and Levine, H. Relationship of selected prenatal factors to pregnancy outcome and congenital malformations. *Amer. J. Public Health*, **55**:268–282, 1965.

11. Frank, C. W., Weinblatt, E., Shapiro, S., and Sager, R. V. Myocardial infarction in men. *J. Amer. Med. Ass.* **198**:1241–1245, 1966.

12. Elveback, L., and Fox, J. P. Illness, oral poliovirus vaccine and interference. *Arch. Environ. Health* **9**:724–726, 1964.

13. Dawber, Thomas R., Kannel, William B., and Lyell, Lorna P. An approach to longitudinal studies in the community: The Framingham Study. *Ann. N.Y. Acad. Sci.* **107**:539–556, 1963.

14. Vital and Health Statistics, Series 1, Number 1, August 1963.

15. Vital and Health Statistics, Series 10, Number 37, May 1967.

16. Vital Statistics of the United States, Vol. 1, 1960, Natality. Washington, D.C.: U.S. Department of Health, Education, and Welfare, Public Health Service.

17. Census of Population, Vol. 1, Part 1, U.S. Summary, 1960.

18. Duffy, E. A., and Carroll, R. E. *United States Metropolitan Mortality, 1959–1961*, PHS Publication No. 999-AP-39. Washington, D.C.: U.S. Public Health Service, National Center for Air Pollution Control, 1967.

19. Kyle, R. A., Nobrega, F. T., Kurland, L. T., and Elveback, L. The 30-year trend of leukemia in Olmsted County, Minnesota, 1935 through 1964. *Mayo Clin. Proc.* **43**:342–353, 1968.

8

Study Design, Sampling, and the Evaluation of Evidence

The design and conduct of epidemiologic investigations of different types will be discussed in Chapter 12. Proper planning and the correct interpretation of results of such studies, whatever the type, depend on the avoidance of faulty study design, the use of appropriate sampling procedures in forming the study groups, and observance of basic statistical principles in both the study design and analysis of the results. These fundamentals will be discussed in the present chapter, with emphasis given to underlying concepts, because detailed methods are the province of more specialized texts.

8-1 Common Pitfalls in Study Design, Execution, and Interpretation of Results

Although errors that may invalidate the results of a study arise in many ways, there are five major sources: improper selection of the study groups (including errors of sampling procedure), improper extrapolation of results, unsuspected biological association, subjectivity in collection and evaluation of information, and errors of response or classification.

Improper selection of the study group In some studies it is possible to select the study group by formal sampling procedures, to be discussed briefly in the next section. Proper adherence to the principles of sampling design are necessary if advantage is to be taken of statistical methods that give measures of the precision of estimates and statements concerning significant differences between population subgroups. Errors may arise either through faulty sampling plan or through failure to adhere strictly to the protocol of an adequate sampling plan.

Several examples of poor sampling procedures have become classic, for example, sampling the residents of a city through the sole use of a list of telephone subscribers or sampling the school age population of a city by the sole use of a list of those attending school. These are examples of failure to sample the entire population under consideration. Equally classic as an example of failure to carry out the specified sampling plan is substitution of the "house next door" for one in which no one is found at home. This leads to the inclusion of a disproportionately small number of persons who are frequently away from home and who, as a class, may be distinguished by such characteristics as marital status (employed single persons), economic status (working mothers), or occupation (traveling salesman) which may be important to the disease under study.

In some epidemiologic studies, even though an adequate sampling plan may be at hand, it may be anticipated that there will be difficulty in securing the cooperation of those selected for study. It is tempting in such cases to rely on volunteers who will, in general, differ in important ways (education, economic status, family size) from nonvolunteers. Indeed, for many studies in which substantial participation is required of the subjects to be studied (e.g., giving of blood or other specimens, submitting to periodic physical examinations, or accepting an inoculation), there is no alternative to relying on volunteers. However, in all such studies careful consideration must be given to any limitations the use of volunteers imposes on interpretation of the results. The extent and severity of such limitations will depend on the nature of the questions asked. In the Francis trial of the Salk vaccine, described in Chapter 1, observations in the "placebo areas" (where the disease experience of volunteers inoculated with placebo or vaccine was compared) revealed a higher rate of disease in the placebo-inoculated volunteers than in nonparticipating children (nonvolunteers) of comparable ages. As emphasized by Brownlee (1), in a highly critical review directed particularly at the large portion of the trial in which the experience of vaccinees was compared with that of "observed controls" (nonvolunteers), this finding made it clear that volunteers differed from nonvolunteers in ways that influenced the occurrence of clinical poliomyelitis. The basic principle to be followed is that, if a study requires the use of volunteers, all of the groups to be compared (experimental and control) must be formed from those volunteering, preferably by the use of some method of randomization.

With mail questionnaires self-selection becomes important when there is a high nonresponse rate. If, for example, the questionnaire deals with smoking habits, nonrespondents may include a higher proportion of heavy smokers than do the respondents. Given a case in which a high non-response rate results, the investigator has several alternatives. Commonly, he first tries to increase the response rate by a second mailing of the questionnaire to the nonresponders. If the nonresponse rate remains high, he may then select a sample of the nonresponders to be tracked to their homes for personal interviews in an effort to estimate the important characteristics of the entire group of nonresponders. The point is that, unless the net nonresponse rate is reduced or the relevant characteristics of the nonrespondents are ascertained, the investigator is not entitled to generalize his observations beyond the population of responders.

Improper extrapolation of results   Whenever sample results are generalized to a population other than that from which the sample was selected, improper extrapolation of results has occurred. Technically, this situation prevails in all studies (such as those illustrated above) in which inadequate sampling procedures are employed. Similarly, the results reported by Hammond and Horn (2) on the relation of smoking to health in nearly 200,000 white males aged 50–69 could not be generalized justifiably to all United States white males in that age group because no adequately defined sampling procedure was used in the selection of their study group. This example is discussed at greater length in Chapter 12. Further examples of improper extrapolation are provided by studies in which it is falsely assumed that hospitalized cases of a disease such as peptic ulcer are representative of all cases or that survivors of myocardial infarction are typical of all cases.

Unsuspected biological associations   Heady and coworkers (3) found support for the hypothesis that coronary heart disease is inversely correlated with physical activity in a study of London bus drivers (who sit while working) and London bus fare collectors (who stand and move about actively). The lesser frequency of heart disease observed among the fare collectors than among the drivers was attributed to their greater physical activity. Critics later pointed out that the drivers tend to be more obese than the fare collectors at the time of employment, that in effect biological selection had predetermined who would sit and who would stand, and that the excess cardiac disease observed among the drivers may have been more related to their obesity than to their relative inactivity. Thus, in this study, obesity represented a biological "third factor" not accounted for, but which also was important with respect to heart disease. Failure to consider obesity in forming the study groups also must be considered an error in study design.

A more subtle example of a hidden biologic association is provided by the early trials of the efficacy of large-scale use of gamma globulin to combat epidemics of poliomyelitis. In a well-designed "double blind" procedure, large numbers of volunteer children were given gamma globulin (containing antibody to all three types of polioviruses) or a gelatin placebo indistinguishable in appearance from the gamma globulin. The significant difference in the frequency of disease in the placebo group versus the gamma globulin group appeared to provide a measure of the protective effect of the gamma globulin (4). In retrospect it was shown by experiments in infected monkeys that the simple inoculation of gelatin would precipitate the occurrence of paralytic disease (5). Thus, the excess disease observed in the placebo group must be explained at least in part by the "provoking effect" of the inoculation of gelatin.

Subjectivity in collection and evaluation of information The influence of nonobjective collection of information is most easily illustrated with clinical or vaccine trials in which the appropriate "double blind" design is not employed. In this case, both the persons studied and the investigator are vulnerable to subjective influences. Let us consider a new drug which may reduce distress resulting from painful menstrual periods. Estimation of its effect is based on a comparison between women receiving and not receiving the medication. Unless a "double blind" procedure involving a placebo is used (neither the subject nor the investigator know during the period of observation who received the drug) the apparent efficacy of the drug may be increased by the psychological relief experienced by the patients who were led to expect it and by a subconscious tendency on the part of the investigator to underestimate the distress reported by the treated women. Similarly, in vaccine trials the occurrence of mild or atypical disease in vaccinees may be underestimated for the same basic reasons unless the "double blind" design is employed.

Less obvious but equally important intrusions of subjective influences may occur in observational studies, especially of the retrospective type. In studies of the relation of smoking to lung cancer, knowledge that patients do have lung cancer may lead the interviewer to probe more diligently for a history of smoking. Conversely, if the patient is aware of the central interest in smoking, his replies may reflect a subconscious desire either to satisfy the interviewer or to minimize his own guilt. In similar fashion, the mothers of deformed infants will try harder to recall experiences such as possible rubella that might explain their tragedy. A related problem may arise when multiple interviewers are employed in that some may be more skillful in eliciting information than others. Although the "double blind" technique employed in experimental trials is rarely applicable in observational studies, subjective influences can be minimized in a number of ways. Wherever possible, objective tests for disease or exposure (e.g., tests for a specific antibody) should be employed. Histories of exposure to suspect determinants can be obtained by use of a standard questionnaire, carefully constructed to include "reasonable" extraneous items which may mask the area of special interest. Whenever possible, interviewers (and subjects) should not be aware of the disease or nondisease status of the subjects interviewed.

Finally, unless treatment groups are formed in experimental studies by randomizing patients to treatment (sometimes approximated by strict adherence to a prestated rule, e.g., experimental drug and the placebo are given to alternate patients admitted to study), the investigator may be subconsciously influenced in his selection or assignment of subjects for inclusion in his experimental and control groups. As rather gross examples, he may form his experimental group from patients in earlier stages of disease (when treatment may be more effective) or assign the more severe cases to the standard treatment, thus prejudicing the results in favor of the experimental drug.

These examples illustrate the necessity of employing formal devices such as randomization, placebo treatments, and "double blind" techniques in order to ensure that subjectivity, conscious and unconscious, has been ruled out.

Errors of response or classification   It is self-evident that invalid conclusions may arise when, because of erroneous information, members of study populations are misclassified as to either exposure or disease status. The common ways in which erroneous information may be developed also are fairly obvious: reliance on memory, unjustified presumption of knowledge, improperly phrased or leading questions, insensitive or imprecise measurement tools, incomplete or inadequate demographic data, and so on. In the following discussion we will consider only a few situations, using disease problems that are used as examples in other chapters of this book.

The question of the relation of maternal rubella to abnormal outcome of pregnancy was introduced in Chapter 1. In attacking this problem, women must be classified as pregnant (or not) and as having experienced rubella (or not) and the outcome of pregnancy must be judged as normal or abnormal. In retrospective studies, comparison groups of normal and abnormal infants are formed as a first step. Whereas classification of obviously abnormal infants is no problem, there is some possibility of failure to recognize abnormality when groups are formed on the basis of information soon after birth; for example, a hearing defect or mental retardation may not become evident until late in infancy. In such case, some abnormal infants would be misclassified as normal and elicitation of histories of rubella during their mothers' pregnancies would lead to overestimation of the prevalence of exposure in the mothers of normal infants. Once the groups are formed, the mothers must be classified as exposed (having experienced rubella) or not. This step is particularly vulnerable to error, because the rash of rubella may be mimicked by many other agents and true rubella infection often is subclinical. Further, unless the mother was medically attended during her suspect illness, reliance must be placed on memory. Such reliance is additionally complicated by commonly existing confusion in the minds of the lay public about the difference between rubeola (measles) and rubella (German measles). In the period when the retrospective studies were conducted, no method existed for the specific etiologic diagnosis of rubella, and one can only suppose that misclassifications of both types (i.e., erroneous assignment as exposed or not exposed) did occur, but tended to offset one another. Presently, rubella virus can be isolated and identified and changes in antibody level demonstrated, so that suspect disease seen during its occurrence can be diagnosed and, if possible exposure is recognized, even subclinical infections can be detected. Even when suspect illness was not studied, some instances of false positive histories can be eliminated when a current serum specimen is found lacking in rubella antibody.

In prospective rubella studies, the exposed (rubella) groups have been formed in two ways. British workers began with women seeking antenatal care in the National Health Service and then sought information as to the occurrence of rubella during pregnancy (6). In most instances this information was obtained in retrospect and, for reasons stated above, undoubtedly led to the inclusion of some unexposed women in the "exposed" group and of exposed women (subclinical infections) in the "unexposed" control group. Investigators in New York City began with currently reported rubella in women of childbearing age and attempted to ascertain pregnancy status (7). Since each case was seen promptly by the investigators (who employed rigorous criteria for clinical diagnosis), the resulting "exposed" group contained few if any unexposed women. However, diagnosis of pregnancy in its earliest stages is notably difficult. The risk here was not of including false pregnancies but the more serious one (for the study objective) of excluding instances of true pregnancy in which early rubella-induced abortions were regarded as normal menses, an error which would lead to underestimation of "disease" prevalence in the exposed group. It should be noted, however, that this error in the New York study was much less than the same error in the British study, which included only women coming to seek antenatal care and, hence, excluded all those with early spontaneous abortions. Similar underestimation of abnormal outcome of pregnancy also would result from failure to maintain observation of live-born infants long enough (at least two years) to ensure detection of all abnormalities.

In Chapters 2 and 12 reference is made to Snow's "Grand Experiment" in which he showed the relation of water supply to cholera (cf. Tables 2-2 and 12-6). His enumeration of the observed high- and low-exposure population groups was based on the records of the Southwark and Vauxhall and the Lambeth Water Companies, respectively, and presumably was free of significant error. To measure the incidence of cholera he relied upon the Registrar-General's lists of death attributed to the disease. Because not all cholera cases died and (probably of lesser importance) because some of the deaths attributed to cholera may have been due to other acute enteric disease (especially in infants), his measure of incidence was undoubtedly imprecise. Cholera deaths reported were assigned to the high- or low-risk population groups, not by checking the records of the water companies (then apparently a nearly impossible task), but by measuring the amount of chloride in water drawn from taps in the homes of the deceased patients. High chloride content (from sodium chloride) was characteristic of water from the Thames river basin (supplied by the Southwark and Vauxhall Company) which was heavily polluted with sewage and at least slightly mixed with sea water. Snow's account suggests that this was a highly reliable method, but some may argue that misclassifications did occur. Fortunately, in this particular study the chances of misclassification as to disease status were equal for both exposure groups and the chance of misclassification of deceased persons as to exposure status was the same for each individual; hence, it is quite unlikely that the errors that existed would invalidate Snow's conclusions.

Finally, we may look briefly at the problem of smoking and lung cancer. Determination of the fact and degree of exposure in all studies was based on interview or questionnaire. The specific information required had to do with when smoking began, the form of smoking, and the amount of tobacco consumed. Although both the framing of the questions (avoidance of leading inquiries) and the context in which they were asked (e.g., before or after lung cancer had been diagnosed, or before or after popular concern about smoking had developed) are important, the major problem here is memory. In particular, smokers are apt to underestimate the amount smoked, for example, a "one-pack-a-day" smoker who eventually admits that he purchases two cartons of cigarettes a week to maintain his regular level of consumption. Determination of disease in the absence of lung biopsy or autopsy is not completely free from error. Incorrect classification as "diseased" may occur because a tumor arising in another unrecognized site spreads to involve the lung or the infrequent adenocarcinoma of the lung (not believed to be influenced by smoking) is not identified as such. Even more surprising, a 1966 British study, in which death certificates completed by physicians for 10,000 hospitalized patients before autopsy were compared with pathologists' findings, suggests that in the absence of autopsy lung cancer would be underdiagnosed by 16 per cent (8).

8-2   Sampling Human Populations

The ideal situation in sampling human populations is that in which the study groups are known to be comparable with respect to all important factors other than that under study. In practice we cannot hope to achieve this ideal and must rely on the use of well-designed sampling procedures. Sampling theory is a highly complex mathematical subject. The sampling design must depend upon the advice of an expert who has knowledge of the wide variety of methods that will enable him to seek the greatest precision within a specified budget (precision required at the lowest cost). The discussion here concerns the simplest and most basic of sampling devices.

The need for formal random sampling devices It has been demonstrated many times and in many fields that honesty, sincerity, and conscientiousness are not adequate guarantees against personal bias in selection. In selecting a sample of 100 students from undergraduates of a given university we could: (1) ask for volunteers; (2) select the first 100 students we encounter in the hall; (3) select all students majoring in history, French, and so on. It is possible to conjecture, as in the preceding section, about the types of errors that might arise from such plans. The basic problem is to find a sampling method which gives the investigator and his readers insurance that personal bias, conscious or unconscious, did not enter into the selection. This can be accomplished only by the use of a formal randomization device, such as tossing coins, pulling numbers out of a hat, or (most appropriate in this case) use of a table of random numbers, to be discussed in a later section. Use of such a device provides still another important advantage in that it justifies the use of standard statistical methods for producing measures of the precision of these estimates.

Some of the most important rules for sampling from a human population are:

1. The population to be sampled must be well defined and the members of that population identifiable.
2. The sampling mechanism must be such that for every member of the population the probability of that person's inclusion in the sample is known and not zero (probability sampling).
3. The sampling plan, which defines these probabilities, must be carried through exactly as planned, without changes which might be tempting for the sake of convenience.
4. Conclusions based on the sample results may be attributed only to the population sampled. Any extrapolation to a larger or different population is a judgment or a guess and is not part of statistical inference.

Defining the population to be sampled Simple as it is to say, defining the population to be sampled requires serious consideration. The definition must be sufficiently clear and precise that, if necessary, each individual member of the population, including those drawn into the sample, can be identified without ambiguity as belonging to the population. Note that if we fail to find and identify as members any individuals (such as people without telephones or school-age children not in school), the probability of their being included in the sample becomes *zero*, which violates rule 2.

The resident population of Manhattan, for census purposes, excludes all persons whose legal residence is elsewhere. There is, however, an effective population that includes large numbers of nonresidents, for example, those who commute to work from outside Manhattan, students present only during the school year, inmates of prisons and other institutions, and visitors who may reside in hotels for days, weeks, or months. The population of students of a university must be defined to indicate whether it includes, in addition to full-time graduate and undergraduate students, students in good standing but out for one semester or attending only on a part-time basis, current degree candidates not presently enrolled in formal classes, persons registered on a special basis or in the extension division, and so on. Defining the population of patients of a hospital on a given day poses different but still comparable problems relating to the inclusion or exclusion of bed patients admitted, discharged or dying on that day, and of patients seen only in the outpatient department.

Sampling plans   In one of the simplest sampling plans the probability of being included in the sample is the same for all individuals in the population. This method is characteristic of taking a single random sample from the entire population, which frequently is not the most efficient method in terms of precision per unit of cost. Other methods which satisfy rule 2, each of which under certain conditions may be more efficient than a single random sample, are illustrated in Table 8-1 as applied to the population of thirty persons in ten families defined below:

WHITE		WHITE		NONWHITE	
FAMILY	PERSONS	FAMILY	PERSONS	FAMILY	PERSONS
1	1, 2, 3, 4	5	11, 12, 13, 14	8	23, 24, 25
2	5, 6		15, **16**	9	26, 27, 28
3	7, 8, 9	6	17, 18, 19	10	29, **30**
4	10	7	20, 21, 22		

The probability of including person 16 (member of white family 5) and person 30 (member of nonwhite family 10) has been computed for each of five sampling plans or methods. The computation is self-evident when either simple random sampling or stratified (white and nonwhite sampled separately) random sampling is employed in drawing samples of size 5. With cluster sampling the sampling unit becomes the family and the probability for inclusion of a specified person is the same as that for the inclusion of his family (i.e., if two of 10 families are to be selected, the probability is 2/10 or 1/5). Cluster sampling with subsampling within the cluster is a two-step procedure; as here applied, the probability for inclusion of a specified person is the product of the probability that his family will be chosen (here 5 out of 10 or 1/2) and of his being selected from his own family (for person 16, whose family contains 6 members, this is 1/6; for person 30 in a family of only two, this is 1/2). The same

TABLE 8-1

Probabilities for inclusion of specified members of a defined population* when different sampling methods are employed

METHOD	DESCRIPTION	PROBABILITY OF PERSON 16 BEING IN SAMPLE	PROBABILITY OF PERSON 30 BEING IN SAMPLE
Simple random sampling	5 persons at random from the entire population	$5/30 = 1/6$	$5/30 = 1/6$
Stratified random sampling	3 persons at random from 22 whites, 2 at random from 8 non-whites	$3/22$	$2/8$
Cluster sampling	2 families at random, and including all persons in the 2 families chosen	$2/10 = 1/5$	$2/10 = 1/5$
Cluster sampling with subsampling	5 families at random and 1 person at random from each family chosen	$5/10 \times 1/6 = 1/12$	$5/10 \times \frac{1}{2} = \frac{1}{4}$
Stratified cluster sampling with subsampling	3 families at random from white population; 2 families at random from nonwhite population; and 1 person at random from each family chosen	$3/7 \times 1/6 = 1/14$	$2/3 \times \frac{1}{2} = 1/3$

*See accompanying text tabulation.

methods of computation apply for stratified cluster sampling (here 3 of 7 white and 2 of 3 nonwhite families) with subsampling.

In the examples used in the foregoing discussion, stratification was based on race. Quite obviously, many other characteristics of human population could serve as readily as the basis for stratification (age, sex, occupation, or other). In many cases, as in the National Health Survey described in Chapter 7, the sampling procedure is very complex and is based in part on area of residence. In a proposed sero-survey for immunity to epidemic typhus in the *altiplano* of Bolivia (to evaluate the need for and guide the application of a vaccine program), the households in the regions to be surveyed would be numbered and located on regional maps. The maps would then be overlayed with a grid, thereby dividing the regions into square areas of equal size within each of which 10 per cent of the included households would be selected at random. Since all members of each chosen household would be bled for serum, the method proposed is stratified (by area of residence) cluster sampling.

Consideration of a problem relating to coronary heart disease (CHD) provides an opportunity to consider the relative merits of different sampling methods. Preliminary evidence has suggested that abnormally high serum cholesterol levels (260 mg per cent or higher) are encountered more often in young adult white males (20–39 years of age) than in Negro males of the same age. If true, this finding may be related to the lesser frequency of CHD among Negro males than among white males, especially in groups forty years old and older. The immediate problem is how best to explore this phenomenon in New York City in which, as of 1960, the population was 85 per cent white and 15 per cent nonwhite. Preliminary data suggested that the proportions (p) with high serum cholesterols were 14 per cent for whites and 7 per cent for Negroes in this age group. The present objective is to obtain the most precise estimates of these values possible within a total sample of 1,000. The basic alternatives are: (1) to draw a single random sample of 1,000 from all males 20–39 years of age; or (2) to draw separate random samples from the whites and nonwhites. In the single-sample method we would expect 850 white and 150 nonwhite subjects. Using the values of p obained in the preliminary study as the basis, the standard deviations (SD) for the resulting estimates would be

$$\text{SD}_{pw} = 3.8 \text{ per cent and } \text{SD}_{pnw} = 6.6 \text{ per cent}$$

indicating that the estimate for the white value would be more precise than that for the nonwhite value. The use of separate random samples makes it possible to predetermine the numbers of whites and nonwhites in such a way that the SDs of each estimate will be approximately the same (650 whites and 350 nonwhites in this example) or that the relative precision of each estimate (SD/p) will be approximately the same (320 whites and 680 nonwhites).

The foregoing suggests that, for the objective desired, separate random sampling would be the method of choice. If we had wished to obtain an estimate of p for all NYC males aged 20–39 years, without regard to race, proper stratification also would yield a more precise estimate than a single random sample but the gain would be slight. Only if p_w and p_{nw} were very different would the gain in precision be substantial.

Unfortunately, use of separate random samples in situations of this type is beset by a major (in the present case, almost overwhelming) difficulty in that the two populations to be sampled must first be listed separately. The city directory ordinarily lists all dwelling units, but without information as to race; the cost of the required separate listing would be high—probably prohibitive. Indeed, even simple random sampling would be confronted with the practical difficulty of persuading all of the individuals included to consent to be bled. For this reason, the investigator would be tempted (perhaps even forced) to sample within an available population, such as males about to get married who must submit to premarital blood tests. In such event, he should sample within each race in the ages 20–39 but would only be entitled to draw inferences concerning the population of newly married persons. Quite clearly, such an investigation could hardly lead to reliable conclusions concerning the relation between serum cholesterol and race in all New York City males in the 20–39 year age group.

Whenever the members of the population to be sampled can be listed and numbered (in any order that is convenient), the most efficient way to obtain a simple random sample is by the use of a *table of random numbers*. Tables of random numbers are prepared by simulation of a simple random experiment (such as coin tossing) by an electronic computer. The Rand Corporation has published a book entitled *A Million Random Digits*. Many textbooks of elementary statistics, such as *Introduction to Statistical Analysis*, by Dixon and Massey (McGraw-Hill, 3rd, ed., 1969), also contain shorter tables of random numbers. A typical page of a table of random numbers might appear as follows:

33557	87793	80692	97614	58949
81167	80647	13062	39712	09542
00740	10721	58531	65814	78731
24405	36647	21967	44386	44652
70011	12237	07828	25969	66743

Consider the problem of selecting a simple random sample of 90 records from a file of 900 records (one for each of 900 patients). First, the records are numbered in whatever order they appear in the file, as 000, 001, 002, ... 899. A page in the random number table is selected arbitrarily (this is sufficient because of the essential random order of the table itself). Suppose the first 25 numbers in the table were those shown above. We would select those records whose numbers matched the first three digits of each random number, rejecting duplications and all numbers greater than 899. The process would continue until 90 records had been selected.

An alternate method for the record file (called systematic sampling) is to make a random selection (using the table of random numbers) of one of the first ten numbers 000, 001, ... 009 and then select this and every tenth following record. If the random start is 004, the sample elements would be 004, 014, 024, ..., 894. *Systematic sampling with a randomized starting point is equivalent to simple random sampling only if the file order itself is strictly random.* This will be strictly true only if it has been randomized through use of a table of random numbers, a process which would be more time-consuming than the selection of a simple random sample. Frequently, however, the sample order is accepted as being unrelated to the characteristic under study. It is important to note that a vast difference exists between a statement to the effect that "there is no known reason for suspecting that the file order is related in any way to the variable under study" and the objectivity achieved by formal randomization. The file order will frequently be alphabetic. It has been argued that this order will group persons of similar ethnic origin. The importance of this factor must be assessed in terms of the purpose of the study. The file order may be chronological. In such case, if the sampling fraction is correct, a systematic sample may give better seasonal coverage than a simple random sample. On the other hand, there is the possibility that, for a certain random start and sampling interval, a disproportionate number in the sample will be for cases seen on Saturday, a group that may have special properties related to age, occupation, and so on. It is important to consider what is known concerning the file order, and recognize the possibility that the estimates may be less precise than those for simple random sampling.

"Representative" samples   The use of probability sampling will not ensure that any single sample will be "representative" of the population in all possible respects. The term "representative" as it is commonly used is undefined in the statistical or mathematical sense; it means simply that the sample resembles the population in some way. If, for example, it is found that the sample age distribution is quite different from that of the population, it is possible to make corrections for the known differences. A common fallacy lies in the unwarranted assumption that, if the sample resembles the population closely on those factors which have been checked, it may be assumed that the sample is "totally representative" and that no difference exists.

The use of probability sampling will allow the investigator to use estimates of known sampling variation and to employ probability statements and tests of hypotheses. In the sections which follow these probability statements will be discussed, as will the nature of the bridge they constitute between the sample results and the population under study. This discussion must be reinforced by a thorough course in statistics before the student can master these concepts.

8-3   Evaluation of Evidence

It is the purpose of this section to illustrate the nature of knowledge in the field of statistics and the usefulness of this knowledge in the interpretation and evaluation of results in experimental and observational epidemiologic studies. Since this knowledge comes basically from the theory of probability—a branch of mathematics that has proved useful in such diverse fields as agriculture, physics, sociology, and medicine—it is best to begin the discussion outside the context of any particular applications.

Some of the early results in probability theory were worked out by mathematicians in response to questions concerning games of chance involving throwing coins or dice and shuffling cards (9). The illustration given here is one of the most basic and far reaching and also one of the simplest.

The binomial distribution and probability   Consider a perfectly balanced die and an experiment performed repeatedly in which the probability that the result of a toss will be a six is exactly 1/6 in every trial. For three fair tosses of the die, the probabilities of 0, 1, 2, or 3 sixes are to be found. Let a six be denoted as a success (S), and any other results as failure (F). Below are listed all possible outcomes and the respective probabilities of their occurrence, as determined by the fundamental theorems of probability (9).

No. of Sixes	Possible Sample Observations	Probability of This No. of Sixes
0	FFF	$\left(\dfrac{5}{6}\right)^3 = 125/216$
1	FFS, FSF, SFF	$3\left(\dfrac{5}{6}\right)^2\left(\dfrac{1}{6}\right) = 75/216$
2	SSF, SFS, FSS	$3\left(\dfrac{5}{6}\right)\left(\dfrac{1}{6}\right)^2 = 15/216$
3	SSS	$\left(\dfrac{1}{6}\right)^3 = 1/216$

For example, in finding the probability of obtaining exactly one six in three tosses, note that the single success can occur on any one of the three tosses, so that the probabilities of each of the results yielding a single six (FFS, FSF, and SFF) must be added. Because the throws are independent, the probabilities multiply, and each of these results has the same probability, $(\frac{5}{6})^2(\frac{1}{6})$ or 25/216.

These results allow statements such as

IF *the die is fair and fairly thrown* (*probability of a six on every throw is* 1/6), THEN *the probability of three sixes in three throws is* 1/216 = .0046.

Armed with this piece of knowledge, imagine yourself in the following situation. A potential opponent in a game of chance, in illustrating the game, begins by throwing three sixes. You must decide whether or not you wish to play and this will depend on your decision as to whether the opponent is using fair dice. You must consider the possibilities: (1) the dice are fair and you just happened to be present at the occurrence of a relatively rare event (but one which is bound to happen sooner or later and is to be expected once in 216 throws of three fair dice); (2) the dice are unfair (the probability of a six is not 1/6).

The knowledge contained in the IF . . . THEN statement above cannot in any way contribute further information to your limited observation on the dice, but only serves to tell you how infrequent the event would be with fair dice. You must now make up your mind on the basis of the knowledge at your disposal and in terms of the penalties you will pay for playing if the dice are unfair or refusing to play if the dice are fair.

As one further step along the way to reality, consider the physician who uses an experimental drug in a situation in which the standard treatment is known to be successful in 1/6 of the cases. He observes success in three patients out of three and proposes to adopt the new drug in all his future cases. Here a new dimension of caution is indicated concerning the method of selection of the three patients. Unless they were randomly selected from the group of patients about whom we wish to draw conclusions, his results may be meaningless. In addition, the penalties of a mistaken decision are more complex and difficult to quantitate. The consequences of an incorrect conclusion consist of (1) using the new treatment when it is not as good as the standard method (in terms of cure rate, side effects, and so on) or (2) continuing to use the standard treatment when the new drug is really superior.

Obviously in both of the examples given it is desirable to have more information from further observation. In practice, decisions must be made at some point, usually on the basis of incomplete information. In no case will application of statistical methods add to the amount of observational information available, but these methods can provide measures of how much information is available and how well estimates can be made or differences between groups detected.

In summary, the mathematician who proved the probability theorems illustrated above was not considering patients' response to treatment or, for that matter, even dice, but merely abstract events of given probabilities. The result of his labor is a series of IF . . . THEN statements. If the THEN part of the statement is to be used in the evaluation of evidence from any study, it is necessary to examine carefully the extent to which the conditions of the study have fulfilled the IF part of the statement. Strictly speaking, the IF part contains a requirement that the study involve some formal experimental devices such as probability sampling or proper randomization procedures.

Tests of significance and confidence intervals   In 1968 Viel and others reported on a study of alcohol use and hepatic damage in residents of Santiago, Chile for whom an autopsy was performed within 24 hours after violent death (10). Their data for males over thirty-five years of age is shown in Table 8-2. As part of their discussion they stated: "Among

TABLE 8-2

Distribution of persons in each drinking habit group according to histopathological findings of the liver

	INTRACELLULAR FAT—NUMBER		TOTAL NUMBER	PERCENTAGE ABUNDANT
	ABUNDANT	SCARCE OR MODERATE		
Normal drinkers	5	168	173	2.9
Inveterate alcoholics	17	116	133	12.8
Total	22	284	306	7.2

Source: Adapted from Viel *et al., J. Chronic Dis.* **21**:157–166, 1968.

males in both age groups the proportion of cases with abundant intracellular fat is greater the more the dependency on alcohol. If the inveterate alcoholic is compared with the normal drinker, regardless of age, there is a greater proportion of cases with abundant fat among those who abuse alcohol. The difference in proportions cannot be explained by chance alone ($p < 0.01$)." The final sentence quoted is equivalent to the statement more frequently found in the literature that "the difference is significant at the 1 per cent level".

The method of testing the significance of the difference between two percentages is described in any elementary book on statistics (11, 12). The discussion here is confined to consideration of the statement that the difference in sample percentages in this case "is significant" or "cannot be explained by chance alone." It is known that different samples randomly selected from the same population will give different results, and the question here is whether or not the observed difference (12.8 per cent − 2.9 per cent) is of a size which would be encountered frequently in repeated pairs of samples taken from populations with identical true percentages. In this example the appropriate calculations based on the sample observations indicate that a difference this large or larger would not be expected to occur more often than once in a hundred such sampling experiments.

It is this fact that leads to the phrase "significant at the 1 per cent level." The possibility that the population percentages are, in fact, equal and the sampling results represent the rare event of unusually large sampling error must be recognized. If this is so, then the conclusion that a difference exists in the population values may be a *type 1 error*, or a false claim of significance. In general, at the 1 per cent level, the investigator would feel justified in seeking some explanation other than sampling error for the observed difference.

If an investigator concludes that the sample difference reflects a real difference in the percentages in the populations, he will then want to know how large this difference is. In the above example, the sample estimate of the difference is $12.8 - 2.9$, or 9.9 per cent, but this statement does not indicate how much information the samples have given us concerning the population percentages. The amount of information given by any sampling experiment will depend on the sample sizes and on the expected sampling variation, and the results are expressed in terms of a *confidence interval* for the population percentage difference. As an example, the *95 per cent confidence interval* is one which is constructed (again by simple calculations from the sample observations) in such a way that in 95 per cent of cases the resulting intervals will include the true population difference (11, 12). In the example here, the results are approximate but permit the 95 per cent confidence interval statement that the true difference in percentage between the populations lies between 1.4 per cent and 18.2 per cent. If a more precise estimate of the difference (a shorter confidence interval) is desired, larger sample sizes are indicated.

In another study, serologic testing for tetanus antibody in drug addicts was undertaken as part of an attempt to explain the higher rate of tetanus in women addicts (13). It was reported that in white addicts the difference between males and females in the proportion with less than 0.1 hemagglutination units (HU) of antibody "*is not significant at the 5 per cent level.*" The abstracted data are given below.

NUMBER WITH HU UNITS OF ANTIBODY

	<.01	>.01	Total	%<.01
Women	5	26	31	16.1
Men	19	38	57	33.3
Total	24	64	88	27.3

In this case the appropriate calculations from the sample observations indicate that sample differences equal to or larger than that observed would be expected to occur rather frequently (in more than 5 per cent) in sampling experiments from populations with identical population percentages. With this result, a common error is to conclude that no difference exists between the true population percentages. The proper conclusion is that it is not possible to determine from these sample observations whether the population percentages are different or equal. Note that here the possibility that the population percentages are equal is accepted, and this may in fact be true. However, if a difference does exist, the samples fail to detect it. This failure is called a *type 2 error*.

In this study the sample estimate of the difference is $33.3 - 16.1$ or 17.2 per cent and the 95 per cent confidence interval estimates the true difference to be somewhere in the interval from -1 to $+35$ per cent. Thus, in this case, the sample observations do not establish the sign (or direction) of the difference or indicate whether it is large or small. Once again, if further information is required, larger sample sizes are necessary. The question is: How much larger? Since large differences are easier to detect than small differences, the answer must be tailored to the investigator's requirements in terms of protection against both type 1 and type 2 errors.

The detecting power of a test of significance and sample size The theoretical determination of the power of a test and the sample size requirements are beyond the scope of this book, but the basic idea is relatively simple and the existing sample size tables are very easy to use (see Tables 8-3 and 8-4).

The investigator may feel that a difference as large as 15 per cent would be of practical importance. He states his requirements as follows:

    a. I would like to limit my chances of making a false claim of significance to not more than 1 per cent.
    b. If a difference as large as $P_1 = 15$ per cent and $P_2 = 30$ per cent exists, then I would like my experiment to have a 95 per cent chance of detecting it.

Luckily, the nonstatistician need not worry about the mathematical calculations involved, but can find the required sample sizes easily by reference to an appropriate table—in this case, Table 8-3. Here we enter the first column headed "the smaller of the two percentages," on the row for 15 per cent and read in the third column for $P_1 - P_2 = 15$ per cent to find that the size of each sample, n_1 and n_2, should be 273. Table 8-4 is for the investigator willing to accept a greater chance (.05) of making a type 1 error, but who still wishes to have a 95 per cent chance of detecting a difference of specified size or, conversely, is willing to accept a 5 per cent (.05) probability of a type 2 error. With P_1 and P_2 remaining at 15 and 30 per cent, respectively, the sample size requirements are reduced to $n_1 = n_2 = 199$. It also can be seen that, if the specified size of the difference to be detected is increased, the size of the samples required is decreased. Thus, if we hold $P_1 = 15$ per cent and read across Table 8-4,

TABLE 8-3

Approximate sample sizes necessary in each of two groups corresponding to various population percentages in order to insure 95% power of the two-tail test at the 1% level

SMALLER OF TWO POPULATION PERCENTAGES	DIFFERENCE IN TWO POPULATION PERCENTAGES									
	5	10	15	20	25	30	35	40	50	60
5	985	318	170	111	79	60	48	39	27	19
10	1555	451	226	139	96	71	55	44	29	21
15	2054	567	273	164	111	80	61	48	31	21
20	2481	665	313	184	122	87	65	50	32	22
25	2837	745	344	200	131	92	68	52	32	21
30	3122	807	368	211	136	95	69	53		
35	3336	852	384	217	139	96	69			
40	3479	879	392	220	139	95				
45	3550	887	392	217						
50	3550	879								

Source: Adapted from Neal W. Chilton and John W. Fertig, The estimation of sample size in experiments, *J. Dent. Res.* **32**(5): 606–612, October 1953.

TABLE 8-4

Approximate sample sizes necessary in each of two groups corresponding to various true percentages in order to insure a 95% power of the two-tail test at the 5% level.

SMALLER OF TWO POPULATION PERCENTAGES	DIFFERENCE IN TWO POPULATION PERCENTAGES									
	5	10	15	20	25	30	35	40	50	60
5	719	231	124	80	58	44	34	28	19	14
10	1135	329	164	101	70	52	40	32	21	15
15	1498	413	199	119	80	58	44	34	22	15
20	1810	485	228	134	89	73	47	36	23	15
25	2070	543	251	145	95	67	49	38	23	15
30	2278	589	268	153	99	69	50	38	23	
35	2434	621	280	158	101	70	50	38	22	
40	2538	641	286	160	101	69				
45	2590	647	286	158						
50	2590	641								

Source: Adapted from Neal W. Chilton and John W. Fertig, The estimation of sample size in experiments, *J. Dent. Res.* **32**(5): 606–612, October 1953.

the n values fall to 119 for a difference of 20 per cent, to 80 for a difference of 25 per cent, and so on.

Sequential experimentation In the preceding discussion the sample sizes are taken as fixed before the beginning of the experiment. In a very important class of experimental designs known as sequential (14, 15, 16) observations are made one at a time and the sequence is continued until a decision is reached. The decision (or test) rule for a preassigned level of significance is set up to give the required detecting power against any specified difference. In sequential tests the sample size is a random variable, but, in general, the average sample size is smaller than that required for the classical test.

Let us return to our example concerning tetanus antibody in which the observed samples did not permit a good estimate of the size of the difference or even the conclusion that a true difference exists. In this case, the investigators might regard a difference of 15 per cent as of practical value and set $P_1 = 15$ per cent and $P_2 = 30$ per cent. In this situation, as described above, we found from Table 8-4 that for a fixed-sample-size experiment we needed $n_1 = n_2 = 199$, if the test is to be made at the 5 per cent level of significance and we are to have 95 per cent power in detecting the difference. The sequential method would be based on selection of a series of pairs of addicts, one male and one female. The antibody tests would be run on each pair and a decision reached on whether or not another pair was needed.

The decision between fixed sample size and a sequential design is governed by consideration of practical difficulties and human values. In the present study, conducted at Beth Israel Medical Center in New York City, accumulation of the study groups and collection of the necessary serum specimens represent a small investment in money and effort and little inconvenience for those studied. In the laboratory, however, substantial gains in cost and convenience would result if sera were held as collected and all were tested at the same time. These latter gains from a fixed sample design probably would outweigh any savings in sample size resulting from use of the sequential design. It requires little imagination, however, to conceive of situations where the smaller sample sizes expected with a sequential design would be advantageous. Examples would include studies of rare diseases in which accumulating enough cases may require much time, studies in which testing procedures are expensive, or studies of therapy in which human lives are at stake.

8-4 Summary

The proper application of statistics to epidemiologic problems frequently involves the integration of knowledge of the medical and disease agent subject matter and appreciation of some rather mathematically sophisticated theorems on probability which, in essence, lie totally outside the medical field. Only infrequently does a single individual have thorough command of both branches of knowledge, and a common effort to establish communication between two experts is usually necessary. The statistician should take part in the original planning of the study design, as well as in the analysis of the resulting data. This effort of cooperation between the epidemiologist and the statistician can be profitable to both and, on occasion, can result in a research method of real and lasting merit.

GLOSSARY

Cluster sampling   A sampling scheme in which each unit selected is a group of persons (all persons in a city block, a family, etc.) rather than an individual.

Detecting power   Frequency with which a true difference of specified size between populations would be detected by the proposed experiment and test rule.

Probability sampling   A formal sampling plan with the property that for every member of the population sampled the probability of being included in the sample is known and nonzero. Cluster sampling, stratification, and systematic sampling can be part of probability sampling.

Statistical significance   In the context of the examples used in this chapter, "statistical significance" refers to the frequency with which a difference as large as that observed would be expected in taking repeated pairs of samples from populations identical with respect to the characteristic studied. If this frequency is less than 5 per cent (or 1 per cent), it is customary to say that the observed difference "is significant at the 5 per cent (or 1 per cent) level."

Stratification   A sampling scheme in which independent sampling plans are used in different, well-defined subdivisions (or strata) of the population.

Systematic sampling   A sampling scheme in which, after a random start, every nth member of an ordered population (such as a card file) is included in the sample.

Type 1 error   The error of making a false claim of significance, or, more precisely of concluding that two populations differ in the value of some parameter when, in fact, they do not.

Type 2 error   The error of failing to detect a true difference, or of making a false conclusion that no difference exists.

95 per cent confidence interval   An interval estimate for a population parameter (or for the difference in two populations) constructed by a method which has the property that the resulting interval will include the true value in 95 per cent of similar sampling experiments.

REFERENCES

1. Brownlee, K. A. Statistics of the 1954 polio vaccine trials. *J. Amer. Stat. Ass.* **50**:1005–1013, 1955.
2. Hammond, E. Cuyler, and Horn, Daniel. Smoking and death rates— report on forty-four months of follow-up of 187,783 men. *J. Amer. Med. Ass.* **166**:1159–1172, 1294–1308, 1958.
3. Heady, J. A., Morris, J. N., Kagan, A., and Raffle, P. A. B. Coronary heart disease in London busmen. *Brit. J. Prev. Soc. Med.* **15**:143–153, 1961.
4. Hammon, William McD., Coriell, L. L., Ludwig, E. H., McAllister, R. M., Greene, A. E., Sather, G. E., and Wehrle, P. F. Evaluation of Red Cross gamma globulin as a prophylactic agent for polio- myelitis. 5. Reanalysis of results based on laboratory-confirmed cases. *J. Amer. Med. Ass.* **156**:21–27, 1954.
5. Bodian, David. Viremia in experimental poliomyelitis. II. Viremia and the mechanism of the "provoking" effect of injections or trauma. *Amer. J. Hyg.* **60**:358–370, 1954.
6. Manson, M. M., Logan, W. P. D., and Loy, R. M. Rubella and Other Virus Infections during Pregnancy. Ministry of Health Reports on Public Health and Medical Subjects No. 101, H.M. Stationery Office, London, 1960.
7. Siegel, Morris, Fuerst, H. T., and Dugan, W. Rubella in mother and congenital cataracts in child. Comparative data in periods with and without epidemics from 1957 to 1964. *J. Amer. Med. Ass.* **203**:116– 120, 1968.
8. Hessman, M. A., and Lipworth, L. Accuracy of Certification of Causes of Death. General Register Office, Studies on Medical and Population Subjects No. 20. H.M. Stationery Office, 1966.
9. Neyman, J. *First Course in Probability and Statistics.* New York: Henry Holt, 1950.
10. Viel, B., Donoso, S., Salcedo, D., and Varela, A. Alcohol drinking habit and hepatic damage. *J. Chronic Dis.* **21**:157–166, 1968.
11. Dunn, Olive Jean. *Biostatistics. A Primer for the Biomedical Sciences.* New York: John Wiley, 1964.
12. Dixon, Wilfred J., and Massey, Frank J., Jr. *Introduction to Statistical Analysis*, 3rd ed., New York: McGraw-Hill, 1969.
13. Cherubin, C. E., Millian, S. J., Palusci, E., and Fortunato, M. In- vestigations in tetanus in narcotic addicts in New York City. *Amer. J. Epidem.* **88**(2):215–223, 1968.

14. Armitage, P. *Sequential Medical Trials.* Springfield, Ill.: Charles C. Thomas, 1960.
15. Elveback, L. Sequential sampling in epidemiology. *Amer. J. Public Health* **52**:1129–1136, 1962.
16. Armitage, P. Restricted sequential procedures. *Biometrika*, **44**:9–26, 1957.

9

Patterns of Disease
Occurrence—Person

The basic premise of epidemiology is that disease does not occur randomly but in patterns which reflect the operation of the underlying causes. A corollary to this is that knowledge of these patterns is not only of predictive value with respect to future disease occurrence, but also constitutes a major key to understanding causation and, hence, to devising methods of control and prevention.

In essence, the pattern of disease in populations is described by the composite answers to three basic questions: Who is attacked? Where does disease occur? When does it occur? In this and the following two chapters we shall consider how these questions can be answered and some implications of answers commonly obtained. First, however, we must consider the basic problems of defining and classifying disease in the individual.

9-1   Health and Disease in the Individual

A goal of medicine is promotion of good health. Conceptually, good health is easy to define: properly integrated functioning of all bodily components to give optimal function of the total individual—mental, emotional, and physical. Practically, "optimum" is not definable, and proof of good health consists of relatively crude evaluations of the overall functional status of the individual as falling within fairly wide limits of "normal" function set by observation of "normal" people coupled with freedom from evident disease. Indeed, a common but more negative definition of good health would be "freedom from disease."

185

Positive health and disease are, by definition, mutually exclusive. Strictly, any deviation from normal function or state (of the total individual or any of his component parts) is a manifestation of disease. However, deviations may often be imperceptible and lead to no immediately evident dysfunction, for example, silent immunizing infection with poliovirus or even a minimal infection with tubercle bacillus, both of which usually result in complete functional recovery. In other instances, equally imperceptible deviations may be precursors of subsequent clearly evident disease, for example, reduced glucose tolerance presaging diabetes or elevated serum cholesterol as a forerunner of arteriosclerosis. Although knowledge of the occurrence of such lesser deviations is of basic importance to full understanding of disease causation, we are forced in practice to define *disease* as clearly perceptible deviation from normal function.

Although simple separation of the healthy from those with disease may be adequate for selecting individuals for military service or life insurance, promotion of good health requires prevention and treatment of disease. These countermeasures are not abstract but take relatively specific forms depending on the nature of the deviations by which disease is manifest and the specific causes of these deviations.

As a working hypothesis, we may postulate that, for a given cause, a specific deviation or set of deviations is reflected in a describable clinical syndrome (the set of clinical manifestations characteristic of a given disease); or, conversely, for a given syndrome, there is a specific underlying cause. Hence, medicine has long been concerned with identifying and describing the many distinct clinical entities that make up the mass of human disease as a necessary first step toward understanding causation and developing methods of treatment.

With its emphasis on defining causation, epidemiology is concerned with describing the impact on man of specific causes or agents. Clinical disease entities, therefore, are of interest as indicators of the occurrence of etiologic disease entities. Unfortunately, the impact of a specific agent only rarely results in a single characteristic and unique (or pathognomonic) disease syndrome, for example, the combination of coryzal onset, Koplik spots, fever, and macular rash which is pathognomonic for measles virus infection.

Much more commonly man's response to a given disease agent varies widely. Thus, with polioviruses there is a gradient ranging from subclinical infection (perhaps 80 per cent) or brief febrile illness with no neurologic signs (about 15 per cent) to more obvious central nervous system (CNS) involvement, including both benign aseptic meningitis (4 to 5 per cent) and the classical paralytic disease which, though occurring in less than 1 per cent of infections, is the really significant outcome. With group B coxsackieviruses, response may vary even more widely. In addition to silent infections, these viruses cause such disparate clinical entities as upper respiratory disease, aseptic meningitis, myocarditis (which in infants is often fatal), and Bornholm's disease (epidemic pleurodynia). Indeed, this is just a fairly modern example of the long-recognized principle that the predominant clinical response to a disease agent is largely determined by the organs or tissues subjected to attack. For some agents like polio or rabies virus there is but a single vulnerable target, in these cases the CNS; whereas for other agents such as the group B coxsackie-viruses and the much longer known spirochete of syphilis or tubercle bacillus, multiple targets exist.

Because the number of possible disease targets in the body is small and the number of potential disease agents is very large, it is hardly surprising that reasonably distinct clinical entities may be caused by more than one agent, sometimes by a large number. In some instances, the clinically similar but etiologically distinct entities are also similar in their salient epidemiologic features, such as mode of spread, reservoir, and seasonal pattern of occurrence. These include not only syndromes such as paralytic poliomyelitis and bacillary dysentery, each caused by three or more distinct but closely similar agent species, but also many respiratory syndromes (common cold, acute pharyngitis, tracheobronchitis, bronchiolitis, pneumonitis, and "influenza"), caused by a large number of agents belonging to such dissimilar groups as rhinoviruses, myxoviruses (influenza, parainfluenza, RS viruses), adenoviruses, mycoplasma (*M. pneumoniae, M. hominis type 1*), and bacteria (group A beta hemolytic streptococci).

In other instances, both the specific etiology and important aspects of the epidemiology of similar clinical entities are different. Clinically indistinguishable epidemic and murine typhus, caused by immunologically related rickettsial agents, are transmitted respectively by human body lice and rat fleas. The clinical entity viral hepatitis may result from fecal-oral spread via various pathways of one or more agents or from syringe transmission (plasma, transfusions, various injection procedures) of still another viral agent. Finally, mosquito-borne yellow fever (caused by a virus) and water-borne Weil's disease (caused by *Leptospira icterohaemorrhagiae*) are sufficiently similar clinically that the noted investigator Hideyo Noguchi spent several years studying the etiology of the latter in the belief that he was investigating yellow fever.

To summarize the foregoing discussion, classification of disease by clinical manifestation is a necessary and useful step in determining causation. Although the same agent may cause more than one clinical syndrome and similar or identical syndromes may be produced by multiple causes, the cause-effect relation is sufficiently constant that the nature of the clinical manifestations of disease constitutes an important clue to causation. For the clinician, it is the basis for establishing a differential diagnosis, that is, a listing of all the known etiologic entities that might include the clinical picture presented by a given patient. For the epidemiologist, similarly, the occurrence of a particular clinical entity reflects the activity of a finite group of potential agents, known or unknown. However, neither the clinician nor the epidemiologist is satisfied with a differential diagnosis. Both ultimately require a specific etiologic diagnosis. Upon this the physician bases his specific treatment and his prognosis and the epidemiologist his description of the occurrence of the etiologic entity, including its full range of possible clinical manifestations, his predictions as to future occurrence, and his prescriptions for disease control.

Recognition of the full range of human response to a given agent is important, epidemiologically, for two main reasons; these reasons are readily illustrated by poliomyelitis. Knowledge of the occurrence of sub-clinical infections and atypical, abortive disease was essential to understanding the mechanisms of virus spread (in the United States largely by contact between young children who only rarely experience disease) without which the less common but important CNS disease could not occur. Further, such knowledge made it possible to describe, within the total occurrence of infection with polioviruses, the pattern of occurrence of paralytic disease in ways that led to the recognition of important factors that predisposed to paralytic disease. Thus, tonsillectomy was recognized as a factor predisposing to bulbar disease, and age, recent inoculations, excessive physical exertion, and pregnancy were found to be factors contributing to paralytic disease in general. The essential principles illustrated are: (1) knowledge of the full extent of human contact with an agent is vital to understanding how it reaches man; (2) the influence of important contributing or modifying factors may be reflected by the patterns of occurrence of clinically different responses to the agent.

9-2   Disease Variation and Attributes of Persons

Persons may differ from one another in respect to a nearly infinite number of attributes, some determined at conception and others subsequently acquired. The former include age, sex, genetic makeup as reflected by race or ethnic origin and membership in familial groups or kinships, and such family-determined attributes as parental age and birth order. Acquired characteristics are far more numerous and fall into several classes. Some are biologic, for example, nutritional state, muscular development, specific immunities, and, for women, parity or number of previous pregnancies. Others are behavioral (personal or cultural) and include dietary choice, extent and nature of physical and recreational activities, religious preference, smoking, sleeping habits, and various personality traits. Still other attributes are social or economic in nature, for example, level of education, occupation or profession, income, and marital status. Each of the characteristics mentioned above (and many more, as well) are variables that may relate to exposure to disease agents or to susceptibility or resistance to the effects of these agents and so to the occurrence, severity, and outcome of disease.

However, some attributes are more useful or important than others. Usefulness depends partly on relevance to the particular disease of interest. More generally, usefulness depends on the ease and reliability with which information about a given attribute can be obtained. For a given individual, particularly a patient, nearly any desired information can be obtained by physical or laboratory examination, interview, and search of relevant records. However, when we want to know the relative frequency of a disease in persons possessing a specified attribute, we must be able to know or estimate the total number of such persons in the population. Census data or other accessible records may make it easy to estimate how many persons there are in groups defined by age, sex, race, occupation, or marital status, but special surveys may be necessary in order to estimate the numbers of persons possessing other attributes such as immunity to rubella, the habit of smoking cigarettes, specific dietary deficiencies, or the regular taking of sleeping pills. Similarly, whereas age, sex, race, and other easily documented characteristics can be ascertained with great reliability, less confidence can be placed in information that derives chiefly from memory, for example, the quantitative aspects of behavioral attributes such as the average use of cigarettes or alcohol or the frequency and amount of consumption of specific dietary items.

The relative importance of personal characteristics to disease description varies in two main ways. First is the strength or degree of association that actually exists between a given attribute and a specific disease. Thus, a cheerful disposition may have a significant negative association with peptic ulcer but none at all with respiratory disease. Or, as with measles, age is strongly associated but sex is not. A note of caution is in order at this point, however. Until the possibility of association has been tested, its existence and its strength remain unknown. Thus, failures to examine the relation between a given attribute and a disease, based on preconceptions as to the improbability of a relation, may result in failures to detect important associations. Who, for example, would have imagined that cigarette smoking might be related to cancer of the urinary tract? The second way in which the importance of an attribute to disease description may vary has to do with the independence or relative interdependence of attributes as variables. The inherent attributes, age, sex, and ethnic origin, are independent of one another, whereas the acquired attributes are almost never independent. As obvious examples, behavioral characteristics such as smoking or the use of alcohol and such social attributes as level of education and profession or occupation are highly interrelated and are strongly correlated with age, sex, and race. In these examples it is usually not too difficult to evaluate the relative influence of the individual interdependent variables. However, the fact that a given acquired characteristic may be determined in part by one or more other characteristics of persons in less obvious or even improbable ways dictates great caution in making inferences from a particular association when association with other, possibly correlated attributes has not been explored.

The gist of the foregoing discussion is that a useful purpose may be served by describing disease occurrence in relation to any attribute of persons that, in practice, may be defined or ascertained. The following discussion, however, will be limited necessarily to the description of disease occurrence in relation to a few of the more important and most commonly used characteristics of persons.

9-3   Age

Disease occurrence in general is more strongly related to age than to any other single personal characteristic. This relation ordinarily is so strong that, until possible differences in age distribution have been taken into account, differences in disease occurrence between population subgroups defined on the basis of other attributes (for example, sex, race, smoking habits) cannot be meaningfully interpreted. It is fortunate, therefore, that age is one of the most readily and reliably ascertained characteristics both of patients with disease and of total membership of the population from which the patients come.

The basic data upon which description of the age pattern of disease rests are simple enumeration of new cases (incidence) and total cases at a point in time, as from a tuberculosis or cancer registry (prevalence) or of deaths (mortality). Such enumerations are commonly summarized in terms of the number and per cent of total cases or deaths falling into sequentially arranged age groups (usually defined in five-year intervals or multiples thereof, for example, 0–4, 5–9, 10–19, 20–39, and so on). Per cent distribution by age of hospitalized poliomyelitis in the United States, 1954–1958, is shown in Figure 9-1 (1). Knowledge of the proportional distribution of cases by age is useful to the clinician and medical care administrators to the extent that special provisions may be indicated for pediatric or geriatric patients. It also is directly useful to the epidemiologist as an indicator of trends in disease risk when data for successive years from the same population area (city, state, nation) are compared, as in the cited example of poliomyelitis which brackets the period when large-scale use of vaccine was introduced. In such cases inferences as to change in relative age-specific risks depend on the assumption that change in numbers and age distributions of the underlying population from one year to the next are slight in comparison with the changes in numbers of cases of disease.

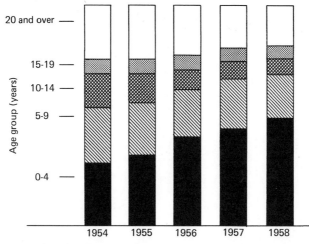

FIG. 9-1 Percentage distribution of paralytic poliomyelitis admissions by age, 1954–1958 (based on hospital notifications received by The National Foundation). (The National Foundation. *Poliomyelitis*, Annual Statistical Review, 1958.)

More often, the relation of disease to age is described by rates that measure the risk of disease in each age group. These age-specific rates (incidence, prevalence, or mortality) are computed by relating the number of cases or deaths recorded for each age group to the total number of persons in the corresponding age segment of the population, as described in Chapter 7. The resulting "age profile" of disease is best visualized in graphic form, as in Figure 9-2, which presents data for two years, 1954 and 1958, for hospitalized poliomyelitis in the United States (1). As the result of widespread use of Salk vaccine in the intervening years, the risk of poliomyelitis decreased greatly in all age groups. However, failure of the less educated (largely Negro) segment of the population to accept the vaccine resulted in a proportionately smaller reduction in the 0–4-year age group within which were contained most of the Negro susceptibles.

Such "age profiles" for a given year reflect with reasonable accuracy the age-related operation of the underlying causes in that year (in the foregoing, infection with wild poliovirus) only when the interval between initiation of cause and disease onset is relatively short. Even when this interval is long (measured in years), a basic relation between age and the operation of the cause can be inferred if, over a period of years, the age profile does not change. However, if the level of activity of a cause with long-delayed effect is not relatively constant, calendar year age profiles may be unduly influenced by the changing activity of the cause. It then becomes necessary to examine the lifetime age-specific disease experience of cohorts (groups of persons born in the same year or five-year period)

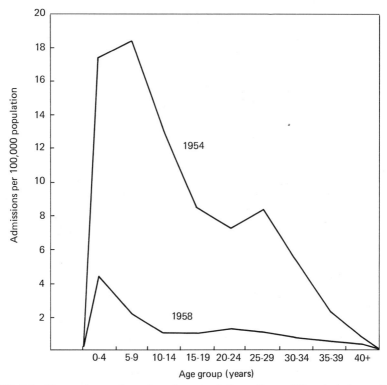

FIG. 9-2 Prevaccine and postvaccine paralytic poliomyelitis admission rates by age group, 1954 and 1958 (based on hospital notifications received by The National Foundation). (The National Foundation, *Poliomyelitis*, Annual Statistical Review, 1958.)

to see whether a relation exists between age and cause. Examples, including tuberculosis (declining exposure) and lung cancer (increasing cigarette consumption), are presented in Chapter 11 in which the use of cohorts is discussed in detail in relation to long-term trends.

There are still other reasons why the age profile of a disease may not accurately reflect the age-related effect of the primary cause. This will be the case if the frequency of recognized disease following contact with the disease agent varies with age. As illustrated schematically in Figure 9-3, which depicts the frequency with age of "serious outcome" of infection occurring in nonimmune persons, risk is relatively high in the first year of life, is least during the remainder of childhood, and then increases progressively with age thereafter. This figure roughly illustrates the situation with poliovirus infection, using "typical" paralytic poliomyelitis to characterize "serious outcome." In the case of measles, the same principle holds in that the risk of the rare, but serious, complication of encephalitis also increases with age. However, since infection results in

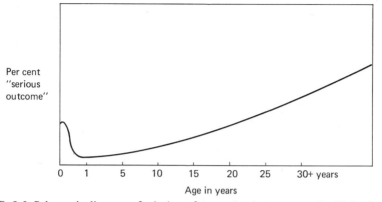
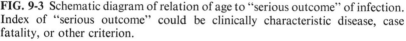

Per cent "serious outcome"

Age in years

FIG. 9-3 Schematic diagram of relation of age to "serious outcome" of infection. Index of "serious outcome" could be clinically characteristic disease, case fatality, or other criterion.

characteristic measles without regard to age, the age profile of typical measles does mirror reliably that of measles virus infection. A second instance in which the age profile may be misleading is when accuracy of diagnosis or completeness of reporting varies with age. Thus, nonparalytic forms of poliomyelitis probably are recognized more often in children than in adults.

Within the limitations suggested, age profiles of acute infectious disease do reflect the age-related activity of the underlying causes and are determined by the relation of age to exposure and to susceptibility. Measles illustrates the case of a commonly prevalent agent, infection with which results not only in disease, but subsequently in lifelong immunity. Infants are usually spared because they are less exposed and because of their maternally derived antibody which disappears after six to eight months of age. Thereafter, the likelihood of exposure increases, reaching a peak at entrance into school. The subsequent decline of incidence rates with increasing age reflects reductions in the proportion of susceptibles and in the risk of exposure. The child who has not experienced infection by age eight or nine may well be spared until he has children of his own because, until then, his contacts will be largely with his age peers, nearly all of whom will be immune. The importance of immunity to the age pattern of measles is most dramatically demonstrated in isolated population groups which are only infrequently invaded by the virus. Where this has been documented as in the Faroe Islands, Tahiti, and Greenland, invasion results in disease with nearly equal high attack rates in all age groups born since the virus was last present and in almost no disease in those born earlier.

A different situation prevails when increasing age is not associated with a marked reduction in the proportion of susceptibles in the population.

Such is the case: (1) when, as with rhinoviruses, a specific serotype is present infrequently and then reaches only a small proportion of the population; (2) when the viral reservoir is in lower animals and, as with most arboviruses, human infection is relatively infrequent; (3) when, as with a number of common respiratory viruses, including influenza, effective postinfection immunity is of short duration; or (4) with most noninfectious disease agents. In these cases the age profile is largely determined by exposure which may be indirectly related to age. Examples include the sharp increase in undifferentiated respiratory disease attendant upon entrance into school, the increased risk of respiratory disease and of such "childhood" diseases as mumps and rubella incurred by parents of young children, and the risk of exposure to zoonotic diseases related to occupations such as tending livestock in the western United States (Rocky Mountain spotted fever) or cutting wood in Brazil (jungle yellow fever).

In the realm of the so-called degenerative diseases such as diabetes, cardiovascular diseases, arthritis, and cancer, incidence and prevalence, and mortality rates increase progressively with age. Although this relation is sufficiently strong and consistent that meaningful comparisons of disease occurrence in different populations can be made only after allowing for differences in age distributions, little is known about either the under-lying causes or their activity in relation to age. Superficially plausible hypotheses would include the cumulative effects of prolonged exposure to unidentified environmental influences, simple degenerative changes ("aging" or wearing out) of tissues which increase susceptibility to disease agents, or a combination of both. That environmental factors play a significant role in most of these diseases is suggested by the fact that incidence rates for corresponding age groups often vary significantly between populations living under differing circumstances. This fact is encouraging with respect to the possibility of prevention, because identifica-tion of noxious environmental influences may lead to countermeasures. No similar hope seems justified in the light of present knowledge for prevention of the aging process as such.

9-4 Sex

With rare (but often well-publicized) exceptions, sex, like age, is an easily ascertained characteristic of both patients and the population at large. Hence, the occurrence of disease in relation to sex is readily described. This description takes its simplest form in the sex ratio for a given disease, that is, the ratio of cases in males to cases in females. Over the years among children, for example, the poliomyelitis sex ratio has been 1.3:1. The implication of this ratio is that the relative frequency of poliomyelitis in boys is 1.3 times that in girls, the assumption being that the population is equally divided by sex.

In point of fact, populations are not equally divided by sex. Among infants born alive in the United States, males exceed females in the proportion of 106:100.* From birth onward, however, in every age group life is harder on males than on females, the death rates for males consistently exceeding those for females in the average ratio for all ages of about 1.5:1. Since the numbers of each sex in childhood are very nearly equal, the sex ratio for poliomyelitis or other diseases among children is a fairly accurate measure of the difference in risk related to sex. From age twenty on, however, the number of females exceeds the number of males of corresponding age and the relative difference increases with advancing age. Not only does the sex ratio become less useful but, in comparing sex-specific rates, the rates must be adjusted for age. For many purposes it is best to compare directly the age profiles for the two sexes (i.e., compare rates for the corresponding age-sex-specific groups), so that possibly important differences in their contour may be seen.

Description of disease patterns by sex is not just an academic exercise, because, aside from strictly sex related conditions, significant though often poorly understood differences are usual and, on the surface at least, contradictory. By whatever index employed (incidence of acute illness, prevalence of chronic illness, frequency of medical consultation, or days confined to bed) females have significantly greater morbidity than males (2.72 versus 2.47 acute illnesses per year, according to the 1957–1958 U.S. National Health Survey); yet, as already noted, the male death rate is 1.5 times that of females. Although the situation is reversed in several specific diseases (morbidity from peptic ulcer and coronary heart disease is more common in men, whereas diabetes deaths are more frequent in women), these general patterns are amazingly consistent and call for understanding.

It is natural to attempt to ascribe differences in the occurrence of illnesses and deaths to the basic biologic differences between the sexes. Diseases related to the reproductive organs and function pose no problem in this respect and one can construct plausible hypotheses based on sex-determined biologic differences to explain the more common occurrence in women of diabetes, hyperthyroidism, and obesity (possibly related to a difference in endocrine status) or of gall bladder and biliary tract disease (possibly secondary to pregnancies). However, a similar biologic basis is less apparent when we consider acute respiratory disease, hypertension,

*In seventeenth-century England, as John Graunt noted, male infants also exceeded females "by about a thirteenth part." This, despite a higher rate of attrition of males due to many causes ("slain in wars, killed by mischance, drowned at sea and die by the hand of justice"), was believed by Graunt to be sufficient "that every woman may have an husband, without the allowance of polygamy." (2)

and arthritis (all more frequent in females) or lung cancer, cirrhosis of the liver, and coronary heart disease (all more common in males). With respiratory and other minor illness, it is possible that disease is equally frequent in the two sexes, but that females seek help more often. However, for major illnesses and deaths the differences are certainly real and relate either to basic biologic differences or to differences in life experiences that characterize the two sexes. In lung cancer and cirrhosis of the liver, male exposure to presumed causative factors such as cigarettes and alcohol probably greatly exceeds that of females. Also, the traditional role of females in caring for the sick in the house may account in part for their reported excess of infectious illnesses. That environmental influences contribute to the general excess of mortality experienced by males and to that attributed to coronary heart disease (CHD) is indicated by the fact that, although both total and CHD-specific mortality rates for each sex have decreased in the past quarter century, the decreases have been greater for females. Until these environmental influences are identified and counteracted, the contribution of sex-related biologic differences to the survival advantage of females will remain unmeasured.

9-5   Racial or Ethnic Origin and Familial Relation

Monozygotic twins excepted, no two members of the species *Homo sapiens* are identical in genetic makeup. These genetic differences are readily evident only insofar as they are reflected in easily observable physical characteristics such as color and texture of hair, skin pigmentation, and color of eyes. Although identification of specific points of similarity or difference that influence disease occurrence depends on greatly increased understanding of the genetic mechanism of man, the Mendelian laws of inheritance permit reasonable assumptions as to the extent of unspecified genetic similarities based on knowledge of the origins of persons and population groups.

The greatest degree of genetic similarity exists between siblings who are the offspring of the same parents and important degrees of similarity exist within familial groups or kinships defined on the basis of known blood relationship extending over several generations. Because variations in disease occurrence between familial groups may indicate the operation of a genetic factor, description of specific disease rates in such groups is of basic epidemiologic interest. In concept, such description involves only two simple steps, listing of the familial group and identifying cases of disease within its membership.

A classical, simple example involving tuberculosis was described by Kallman and Reisner (3). Index cases were twins and the familial groups were restricted to members of the immediate families of the twins. These were readily identified and their disease status ascertained. Special interest pertained to the fact that disease prevalence increased directly with the degree of genetic similarity, namely, spouses, parents, dizygotic co-twins and other siblings (the same), and monozygotic co-twins. As another simple example, already alluded to in Chapter 5, the readily verified occurrence of paralytic poliomyelitis was determined for the preceding five-year period among close living relatives (immediate family, aunts, uncles, and first cousins) of current-year polio patients. Finally, offspring of mothers dying of breast or uterine cancer have been followed for the occurrence of cancers of all types with observed incidence well above that "expected" on the basis of the experience of the general population.

The problem becomes greater as the familial group is expanded to include more generations. Not only may it be difficult to develop a genealogic chart or "family pedigree" that extends backward for more than three generations but, when this is possible, determination of disease status of long-deceased persons may be unreliable or impossible unless reliable medical records exist or, as with some rare truly heritable conditions (hemophilia, Huntington's chorea), disease is reflected by highly characteristic manifestations. For more common important diseases (diabetes, arteriosclerosis, arthritis), construction of a family pedigree may be very important with respect to identifying a living cohort of related persons (comprising two or three generations) whose past disease experience can be well documented and whose future disease experience can be observed. A major effort of this type is being undertaken in an important contemporary long-term study of noninfectious diseases in a total community (4).

Grouping of persons by race or ethnic origin brings together individuals possessing a much smaller, but still significant, degree of similarity in genetic constitution which derives from their remote common origin and the predominance over countless generations of mating within the group. The concentration within ethnic groups of certain heritable diseases involving major genes (amaurotic family idiocy among persons of Semitic origin, anemias due to abnormal hemoglobins such as sickle cell disease among Negroes, and thalassemia among the Thai and certain Mediterranean peoples) represents readily visible consequences of the preservation of genetic distinctness and supports the possibility that ethnic groups may also differ in genetically determined susceptibility or resistance to infectious or other environmental causes of disease.

Although complicated by an increasing frequency of mixed marriages between persons of different ethnic or national origin, especially in the United States, it is reasonably easy to characterize individual patients by racial or ethnic group. Also, information as to race and native origin for the United States population at large is collected during the census. Persons of mixed racial parentage are classified by the race of the nonwhite parent or, if both are nonwhite, by that of the father. Persons of foreign birth are classified by country. Native-born children of foreign-born parents are also identified as "foreign stock," the birthplace of the father governing in the case of mixed marriages. Thus, on the basis of census data (published for larger areas or obtainable on request for smaller areas), estimates can be made for United States populations of subgroups belonging to various "races" (white, Negro, American Indian, Chinese, Japanese, Filipino) or "foreign stocks" (including both foreign born and first generation).

Within the United States population differences in the occurrence of many diseases have been noted between population subgroups defined by racial or ethnic origin. Such disparate diseases as tuberculosis, essential hypertension, and rickets are more common among Negroes than among whites who, in turn, are more often afflicted with coronary heart disease (CHD) and skin cancer. Gastric cancer (a peculiarly disappearing entity in the United States) is more common among foreign-born persons (especially those from Scandinavian countries), and cancer of the cervix is relatively uncommon among Jewish women.

Knowledge of such differences is useful in a practical way in case-finding efforts and application of specific preventive measures. Explanation of the differences is important to full understanding of the causation of disease; indeed, their mere existence may provide important clues to such understanding. Do they reflect the operation of some genetically deter-mined and, hopefully, identifiable characteristic? Are they the result of environmental factors (again hopefully identifiable) that affect different ethnic or racial groups unequally because of voluntary or involuntary differences in their behavior and pattern of living?

Skin cancer and rickets exemplify the operation of a genetically deter-mined attribute, skin pigmentation. The heavy pigmentation of the Negro skin limits adsorption from solar radiation of the ultraviolet spectrum which promotes the occurrence of skin cancers and the natural synthesis of rickets-preventing vitamin D. The excess of tuberculosis among Negroes, a constantly controversial question, is obviously related in large part to deprivation. However, Negroes as a racial group have had only brief experience (perhaps three centuries) with this lethal disease, whereas Caucasians have had countless centuries of experience during which natural selection for resistance has been operating.

The relative freedom of Jewish women from cervical cancer illustrates a situation in which a very specific environmental factor, the ritual cir-cumcision of the male, provides both a plausible explanation for the difference and a possibly important clue to the basic etiologic mechanism. Of similar import, the lesser frequence of elevated blood cholesterol among young adult Negro males as compared with whites (presumably attribut-able to economically determined dietary differences) has been advanced as a partial explanation for the lesser occurrence of CHD among Negro males in middle age and so, by inference, supports the idea that prolonged exposure to elevated blood cholesterol is an important cause of CHD.

In the case of the other diseases mentioned, essential hypertension and gastric cancer, causation remains even more obscure, but the fact of differences associated with race or ethnic group provides a point for departure. The gastric cancer problem illustrates one way in which this fact is being exploited. Japan is a country with a very high incidence of gastric cancer. Hawaii and the mainland United States contain substantial populations of Japanese background, including many born in Japan. Japanese culture, including dietary practices, has been retained to a greater extent in Hawaii than in the mainland United States. The occurrence of gastric cancer among immigrants overall is less than in Japan, is less in mainland United States than in Hawaii, and in both varies inversely with the time elapsed since immigration. Among United States (including Hawaii) born Japanese, the incidence differs little from that among United States natives overall. Clearly, an important specific cause of gastric cancer must be environmental, probably dietary. (5) Current comparative studies should reveal its nature.

9-6   Parental Age, Birth Order, and Family Size

By being born into a family, an individual involuntarily assumes family-determined but nongenetic attributes. Parental ages and birth order are determined as of birth and become a matter of record on the birth registration certificate. Total family size cannot be established until the mother has reached the menopause, although the size at any given moment can be known and the distribution of the population by sibship size can be estimated from birth registration and census data. Thus, for a given abnormality or disease state, the frequency of occurrence among persons classified by these attributes can be estimated and the degree of association between disease occurrence and individual attributes can be examined. Since the attributes in question, particularly parental age and birth order, are closely associated, considerable caution is necessary in interpreting associations observed. For an excellent discussion of the methods for handling such data, the reader is referred to MacMahon, Pugh, and Ipsen (6).

The ways in which these family-determined variables may affect the health of the individual are too numerous to describe completely. Some depend on purely biological mechanisms and others upon correlated social circumstances. Mongolism (Down's syndrome), a major example of mental retardation, is typically associated with an extra chromosome of number 21, a form of chromosomal nondisjunction directly related to maternal age. Overall, Mongolism occurs with a frequency of 1.5 per 1,000 births, but the range is from 0.2 for maternal ages under thirty years to 15.0 for ages 40–44 years and over 20.0 for still older maternal ages. Hemolytic disease of the newborn due to Rh incompatibility illustrates nearly complete dependence on birth order. An Rh-negative woman (whose red cells lack the Rh antigen) married to an Rh-positive husband may conceive an Rh-positive fetus. Rh antigen from such a fetus induces formation in the mother of anti-Rh antibody, which then can enter the fetal circulation via the placenta. The first such fetus is ordinarily unaffected (unless the mother has been sensitized by a prior transfusion with Rh-positive blood), because the maternal antibody response is both delayed and of low magnitude. The risk increases, however, for subsequent Rh-positive fetuses, which restimulate the already sensitized mother to develop levels of antibody which, transferred via the placenta to the fetal circulation, are sufficient to cause significant destruction of fetal red cells. A converse example, decreasing risk with increase in birth order, is provided by congenital hypertrophic pyloric stenosis, which, for reasons not known, occurs most commonly among first-born infants.

Another aspect of birth order is the influence it has upon the age and the overall probability of acquiring infections that are transmitted by contact. Contact between family members is particularly close so that, when one member becomes infected, he typically shares it with those not already immune. As a corollary, the larger the family, the greater is the probability that one member will bring an infection home. Also, the higher the birth order (i.e., the younger the child), the greater is the probability of contracting an infection at an early age from an older sibling. The importance of such timing of infection depends on the relation that exists between age and the consequences of infection. At one extreme is the early intrauterine phase of fetal life when infection with rubella virus, acquired transplacentally from the mother, may lead to fetal death and abortion or to the development of serious congenital defects. In this case, the risk of maternal infection is increased by the presence of previously born children in the home. As pointed out in Chapter 5 and again in this chapter, the risk of serious consequences of infection often increases gradually with age, particularly after early childhood. This phenomenon is a special problem of only children who, lacking the assistance of siblings, may have their first intrafamilial exposure when their own children bring home infections with measles, mumps, or polioviruses acquired at nursery school or kindergarten.

Family size and, hence, both birth order and parental age also reflect reproductive patterns that are characteristic of social classes as defined by cultural or religious bases or economic status. The influence of these attributes or variables is considered in the following section. However, it may be noted that many forms of birth control are not sanctioned by the Roman Catholic Church and that, in the Western Hemisphere, frequency of reproduction varies inversely with economic status. Thus women in the lower economic stratum contribute disproportionately to births of higher orders and at younger maternal ages. Finally, it should be recognized that, within a sibship, family income, the social status of parents, and the standards of parental discipline may well shift as parental age and the size of the sibship increases.

9-7 Acquired Attributes of Persons

Important acquired personal attributes substantially outnumber those determined by or at birth. In Chapter 5 these were reviewed systematically to illustrate how they may influence disease occurrence. Although describing disease occurrence in relation to certain acquired attributes is administratively useful for guiding control activities or planning for medical services, it is most important as a first step in determining the extent to which a given attribute influences the occurrence of a particular disease. This determination is typically complicated by the fact that acquired attributes are not independent variables, a point that will be illustrated as we look at particular attributes. The few we will examine have been chosen because they illustrate the importance of acquired attributes to disease occurrence and because information about their prevalence in the general population is readily available, chiefly from the census data. It should be emphasized again, however, that prevalences of potentially important attributes not reported in census tabulations, such as specific immunities, elevated serum cholesterol, consumption of alcohol, or use of cigarettes, can be estimated from special surveys.

Marital status is a relatively independent variable routinely recorded in census records and on death certificates and readily ascertainable with respect to individual patients. It also is one of the attributes routinely recorded in the National Health Survey. However, published data relating marital status and disease prevalence from the Survey are limited. Observations from the 1960–1962 tabulations include: (1) less than expected oesteoarthritis among "never married" for both sexes; (2) rheumatoid arthritis was high for "never married" men, but less than expected for widowed men and "never married" women; (3) widowed or divorced men have less definite coronary heart disease than expected; and (4) complete freedom from any chronic condition, on an age-adjusted basis, was more common among "never married" (51 per cent) than "ever married" (40.5 per cent).

In view of the foregoing data it is surprising that age-adjusted mortality rates for all causes (Table 9-1) for both sexes and for each sex are lowest for married persons and, within each sex, highest for widowed and

TABLE 9-1

Age-adjusted* mortality rates by marital status for males and females aged twenty years or more, United States, 1960 (per 1,000 population)

MARITAL STATUS	BOTH SEXES	MALES	FEMALES
Single	17.55	23.17	12.61
Married	10.97	14.73	8.75
Widowed	16.76	28.11	14.70
Divorced	26.29	39.77	15.19
Total	14.24	17.62	11.27

*Rates are standardized to the age distribution of the total United States population aged twenty and over in 1960.

Source: Data from *Vital Statistics of the United States*, 1960.

divorced persons in that order. Most disease-specific mortality rates also are higher for single than married persons. Examples of particularly great differences, given as the ratio of 1949–1951 mortality rates for single persons to those for married persons, include respiratory tuberculosis (4.3 and 2.2, respectively, for males and females), all forms of cancer (1.3 and 2.6), influenza and pneumonia (2.7 and 1.9), and accidents (2.0 and 1.2) (National Office of Vital Statistics, 1956).

How marital status influences mortality is uncertain. The principal explanations advanced are: (1) persons with persistent illness are unlikely to marry; (2) adventurous persons who seek risks rather than avoiding them also are less likely to marry; and (3) unspecified differences in the living patterns of single and married persons influence the occurrence of some diseases. The most obvious of these differences relate to such marital functions as sexual intercourse and reproduction. These are currently advanced to explain, respectively, higher rates for cancer of the cervix and lower rates for breast cancer in married than in single women.

Finally, occurrence of a given disease in both husband and wife is a phenomenon of great potential interest. Excluding diseases resulting from known transmissible agents where concordance can be attributed to close contact, the excess occurrence of cancer and of such chronic illnesses as arthritis and hypertension among spouses of index persons similarly afflicted has been noted. Such evidence argues for causative factors either of heretofore unsuspected infectious nature or within the maritally shared environment.

Information as to *occupation* is regularly collected for the census, the National Health Survey, death certificates, and many other useful records. Because of its close association with such attributes as level of education, family income, and social standing, occupation is often used as an index of social class, especially by the British. Occupation also relates to the working environment within which more or less specific influences on health may operate. A number of classical examples of specific occupational hazards, as well as occupational associations with particular racial or ethnic groups, were described in Chapters 5 and 6. Differences in disease occurrence between occupational groups are still being studied actively in the hope of identifying additional environmental causes of disease. Hueper, for example, has shown significant association between lung cancer and occupations entailing exposure to motor exhaust fumes (7). Of special interest is evidence suggesting that sedentary occupations are associated with increased risk of coronary heart disease. An early example was the observation by Morris and coworkers (8) that drivers of London buses had a higher risk than the very active conductors of the buses. Pointing in the same direction are 1960–1962 National Health Survey data which show that the prevalence of CHD among workers in agriculture, forestry, and fisheries (1.9 per cent) is markedly less than that expected if disease occurs equally in all occupational groups (4.2 per cent), whereas for the wholesale and retail trade the situation is reversed (4.5 per cent versus 2.9 per cent).

Socioeconomic status represents a complex of attributes which includes the intangible attribute of "social standing" and the more readily definable attributes of level of education (expressed in terms of years of school completed) and income (usually family income). Information for both of these is collected during the census and in relation to the National Health Survey, but would have to be specially ascertained for individual patients and members of special study groups. Although education and income are closely associated, their separate use does not always result in description of similar disease patterns. In the case of periodontal disease, NHS data for 1960–1962 show parallel inverse correlations between prevalence of disease and both income and level of education. However, lack of parallelism was true of CHD. Lower than expected CHD prevalence was observed in the lowest stratum as measured by education (under five years of schooling), and in the highest stratum as measured by income (at least $10,000 per year).

Another indicator sometimes used in the United States is based on area of residence as classified by median income or other criteria. This information is available from census data by census tract. Its usefulness is restricted to tracts of fairly homogeneous character. In studies in New Haven, Connecticut it was shown that prevalence of immunity to measles on admission to first grade varied inversely with class of neighborhood (9). Neighborhoods also can be classified by measures reflecting housing standards such as average number of persons per room or type and abundance of sanitary plumbing.

However, the single attribute which perhaps most closely reflects socioeconomic status is occupation, on the basis of which the British have defined five broad classes. Such a classification is directly applicable to males in the ages of employment and can be extended to cover their dependants. An interesting application of this classification involves mortality due to cirrhosis of liver in which apparently contradictory observations were made in Britain (Table 9-2) and the United States (Table 9-3) (10.) Standardized mortality ratios (SMR) significantly higher

TABLE 9-2

Standardized mortality ratios, cirrhosis of the liver, men age twenty to sixty-four years by social class, England and Wales, 1949–1953

SOCIAL CLASS		STANDARDIZED MORTALITY RATIO
I.	Professional occupations	207
II.	Intermediate occupations	152
III.	Skilled occupations	84
IV.	Partly skilled occupations	70
V.	Unskilled occupations	96

Source: Terris, Milton. Epidemiology of cirrhosis of the liver. National mortality data. *Amer. J. Public Health* **47**: 2076–2088, 1967.

TABLE 9-3

Standardized mortality ratios, cirrhosis of the liver, men age twenty to sixty-four years, by occupation level, United States, 1950

OCCUPATIONAL LEVEL		STANDARDIZED MORTALITY RATIO		
		TOTAL	WHITE	NONWHITE
I.	Professional workers	90	—	—
II.	Technical, administrative, and managerial workers, except farm	88	88	—
III.	Clerical, sales, skilled workers	105*	107*	54
IV.	Semiskilled workers	118*	122*	85
V.	Laborers, except farm	148	158*	121
	Agricultural workers	51	51	54

*Standardized mortality ratio significantly higher than 100.
Source: 1. U.S. Dept. of Health, Education and Welfare. Mortality by occupational level and cause of death, U.S., 1950. Vital Statistics Special Reports, **53**:5, September 1963. 2. Terris, Milton. Epidemiology of cirrhosis of the liver, National mortality data. *Amer. J. Public Health* **47**: 2076–2088, 1967.

than 100* were observed in classes I and II in Britain, but in classes III, IV, and V in the United States. These data were used to support the hypothesis that consumption of distilled spirits and wine, rather than beer and ale, is a major determinant of liver cirrhosis. In Britain the high cost of whiskey and gin virtually restricts the lower classes to beer, whereas, in the United States, the wage-price balance is such that the form of consumption of alcohol is governed more by personal preference and social attitude.

9-8   Summary

"Disease" is a state of evident disturbance of normal function. Because of the common relation between specific cause and clinical effect, descriptions of disease occurrence based on clinical features help define human contact with specific disease agents. Such descriptions are in terms of who is attacked (person), where (place), and when (time).

Variation of disease among persons is described in terms of many attributes, some determined at birth (e.g., age, sex, genetic makeup, birth order) and many more acquired later (e.g., immunities, behavior, aspects of social class, and economic status). Nearly any attribute of an individual (patient) can be readily ascertained. However, the prevalence of an attribute in the population must be estimated from special surveys, unless it is a matter of record (e.g., included in census information). Although ready availability of prevalence data enhances the usefulness of an attribute, its importance depends on how strongly it is associated with disease and on its degree of independence of other attributes. The common interdependence of attributes requires that, when the influence of an attribute is being evaluated, the influence of possibly correlated attributes be taken into account.

The personal attribute most widely and strongly correlated with disease is age. Hence, differences in age composition must be taken into account before populations defined by other attributes can be meaningfully compared. Age influences disease by its relation to susceptibility and exposure. The age pattern of disease is described in terms of incidence, prevalence, or mortality rates calculated for sequential age groups in the population (age-specific rates). The resulting age profile for acute diseases reflects the age-related operation of the underlying causes, unless occurrence of disease following contact with the agent (e.g., infection) varies markedly with age. For degenerative diseases the age profile (occurrence typically increasing with age) less clearly reflects the parallel activity of causes,

---

*SMR of 100 means that the observed deaths in a group equalled exactly those expected when the age- and sex-specific rates in the general population were applied to the group (discussed in Chap. 7).

but differences in corresponding age-specific rates between populations living under different circumstances suggests the influence of environmental factors.

The relation of sex to disease occurrence is best described in terms of age- and sex-specific rates. However, males and females under age twenty are present in nearly equal numbers and the sex ratio (of cases in males to those in females) is useful. Annual death rates for males average one and a half times those for females, a fact which emphasizes the major relation of sex to disease. This relation does not hold for all diseases and, for some diseases, has changed with time, presumably because of changes in environmental influences. The relative extent to which basic biologic differences and differences in life experience (environment) contribute to sex-related differences in disease is known for few, if any, diseases.

Genetic makeup is determined by membership in families (kinships) and in racial or ethnic groups. When important differences deriving from environment can be adequately taken into account, differences between kinships or ethnic groups in disease occurrence can be attributed to genetic influences. Conversely, when groups similar genetically differ in place of residence (e.g., Japanese in Japan and in the United States), differences in disease experience must reflect environmental factors.

Parental age, birth order, and family size are attributes determined at or by birth and are matters of record (birth registration, census). They are closely interrelated and greatly influenced by religion or culture, social class, and economic status. Description of disease in relation to these attributes is important to understanding of both biologic mechanisms and the influence of the associated socioeconomic factors.

Description of disease in relation to the many personal attributes acquired after birth is useful both administratively (e.g., in planning for medical care) and in estimating the influence of individual attributes on disease occurrence. Examples of important acquired attributes include marital status (married persons live longer than single persons); occupation (related to social class, economic status, and specific hazards in the working environment); and the many facets of socioeconomic status (level of education, income, type of neighborhood, and social class) that are significantly related to many diseases.

GLOSSARY

Arthritis (rheumatoid arthritis, oesteoarthritis) Inflammation of joints (involving joint tissues, or bony structures).

Aseptic meningitis Nonbacterial (usually viral) inflammation of the meninges (the covering layer of the brain and spinal cord).

Cirrhosis of the liver Disease associated with great increase of fibrous tissue throughout the liver (usually following acute destruction of liver cells).

Clinical syndrome   Combination of symptoms and physical signs which accompany disease.

Hypertension (essential hypertension)   High blood pressure (without preceding other disease).

Monozygotic (dizygotic)   As applied to twins, from a single ovum (from two ova).

Myocarditis   Inflammatory disease of the heart muscle (myocardium).

Periodontal (disease)   Of the bony and soft tissues surrounding the teeth.

Reproductive pattern   Described in terms of parental age and spacing and total number of children.

Rhinovirus   From *rhino*, meaning nose; large group of viruses antigenically distinct (over 60 serotypes) but similar in small size, chemistry (RNA), and ability to cause common colds (coryza) in man.

REFERENCES

1. Poliomyelitis Annual Statistical Review. New York: The National Foundation, 1958.
2. Wilcox, W. F., ed. *Natural and Political Observations Made upon the Bills of Mortality by John Graunt* (a reprint of the first edition, 1662). Baltimore: Johns Hopkins Press, 1937.
3. Kallman, F. J., and Reisner, D. Twin studies on the significance of genetic factors in tuberculosis. *Amer. Rev. Tuberc.* **47**:549–574, 1943.
4. Francis, Thomas Jr., and Epstein, Frederick. Studies of a Total Community, Tecumseh, Michigan, in *Comparability in International Epidemiology*. Roy M. Acheson, ed. New York: Milbank Memorial Fund, 1965, pp. 333–342.
5. Haenszel, William, and Kurihara, Minoru. Studies of Japanese migrants. 1. Mortality from cancer and other diseases among Japanese in the United States. *J. Nat. Cancer Inst.* **40**:43–68, 1968.
6. MacMahon, Bryan, Pugh, T. F., and Ipsen, J. *Epidemiologic Methods*. Boston: Little, Brown, 1960, pp. 187–209.
7. Hueper, W. C. Environmental causes of cancer of the lung other than tobacco smoke. *Dis. Chest* **30**:1–19, 1956.
8. Morris, J. N., Heady, J. A., Raffle, P. A. B., Roberts, C. G., and Parks, J. W. Coronary heart-disease and physical activity of work. *Lancet* **2**:1053–1057, 1111–1120, 1953.
9. Black, Francis L., and Davis, Dorothy E. M. Measles and readiness for reading and learning. II. New Haven study. *Amer. J. Epidem.* **88**:337–344, 1968.
10. Terris, Milton. Epidemiology of cirrhosis of the liver. National mortality data. *Amer. J. Public Health* **57**:2076–2088, 1967.

10

Patterns of Disease Occurrence—Place

10-1 General Implications of Place

Place is a geographic concept described technically in terms of latitude, longitude, and altitude relative to sea level. It is visualized with the aid of maps which may vary greatly in scale, for example, from the global view of an orbiting astronaut to the most local view of the pilot of a low-flying helicopter who identifies individual dwellings in a city block. Epidemiologically, place is of interest to the extent that it is occupied by man. In the discussion that follows, unless specifically indicated as referring to work, recreation, or travel, "place" is assumed to mean location of residence.

Place thus is the basis for describing the spatial distributions of populations and diseases, commonly in terms of hemisphere, region, nation, or smaller political subunits. Places also can be usefully classified by a variety of environmental characteristics. These include climate, geologic and other physical features, type of vegetation and fauna, level and type of economic development, such aspects of population as race or ethnic group, density, and, most commonly, urban or rural nature. However place is classified, variations in disease occurrence with place reflect parallel variations in the operation of causative factors.

Observation of disease variation with place raises an important general question. Are the operating causative factors to be found in the characteristics of the physical and biologic environment inherent to place or in characteristics of the inhabitants? True association with place is suggested when age-adjusted risk of disease increases for immigrants and decreases for emigrants, when all ethnic groups present are at similar

209

high risk and when similar ethnic groups residing elsewhere are at lower risk. Finally, one should remember that spurious associations of disease with place may be the product of differences in the reliability and completeness of disease recognition and reporting.

10-2   Variations Between Regions and Nations

Comparability of data   On the global scale, the official sources of information concerning disease occurrence are the statistics collected routinely within nations for morbidity from notifiable (and notified) infectious diseases and for causes of death. These are gathered and published periodically by the World Health Organization (WHO) for many countries. Unfortunately, there are great variations between countries with respect to the quality, availability, and distribution of medical care which directly influence the reliability of diagnosis and the completeness of reporting and recording of diseases, births, and deaths. Europe (including Great Britain), New Zealand, Australia, Canada, and the United States are comparable in terms of basic demographic data, availability and quality of medical care, and vital statistics, so that both numbers (cases or deaths) and rates can be compared. In less developed countries, the available physicians and medical care facilities are concentrated in the cities, so that illness and death in the large rural populations typically are not medically attended. Although many unattended deaths are ultimately recorded, their causes usually remain unknown. Even in urban populations (the small upper class excepted) births are commonly attended by midwives (often untrained) and birth registration is so incomplete that many persons first appear in the population rolls on entry into school or military service. In this situation, infant mortality rates are particularly unreliable, since reporting is more complete for infant deaths than for births.

Usefulness of comparative data   Despite the limitations just emphasized, differences between countries in the recorded frequencies of disease remain of great interest, particularly in the case of many chronic diseases for which causation is at best incompletely elucidated. Age-adjusted death rates for coronary heart disease are highest in the United States and unusually low in Italy, Spain, Portugal, and Japan. The last-named country, peculiarly, records exceptionally high frequencies of hypertension and cerebrovascular accidents. Differences of this sort have prompted international studies aimed at both verifying the fact of difference and seeking explanations which might incriminate specific environmental factors (especially, dietary) as causative. To exclude the possible effect of genetic influences related to ethnic group, some investigators have made comparative studies of corresponding emigrant populations (and their progeny) residing in the United States. An example of this type of study, related to gastric cancer among Japanese, was cited in Chapter 9. Similar studies with respect to CHD, hypertension, and cerebrovascular disease in Japan and in United States residents of Japanese stock also are being conducted. As with gastric cancer, the pattern of occurrence of these diseases among Japanese in the United States (mainland and Hawaii) apparently is shifting in the direction of the overall United States patterns, thus supporting the existence of causative factors among the environmental characteristics inherent in place. (See Ref. 5, Chap. 9)

With infectious and parasitic diseases, comparisons of disease frequency are less important than qualitative knowledge of disease distribution and spread which guides the application and enforcement of international quarantine and control measures. With such important diseases as smallpox, bubonic plague, cholera, and yellow fever, a few sporadic cases in rural areas could easily escape notice, but substantial numbers of cases will almost certainly come to attention because of their high fatality and characteristic clinical pictures. However, even when information exists that a disease such as cholera is occurring within a nation, this knowledge may not be made generally or promptly available. Communist China, for example, does not belong to or release figures to the WHO, and some countries, hopeful that a new disease outbreak will be soon controlled, may withhold information which might discourage tourists upon whom they are economically dependent.

Hazards of foreign travel   Knowledge of geographic distribution and variation in the risk of important infectious and parasitic diseases has become of great practical importance in this era of extensive international travel and, in the case of the United States, worldwide deployment of military forces and Peace Corps volunteers. The usual tourist or civilian business traveler typically limits his visits to larger population centers and popular tourist attractions such as the Egyptian pyramids, the Taj Mahal, or the Inca ruins at Machu Picchu in Peru. For him, application of this knowledge takes the form of immunoprophylaxis (vaccinia, typhoid, cholera, yellow fever, polio, and typhus vaccines and gamma globulin for infectious hepatitis), a supply of medicines (chloroquin for malaria prophylaxis, kaopectate and paregoric for diarrhea, halogen tablets to put in drinking water), and advice about food such as "consume only what has been cooked or peeled." The specific combinations of the above are tailored to combat the known hazards in the regions to be visited. For military troops, Peace Corps workers, and others whose activities will take them off beaten paths and into more intimate contact with the people and the biological environment, supplementary measures usually are indicated. For areas such as southeast Asia (especially Thailand and Viet Nam), India, and Andean South America where rabies is highly prevalent among the abundant stray dog population, a primary course of duck embryo rabies vaccine may be added to the immunization regimen. For regions where scrub typhus exists (including all of southeast Asia), chemically impregnated clothing is issued to troops to protect them against the mite vector.

As a note of caution, the recognized occurrence of disease among indigenous populations does not always provide an adequate measure of the risk for a newcomer. In West Africa the risk of fatal yellow fever is much greater for Caucasians, who usually arrive as adults, than for indigenous Negroes. Prior immunity to antigenically related dengue virus which also is endemic, or young age at the time of yellow fever infection are believed responsible for the usually milder course of this disease in Africans. In Ceylon scrub typhus undoubtedly has been occurring in sporadic fashion among field workers for many years, but its presence was not recognized until World War II when contingents of troops from Africa underwent field training in division strength and over 700 cases occurred in a brief time (1). Finally, both poliomyelitis and infectious hepatitis viruses cause infrequent typical disease in the indigenous populations of underdeveloped areas, presumably because nearly everyone becomes infected at a very early age when most infections remain silent. However, the viruses are sufficiently abundant in the environment that newcomers from temperate zones, including troops and tourists, incur great risk.

Global patterns of distribution and spread   Whereas information about worldwide distribution of disease derives from national sources, disease occurrence is less influenced by political boundaries than by important geographically determined environmental factors (climate, altitude, flora and fauna, and so on). Hence, for depicting the global distribution of a particular disease it is useful to divide the world into regions defined on the basis of the presence of those factors known (or believed) important to disease occurrence. Figure 10-1 portrays the worldwide distribution, during World War II, of two clinically similar diseases, epidemic and murine typhus, the rickettsial agents of which are closely related antigenically but depend on very different transmission and reservoir mechanisms (2). *R. prowazekii* (epidemic typhus) infects only man and the human body louse which lives and propagates only in clothing worn for long periods without laundering. Louse infestation is engendered by a combination of cool climate and poverty (found in underdeveloped temperate zone areas or at higher altitudes in the tropics and subtropics) or culture (Arabs of North Africa and the Middle East). Murine typhus requires domestic rats and the rat flea, *Xenopsylla cheopis*, which needs a warm climate to achieve real abundance. Despite these different climatic requirements, some overlap is seen in the distribution of these two diseases, notably in mainland China, North Africa, and Mexico. Similar maps have been or could be prepared for many other diseases. In the case of

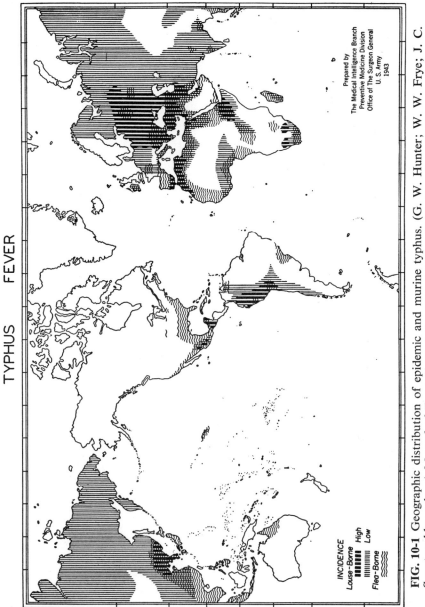

TYPHUS FEVER

INCIDENCE
Louse-Borne
High
Low
Flea-Borne

Prepared by
The Medical Intelligence Branch
Preventive Medicine Division
Office of The Surgeon General
U. S. Army
1943

FIG. 10-1 Geographic distribution of epidemic and murine typhus. (G. W. Hunter; W. W. Frye; J. C. Swartzwelder, eds. *A Manual of Tropical Medicine.* Philadelphia: W. B. Saunders, 1960.)

213

malaria and smallpox, WHO-supported programs for worldwide control
or eradication are guided by such maps of distribution.

The global patterns of spread of major epidemic diseases also are
important. In the pre-Pasteur era, John Snow noted that cholera spread
only along routes of human travel and with a speed not exceeding that
of the mode of transport employed. He used this fact to support his then
radical concept that cholera was communicable from man to man rather
than generated by local miasmas. Today, cholera still erupts periodically
from its endemic reservoirs in Indonesia and India (3) and its spread is charted
(see Figure 10-2 which depicts the situation in 1967) on regional maps

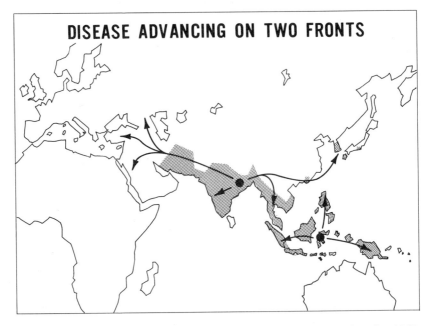

FIG. 10-2 Spread of cholera from endemic reservoirs. Situation in 1967.
(Cholera flare-up poses new threat. *Med. World News* **8**: 1967.) Reprinted with
permission of *Medical World News*.

so that populations lying in the paths of spread may be forewarned.
Because of its fecal-oral mechanism of spread, cholera is a threat only
in countries where sanitary control of the environment is deficient.

A different situation prevails for infections depending on airborne transmission to the respiratory portal. Even the most highly developed nations
remain vulnerable to such agents unless their populations are effectively
immune. For many diseases so transmitted, including diphtheria, pertussis, measles, and mumps, natural occurrence of infection or widespread
childhood immunization has maintained adequate herd immunity in all
but the most isolated populations. Because smallpox is both highly

infectious and frequently fatal, there is constant concern about its spread, especially in Britain where vaccination is no longer mandatory. This concern is reflected in the uniform requirement of a valid smallpox vaccination certificate for all international travelers. Fortunately, the availability of effective vaccine makes it possible to localize rapidly the inevitable but sporadic importations of the disease into the vast regions where it is no longer endemic.

Influenza remains one disease with the potential for causing worldwide epidemics (or pandemics) for which fully effective methods of control remain to be developed. Its potential for both a very high attack rate and significant case fatality rate was indelibly recorded in the 1918–1919 pandemic. Influenza viruses of three antigenically unrelated types, A, B, and C, are widely distributed throughout the world. Because they are nearly as infectious as measles, primary infection occurs typically early in life and the population thereafter possesses immunity. However, as described in Chapter 4, influenza viruses A and B undergo progressive changes in antigenic character and so are able to reinfect and cause disease in persons immune to the previously prevalent virus strains. When and where new mutants arise are unpredictable but, wherever they occur, they usually succeed in spreading throughout the world. This is particularly true when, after a major change, the entire population of the world constitutes a virgin soil for the mutant strain. The 1918–1919 pandemic undoubtedly resulted from such a major change, but the 1957 pandemic of Asian influenza is the first such episode fully documented. The pattern of spread proceeding around the world in both directions from a source in mainland China, is shown in Figure 10-3 (4). In contrast to the 1918–1919 episode, the 1957 pandemic covered the globe within little more than six months, no doubt greatly assisted by air travel. Influenza vaccine can be made, but, to be reasonably effective, it must contain virus antigenically close to the prevalent strain. For this reason, WHO supports regional laboratories throughout the world which receive isolates from current cases and characterize them antigenically. This constant surveillance makes it possible to recognize new mutant strains, to chart their spread, and to distribute prototype material for vaccine production in regions not yet affected.*

Spread of disease along paths of human travel does not always indicate that man is directly involved in transporting the agent. Livestock and household pets move along the same paths and may carry zoonotic agents that can affect man. In recognition of this fact, countries such as England and Australia which are free of rabies forbid importation of dogs and

*In Hong Kong in August 1968 a strain of influenza A virus was recovered which represents another major mutant and provided the first real test of the value of the WHO surveillance effort. In this instance, monovalent vaccine containing the new strain was commercially available by December, 1968 in the United States.

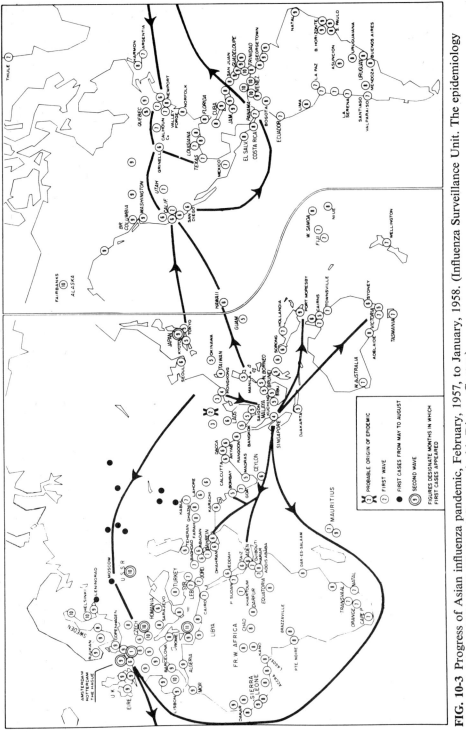

FIG. 10-3 Progress of Asian influenza pandemic, February, 1957, to January, 1958. (Influenza Surveillance Unit. The epidemiology of Asian influenza 1957–1960. National Communicable Disease Center.)

cats unless they have been held in quarantine for many months. Rats, together with their fleas, are notorious fellow travellers of man, especially on ships. Guards are routinely placed on mooring lines of newly arrived ships to prevent the disembarkation of rats and the possible introduction of bubonic plague. Also, arthropods harboring such agents as the viruses of yellow fever or Japanese B encephalitis may travel uninvited aboard transport vehicles. The periodic introduction of yellow fever into the port cities of Europe and the United States (see Figure 10-4) in the nineteenth century is recognized, in retrospect, as an example of this phenomenon (5). Presumably because the danger has been long recognized and precautionary measures strictly enforced, no modern examples of disease spread by this means can be cited.

10-3   Variations Within Nations

Reliability and availability of data   Death records and the reports of notifiable diseases remain the usual sources for data concerning the distribution of diseases within nations. Within the more highly developed nations, comparisons may be made with little concern about variation in standards of medical care and reliability and completeness of reporting. Variations in ethnic composition and cultural aspects of the population and in the important environmental characteristics inherent in place are less within than between nations. Finally, the political subunits for which health statistics are available often are small enough to be homogeneous with respect to some environmental and population variables and yet contain sufficient population to permit reasonable estimates of disease frequencies.

The United States is a country of sufficient size that variation in environmental factors inherent in place is still substantial. The sources of health information have been described in Chapter 7. Very briefly, basic demographic data are provided by a decennial census, and annual tabulations of deaths by cause and by age, sex, race and residence are published. Incidence figures for notifiable diseases are similarly available and, from the National Health Survey, information concerning many other types of illness can be obtained. In addition, the National Center for Health Statistics publishes periodic summaries of disease-specific mortality rates for various segments of the population. Not regularly available, however, are figures reflecting geographic variations in risk of disease adjusted to take account of the substantial variations with place in such population characteristics as age and race. Such adjustment is imperative when one is seeking to relate observed variation to place-determined aspects of the environment and when, as with many of the presumably noninfectious

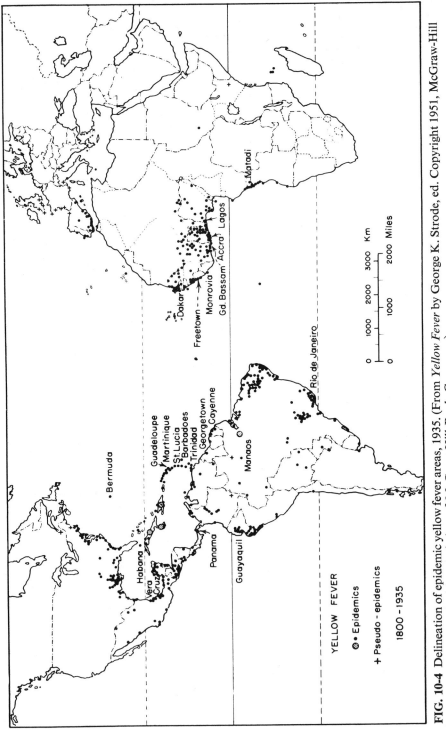

FIG. 10-4 Delineation of epidemic yellow fever areas, 1935. (From *Yellow Fever* by George K. Strode, ed. Copyright 1951, McGraw-Hill Book Company. Used with permission of McGraw-Hill Book Company.)

YELLOW FEVER

⊘● Epidemics

+ Pseudo - epidemics

1800 - 1935

diseases in particular, age and race are known to be strongly associated with disease occurrence.

Some patterns of disease occurrence Marked variations within the United States exist in the physical and biologic environment which, in turn, are reflected in major variations in the frequency of zoonotic diseases. Murine typhus has been restricted to the South Central and Southeastern states (see Figure 10-5), not because rats are absent elsewhere, but because the warm, humid climate insures an abundance of rat fleas (6). Scrutiny of the lower right corner of Figure 10-5, incidentally, indicates that complete

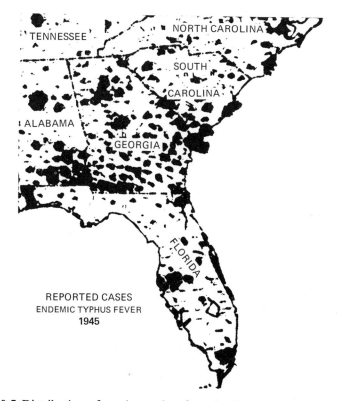

REPORTED CASES
ENDEMIC TYPHUS FEVER
1945

FIG. 10-5 Distribution of murine typhus fever in Southeastern corner of the United States, 1945.

confidence in the comparability of case finding and reporting within a country may be misplaced. Although the map suggests that the state line prevented typhus from spilling over into Florida from Georgia, special serologic surveys proved this distributional peculiarity to be an artifact. The rickettsiae of Rocky Mountain spotted fever (RMSF) depend on certain species of ticks and various small wild animals and are particularly abundant where the ecologic conditions favor these requisite hosts.

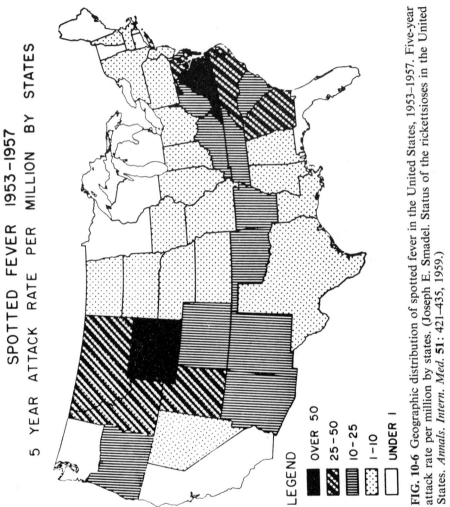

SPOTTED FEVER 1953–1957

5 YEAR ATTACK RATE PER MILLION BY STATES

LEGEND

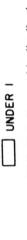

OVER 50
25–50
10–25
1–10
UNDER 1

FIG. 10-6 Geographic distribution of spotted fever in the United States, 1953–1957. Five-year attack rate per million by states. (Joseph E. Smadel. Status of the rickettsioses in the United States. *Annals. Intern. Med.* **51**: 421–435, 1959.)

Although RMSF has been recognized in man in most states, there are marked concentrations of cases in certain areas (Figure 10-6) determined by both underlying ecologic requirements and density of human population (6). Similar considerations also govern the overall distribution and the typically focal nature of outbreaks of arbovirus diseases such as St. Louis encephalitis and eastern and western equine encephalomyelitis.

Infections dependent entirely on man do not occur uniformly throughout the United States. To some extent, this is a matter of time. The great wave of rubella that peaked on the East Coast and in the Midwest in the spring of 1964 did not affect the West Coast until the following year. Also, the roughly three-year cycle of peaks in measles that is characteristic of larger metropolitan areas is not synchronized throughout the country, the peak year in each such area depending on the local buildup of susceptibles.

A more fundamental difference in long-term frequency of disease dependent on man is seen in infectious hepatitis and poliomyelitis. Lobel and McCollum (7) noted an inverse relation between population density and incidence rates for infectious hepatitis over the period 1954–1962. Average annual rates per 100,000 population were 12.8, 8.1, and 6.0, respectively, for states with population densities per square mile of under 10, 10–19, and 100 or over. In Figure 10-7 relative frequency of the disease by state is shown in three epidemiologic years, 1962–1965. These data suggest a regional variation not entirely dependent on population density in that relative sparing is seen in sparsely populated states such as Nevada, Texas, Nebraska, and Minnesota, whereas such populous states as California, New York, and Massachusetts and the island of Puerto Rico experienced high attack rates. With poliomyelitis, sharp contrasts have been noted (in the prevaccination era) between Southeastern states and Northern states, the latter experiencing more frequent and severe epidemics and higher average annual rates. Both hepatitis and poliomyelitis depend basically on fecal-oral transmission. Indirect transmission is favored by less adequate environmental sanitation (as has characterized the Southeastern states) and contact spread is favored by greater population density. As noted elsewhere, where spread of an infectious agent is facilitated, infection tends to occur at an earlier average age when, at least with polio and hepatitis, overt and serious disease is less apt to result.

One difficulty with using area maps to depict geographic variation in frequency of disease is that population density varies widely and the area of a state or other subdivision bears no direct relation to the size of the population at risk. It is possible, with some ingenuity, to develop demographic base maps in which area of administrative units is proportional to population and contiguity of geographical boundaries is reasonably maintained. Although such maps have been made for the United States, they have not often been used to depict variations in health status. Forster

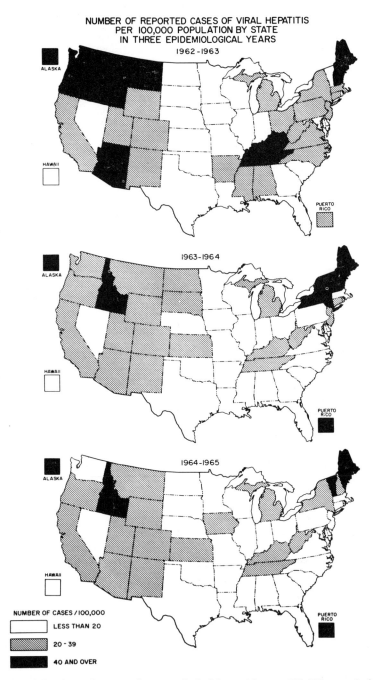

FIG. 10-7 Number of reported cases of viral hepatitis per 100,000 population by state in three epidemiological years. (Hepatitis Surveillance Unit. Hepatitis Surveillance Report No. 24. National Communicable Disease Center.)

(8) has used average mortality rates, 1959–1963, for all causes among
females, 45–54 years of age, in Scotland to illustrate this method. A basic
cartogram for the Public Health districts in Scotland was developed on
the basis of the 1961 census. Figures 10-8 and 10-9, respectively, show the
very marked variations between districts on a conventional map and on
the cartogram. From the latter it is clear that the highest rates apply to

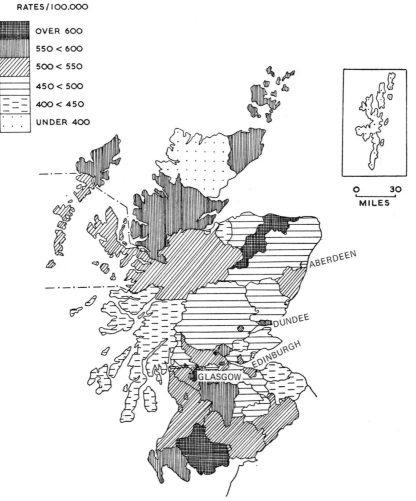

RATES / 100,000

OVER 600
550 < 600
500 < 550
450 < 500
400 < 450
UNDER 400

0   30
MILES

ABERDEEN
DUNDEE
EDINBURGH
GLASGOW

—Average mortality rates 1959–63, all causes of death. Females aged 45 to 54 years. (Conventional map).

FIG. 10-8 Average mortality rates 1959–1963, all causes of death in Scotland
by public health districts. Females aged 45 to 54 years. (Conventional map.)
F. Forster. Use of a demographic base map for the presentation of areal data in
epidemiology. *Brit. J. Prev. Soc. Med.* **20**:165–171, 1966.) Reprinted by permission of the author and editor.

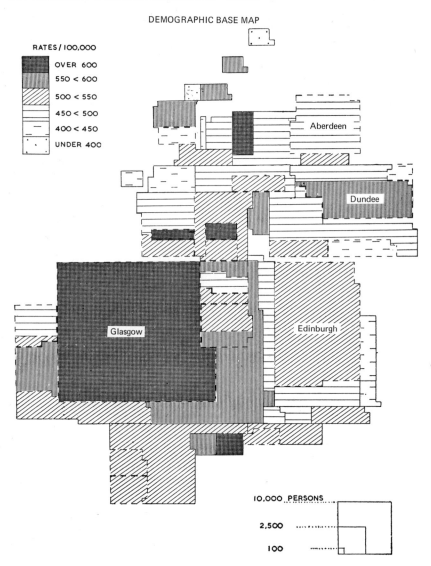

DEMOGRAPHIC BASE MAP

RATES / 100,000

OVER 600
550 < 600
500 < 550
450 < 500
400 < 450
UNDER 400

Aberdeen

Dundee

Glasgow

Edinburgh

10,000 PERSONS
2,500
100

FIG. 10-9 Average mortality rates 1959–1963, all causes of death in Scotland by public health districts. Females aged 45 to 54 years. (Cartogram.) F. Forster. Use of a demographic base map for the presentation of areal data in epidemiology. *Brit. J. Prev. Soc. Med.* **20**:165–171, 1966.) Reprinted by permission of the author and editor.

a much larger population than is suggested by the conventional map.

The marked geographic variation in age-specific mortality of Scottish women presumably reflects parallel variation in the chronic diseases that are the principal causes of death after age forty-five. Data for the United

States suggest that the frequency of many presumably noninfectious diseases varies geographically without relation to population age. One example is shown in Table 10-1 which presents age-specific death rates for congenital malformations for United States white children, 1945–1951, by region. For reasons not obvious but presumably place-associated, impressively low rates were produced by the Pacific and three southern groups of states. Death rates for selected chronic diseases and for all causes for the United States, 1959, are shown by region in Table 10-2. These data are not adjusted for age or for race, but the variation in death rates for all causes suggests that the age composition of the underlying populations varies substantially, the Southern, Mountain, and Pacific states having younger populations than the Northern states. Since the causes of death selected are strongly age-associated, it is not surprising to find that the cause-specific death rates for the Northern states, without exception, exceed the corresponding rates for the other states. However, some underlying effect of place is suggested in most instances by the much greater variation manifested by the cause-specific rates than by the rates for all causes. This is most evident for digestive cancers, diabetes mellitus, and arteriosclerotic heart disease. For the latter, significant differences persisted after age-adjustment of the 1950 death rates for white males; the highest were 360 and 330 per 100,000 for the Middle Atlantic and New England states, respectively, as compared with 250 for the West North Central, Mountain, and West South Central, and 220 for the East South Central states.

TABLE 10-1

Average death rates (per 100,000) for congenital malformations for United States white population by selected age groups and region, 1949–1951

REGION	UNDER 1 YEAR	1–4 YEARS
New England	503.4	12.0
Middle Atlantic	494.3	12.0
East North Central	511.3	12.0
West North Central	506.4	12.4
South Atlantic	455.8	11.5
East South Central	461.0	10.8
West South Central	431.1	10.8
Mountain	486.8	12.3
Pacific	409.0	11.3
United States	477.4	11.7

Source: Vital Statistics, *Special reports* **49** (56): Aug. 13, 1959.

TABLE 10-2

Death rates (per 100,000) for selected causes, United States, by region, 1959 (both sexes, all ages and races)

REGION	MALIGNANT NEOPLASMS					DIABETES MELLITUS (260)	ARTERIO-SCLEROTIC HEART DISEASE (420)	ALL CAUSES
	ALL (140–205)*	DIGESTIVE (150–156A, 157–159)	RESPIR-ATORY (160–164)	BREAST (170)	LEUKEMIA (204)			
New England	181.4	66.0	25.0	16.9	7.8	19.8	355.7	1070.6
Middle Atlantic	178.8	66.4	26.5	17.1	7.4	20.3	347.7	1048.5
East North Central	150.2	53.4	20.9	13.6	7.0	18.9	280.7	933.9
West North Central	155.0	54.6	19.8	13.4	8.4	16.6	284.7	988.5
South Atlantic	122.2	37.5	18.7	10.2	5.6	12.7	207.1	868.3
East South Central	123.0	38.6	16.5	9.2	6.4	12.7	202.3	917.6
West South Central	126.3	39.6	19.5	9.6	6.4	13.4	205.8	842.1
Mountain	109.7	37.4	14.2	9.1	6.4	10.8	193.2	809.0
Pacific	143.9	46.9	21.8	13.7	7.4	10.5	254.7	889.1
United States	147.4	50.7	21.2	13.1	7.0	15.9	268.8	939.1

*Numbers in parentheses indicate category of the Seventh Revision of the International Lists of Causes of Death, 1955.
Source: Vital Statistics, *Special reports* **54** (4): 1961.

10-4   Local Patterns of Disease Occurrence

In the United States, the smallest area for which demographic data are readily available is the census tract. Political units such as counties and cities may contain several to many census tracts, for each of which disease frequencies can be calculated if the numbers of cases warrant it. Thus, variation in disease risk within a community can be depicted in reasonable detail. Since census tracts often can be characterized in terms of median income level (or other index of socioeconomic status) and racial or ethnic group, variation between census tracts may reveal association of disease with these characteristics, as discussed earlier in this chapter.

Calculation of disease frequencies often is either not appropriate or not required for the immediate purpose to be served. In such instances, local distribution of disease is typically shown by spot maps. In the case of relatively rare diseases, such as leukemia or sudden deaths in infancy, cases occurring during one or even several years in any one census tract

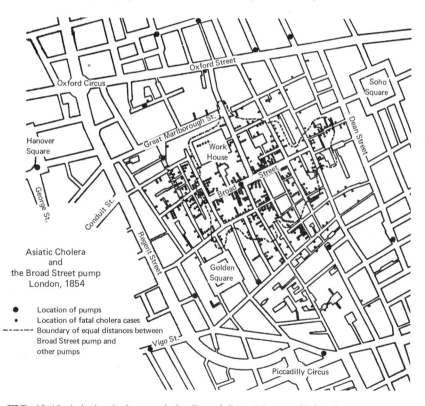

FIG. 10-10 Asiatic cholera and the Broad Street Pump. (John Snow. *Snow on Cholera.* New York: The Commonwealth Fund, 1936.)

may be so few that actual calculation of frequency would have little meaning. Nonetheless, visualization of their geographic distribution may be of great interest, particularly in that any tendency for clustering might suggest some common link such as an infectious agent or environmental factor. Interpretation of such distributions, however, requires knowledge of the distribution of the population within which the cases have occurred.

Spot maps are almost universally used in relation to outbreaks of acute disease. As the outbreak evolves, new pins may be placed in the map to mark the residences of newly reported cases (sometimes different colors are used for successive time intervals), so the geographic progression of the outbreak can be observed. Distribution of disease so visualized can greatly aid in investigations of the immediate cause. A classic example of spot mapping is the 1854 outbreak of cholera in the Golden Square

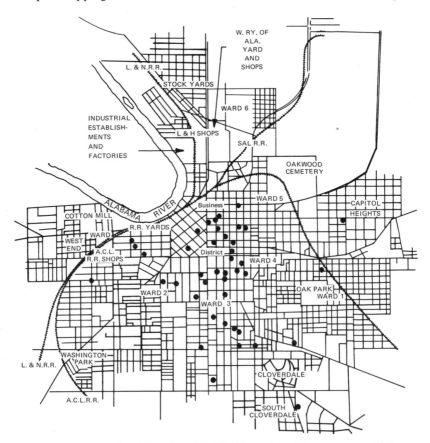

FIG. 10-11 Cases of mild typhus (Brill's disease) in Montgomery, Alabama, 1922–1925, spotted according to residence. (Kenneth F. Maxcy. An epidemiological study of endemic typhus (Brill's disease) in the Southeastern United States. *Public Health Rep.* **41**: 2967–2995, 1926.)

district of London (9). This was described by John Snow, who located each fatal case on a map, as shown in Figure 10-10. The concentration of cases about the pump on Broad Street focused his attention on this pump, which was convincingly incriminated as the source by Snow's rapid but carefully detailed further investigation. In similar fashion, distributions of disease conforming to portions of water distribution systems, to milk routes, or to areas served by a school or a local delicatessen may provide clues to common sources or vehicles of infection.

Place of residence, of course, is not always a guide to source of infection. In a classical study of murine typhus in Montgomery, Alabama, Maxcy (10) plotted cases by place of residence (Figure 10-11) and by place of work (Figure 10-12). The latter, showing concentration in relation to feed

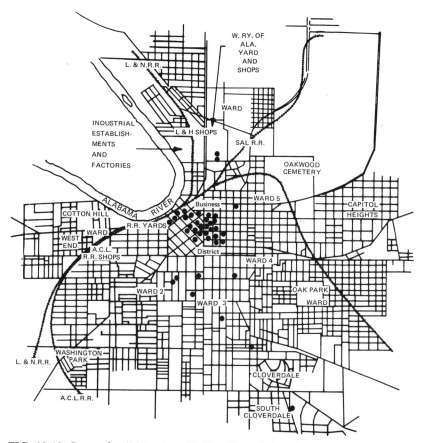

FIG. 10-12 Cases of mild typhus (Brill's disease) in Montgomery, Alabama, 1922–1925, spotted according to place of employment or, if unemployed, according to place of residence. (Kenneth F. Maxcy. An epidemiological study of endemic typhus (Brill's disease) in the Southeastern United States. *Public Health Rep.* **41**: 2967–2995, 1926.)

stores and food-handling establishments, all heavily rat infested, led Maxcy to studies which conclusively demonstrated the basic role of the rat and the rat flea in murine typhus.

Sometimes the pattern of disease distribution changes with time. This is illustrated in the case of poliomyelitis in Figure 10-13 which utilizes both the spot-map technique and census tract information in showing the distribution of disease in Kansas City, Missouri in three different epidemic years (11). More cases occurred in 1952 than in 1946, but in both these years the entire city was affected, including, especially in 1952, the upper-class section in the southwest part of the city. After 1955, Salk vaccine was widely offered but was more often accepted among the white population. The 1959 outbreak is notable for its sharp concentration in the portion of the city occupied by the less vaccinated Negro population.

Contact-transmitted diseases often begin in one small area and then spread. This is particularly easy to demonstrate with diseases of lower infectivity and relatively long incubation, such as infectious hepatitis. Albany County, New York, experienced a two-year epidemic in 1962 and 1963 of sufficient intensity that calculation of incidence rates was warranted. As shown in Figure 10-14, the epidemic began in lower-economic central Albany and slowly spread to involve all but one small segment (A) with annual incidence rates of 51 per 100,000 or higher (12).

10-5   Urban–Rural Differences

The usefulness of classifying places according to salient environmental characteristics has been discussed already and illustrated by the world-wide distribution of murine and epidemic typhus in relation to climatic factors. Another characteristic, useful in both international and within-country comparisons and independent of geographic contiguity, is urbanization. In the United States census the population is classified by residence as rural-farm, rural-nonfarm, and urban according to land use and population density. Further, in recognition of the pattern of population concentration in contiguous areas surrounding major cities, the Census Bureau as of 1960 had defined some 212 Standard Metropolitan Statistical Areas (SMSA) comprising county units containing or clustered about cities. Such SMSA counties contain about three fifths of the United States population and are predominantly urban in character. Areas so classified differ substantially with respect to many factors, including population density, water supply and waste disposal, level of industrialization, many aspects of the biologic environment, and bussing of school children. They also differ in respect to the occurrence of many diseases. Information as to cause-specific death rates and the prevalence and incidence of many

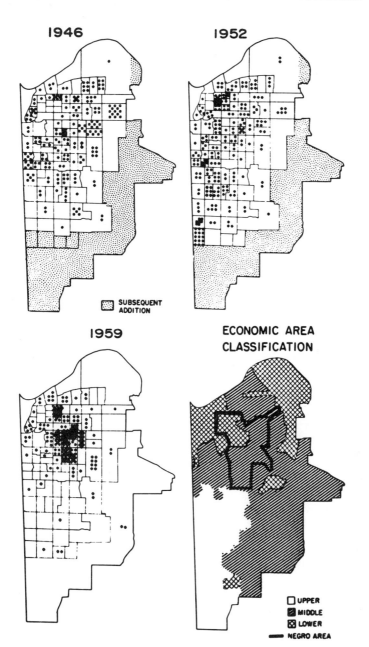

FIG. 10-13 Distribution of reported poliomyelitis cases, by census tract, Kansas City, Missouri, epidemic years 1946, 1952, and 1959. (Tom D. Y. Chin and William W. Marine. The changing patterns of poliomyelitis observed in two urban epidemics, Kansas City and Des Moines, 1959. *Public Health Rep.* **76**:553–563, 1961.)

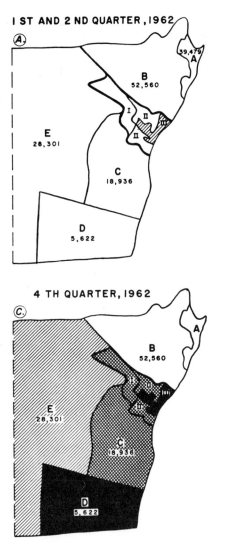
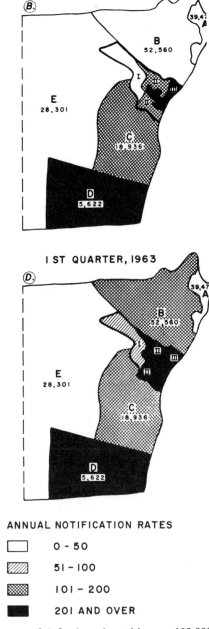

I, II, III :
SOCIO ECONOMIC LEVEL
OF CITY AREAS

A – E :
TOWNS AND COMBINATIONS
OF TOWNS, WITH POPULATION
OF ALBANY COUNTY, OUTSIDE
OF ALBANY CITY

ANNUAL NOTIFICATION RATES

☐   0 – 50

▨   51 – 100

▧   101 – 200

■   201 AND OVER

FIG. 10-14 Reported annual number of cases of infectious hepatitis per 100,000 population in successive periods of 1962 and 1963, Albany County, New York. (Hans O. Lobel and Roger F. Robison. Epidemiologic aspects of an outbreak of infectious hepatitis in Albany, N.Y. *Amer. J. Public Health* **55**:1176–1182, 1965.)

disease conditions by SMSA and nonmetropolitan counties and by urban or rural residence is available in many publications of the National Center for Health Statistics. However, interpretation of any differences requires that full account be taken of the differences in age and racial composition of the urban and rural populations.

Historically, cities were notoriously unhealthy places, largely because population density made them particularly vulnerable to the great epidemic diseases such as cholera, yellow fever, and smallpox and to tuberculosis, all of which were major causes of death. As a result death rates typically exceeded birth rates and cities grew only because of a continuing influx of persons from the surrounding countryside. In New Orleans, deaths exceeded births as recently as 1900. The belief persists to this day that country living is healthier than urban living, but the difference, if any, is hard to measure, at least in terms of death rates. For 1960 crude United States death rates (per 1,000 population) were 9.5 overall, 10.3 for urban areas, and 8.4 for rural areas. However, for the SMSA counties the average death rate was 9.3 as compared with 10.0 for the nonmetropolitan counties. Comparison of age-specific death rates in Table 10-3 suggests that, as measured by death rates, the urban or metropolitan counties are healthier only for persons under forty-five and over eighty-five years of age. The moral, perhaps, is to move to the country at age forty-five.

Popular opinion would concur that the least healthy area in the country

TABLE 10-3
Age-specific death rates (all causes) for metropolitan and nonmetropolitan counties, United States, 1960

Age (years)	Metropolitan Counties	Nonmetropolitan Counties
Under 1	26.0	28.7
1–4	1.0	1.3
5–14	0.4	0.5
15–24	0.9	1.3
25–34	1.4	1.6
35–44	3.0	3.1
45–54	7.8	7.1
55–64	18.0	16.3
65–74	39.6	36.0
75–84	89.0	85.3
85+	196.0	200.7
All	9.3	10.0

Source: Vital Statistics of the United States, 1960.

would be the largest SMSA, New York City, the crude death rate for which (10.45) does exceed that for the United States as a whole. However, the New York SMSA contains a slightly larger proportion of nonwhites (12 per cent versus 11.4 per cent) for whom the United States age-adjusted death rates (using the United States 1940 population as the standard) was 10.4 as compared with 7.3 for whites. The New York SMSA population also is somewhat older than the United States average. After adjustment for differences in age and race composition, the death rate for the New York SMSA turns out to be 9.9, only slightly greater than that (9.5) for the United States as a whole.

Population density, level of sanitation, and biological environment are the major aspects of difference between urban and rural residence that influence the occurrence of infectious and parasitic diseases. Diseases transmitted from animal to man, including those involving arthropod vectors, are more frequent in rural areas or the suburban outskirts of cities. St. Louis encephalitis, spread by culex mosquitos from avian sources, illustrates particularly well the vulnerability of the semirural suburbs with substantial population density. In the original 1933 outbreak the attack rate was 252 per 100,000 population in St. Louis County as compared with 66 in the city of St. Louis (13). This pattern has been repeated in many subsequent outbreaks. Hookworm, acquired by walking barefoot on soil contaminated with human feces, is a special problem of rural Southeastern United States (fortunately decreasing as rural sanitation has improved).

Infections spread by contact or by airborne droplets flourish in direct proportion to population density. As a result, they are acquired by rural residents later in life (if at all) than by city dwellers. As one consequence of this, military recruit camps notoriously entertain epidemics of measles and other childhood diseases which spread among recruits from rural areas. For infections that are more often inapparent when acquired early in life, rural populations are at a particular disadvantage. Earlier in this chapter, attention was called to the inverse relation between population density of states and the average annual attack rate for infectious hepatitis. As seen in Figure 10-15 which shows annual attack rates for New York State from 1954 to 1963, rural populations are especially affected during epidemic periods (7).

Conditions not obviously resulting from infectious causes also differ in frequency between urban and rural populations. Largely because of farm situations, accidents of all types are somewhat more frequent among rural residents. However, such factors as stress of living, reduced opportunity for physical activity, and air polluted by industry or automobiles weigh measurably against the city dweller. Haenszel and Shimken (14) showed that age-adjusted rates for lung cancer were nearly twice as high among urban as among rural males. A similar relation prevails for deaths

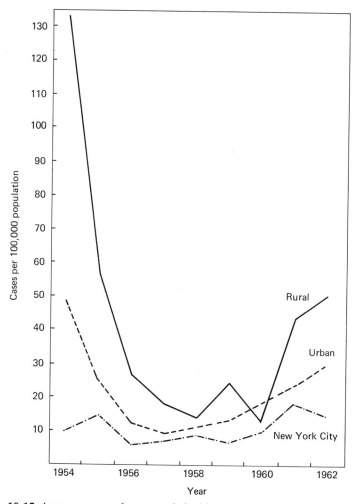

FIG. 10-15 Average annual reported incidence of infectious hepatitis per 100,000 population in New York City and in rural and urban counties of up-state New York, 1954–1962. (Hans O. Lobel and R. W. McCollum. *Bull. WHO* **32**:675–682, 1965.)

attributed to cirrhosis of the liver, presumably reflecting the greater urban prevalence of alcoholism. Finally, age-adjusted death rates for arterio-sclerotic heart disease are 20 per cent higher for urban residents of SMSA counties than for nonmetropolitan counties. However, in the case of the largest United States city, New York, 1960 age-adjusted death rates for CHD for both whites and nonwhites are lower than the corresponding United States race-specific rates, although only slightly lower in the case of whites.

10-6   Summary

Place as a geographic concept is useful in describing spatial distributions of people and disease. Places also are classified by characteristics of physical and biologic environment and of human inhabitants. When disease varies with place, it reflects the operation of factors either inherent in place environment or relating to the populations.

Because of differences in completeness and reliability of information, data concerning disease occurrence vary greatly in quality between nations. Nonetheless, comparative studies of chronic diseases offer much promise for elucidating important environmental causes. For serious acute diseases such as smallpox or cholera simple qualitative information as to distribution and spread suffice to guide international control measures. Such information also is important to foreign travelers and, particularly, military and other personnel whose activities result in maximum contact with foreign environments. Some disease agents, for example, polio and hepatitis viruses, are widely prevalent without causing much overt disease in indigenous populations.

Global patterns of zoonoses are determined largely by physical and biologic features of the environment. Patterns for diseases resulting from infectious agents restricted to man depend on population density (airborne transmission) or on environmental sanitation (fecal-oral transmission). For the former, the immunity in populations is the major factor restricting spread. Global and regional maps of disease distribution and spread, coupled with knowledge concerning aspects of the environment and populations, contribute to understanding of disease occurrence and are vital to international control activities. Spread along routes of human travel is consisent with human carriage of agents, but also occurs when infected animals or arthropods travel with man.

Within nations, disease may vary with place and comparisons are less affected by variation in completeness and reliability of data (death records, birth registrations, reports of notifiable diseases). In the United States such information is supplemented by special information collected by the National Health Survey. Differences in physical and biologic environment and in population characteristics are still great enough to influence the occurrence of both zoonoses and purely human infectious diseases. Some chronic and noninfectious diseases show greater variation related to region than can be explained by differences in age and racial composition of the populations. Demographic base maps (area proportional to population) provide a device for visualizing both geographic variations in disease frequency and the size of the affected populations.

Locally, demographic data are usually available for small political units or, in the United States, for census tracts. Because of their socioeconomic homogeneity, census tracts are useful in revealing disease associations with socioeconomic variables. Local distributions of disease are often depicted with spot maps to reveal clustering, patterns of spread, and changes of distribution over extended periods of time.

The most important example of classifying place by environmental characteristics is in relation to urban and rural residence. In the United States, such classification is supplemented by defining larger Standard Metropolitan Statistical Areas about major cities for which special tabulations are available. Analysis of mortality data indicates that rural living is, overall, no longer much healthier than urban living. However, the distribution of diseases by residence reveals important differences in risk of specific diseases related to urban or rural living.

GLOSSARY

Congenital malformation Defect occurring during embryonal or fetal development.

Quarantine Measures to prevent contact between persons suspected of being infected (because of known or suspected exposure) and unexposed persons, e.g., detention of ships or passengers coming from ports where a feared disease is prevalent.

Vaccinia Pox virus used as live virus vaccine against smallpox (commonly thought to have originated from cowpox as described by Jenner).

REFERENCES

1. Maxcy, Kenneth F. Scrub Typhus (Tsutsugamushi Disease) in the U.S. Army during World War II, in *Rickettsial Diseases of Man*. Forest R. Moulton, ed. Washington, D.C.: American Association for the Advancement of Science, 1948, pp. 36–46.
2. Fox, John P. Epidemic Typhus, in *A Manual of Tropical Medicine*, 3d ed. George W. Hunter, William W. Frye and J. Clyde Swartzwelder, eds. Philadelphia: W. B. Saunders, 1960, pp. 70–79.
3. *Med. World News*, **8**:32–33, 1967 (July 7).
4. Epidemiology Branch, Communicable Disease Center. *The Epidemiology of Asian Influenza* 1957–1960. Atlanta: Communicable Disease Center, 1960.
5. Taylor, Richard M. Epidemiology, in *Yellow Fever*. George K. Strode, ed. New York: McGraw-Hill, 1951, p. 528.
6. Smadel, Joseph E. Status of the rickettsioses in the United States. *Ann. Intern. Med.* **51**:421–435, 1959.
7. Lobel, Hans O., and McCollum, Robert W. Some observations on the ecology of infectious hepatitis. *Bull. WHO* **32**:675–682, 1965.
8. Forster, F. Use of a demographic base map for the presentation of areal data in epidemiology. *Brit. J. Prev. Soc. Med.* **20**:165–171, 1966.

9. *Snow on Cholera*, being a reprint of two papers by John Snow, M.D., together with a biographical memoir by B. W. Richardson and an introduction by Wade Hampton Frost. New York: Commonwealth Fund, 1936, Map No. 1.

10. Maxcy, Kenneth F. An epidemiological study of endemic typhus (Brill's disease) in the southeastern United States. *Public Health Rep.* **41**:2967–2995, 1926.

11. Chin, Tom D. Y., and Marine, William M. The changing patterns of poliomyelitis observed in two urban epidemics, Kansas City and Des Moines, 1959. *Public Health Rep.* **76**:553–563, 1961.

12. Lobel, Hans O., and Robison, Roger F. Epidemiologic aspects of an outbreak of infectious hepatitis in Albany, N.Y. *Amer. J. Public Health* **55**:1176–1182, 1965.

13. Lumsden, L. L. St. Louis encephalitis in 1933: observations on epidemiological features. *Public Health Rep.* **73**:340–353, 1958.

14. Haenszel, William, and Shimkin, Michael B. Smoking patterns and epidemiology of lung cancer in the United States: Are they compatible? *J. Nat. Cancer Inst.* **16**:1417–1441, 1956.

11

Patterns of Disease
Occurrence—Time

In the foregoing discussions of patterns of disease occurrence with reference to person or place, time, specified or implied, has been an essential element. Conversely, as we examine variations with time, the affected population must be defined at least by place. Variation of disease with time is of interest because it reflects temporal variation in the activity of the cause(s). Thus, time is another important variable in testing the association of possible causative factors with disease.

11-1 General Considerations

Several general points must be stated before we can systematically consider how to describe disease occurrence in time. First, time can be divided into units varying from minutes or hours to centuries, the choice depending on the detail desired and the span of time over which comparisons are made. In a food poisoning outbreak, hours are important. A median incubation period of three to six hours suggests staphylococcus etiology, whereas twelve to fourteen hours points to salmonella. For chronic diseases, on the other hand, decades may be required to discern trends in occurrence. Second, when the time span exceeds one or two decades, problems arise as to comparability of data, especially with respect to standards of diagnosis and reporting. This problem arose notably with poliomyelitis in the United States when reporting was extended in the 1940s to include cases with minor paralysis or nonparalytic disease.

Third, several requirements must be satisfied if mortality is used as an index of time trends in disease occurrence. Most important, the disease must result in fatal outcome with uniform and significant frequency. When death occurs in less than 5 per cent of cases, or, as with measles, only once in 1,000 or more cases, mortality is an insensitive index of disease frequency. It is an unreliable index when improved treatment reduces case fatality, as with typhoid fever after chloramphenicol became available or with coronary heart disease (CHD) since the introduction of intensive cardiac care units in many hospitals. Also important, the interval between disease onset and fatal outcome must not vary excessively. Mortality is a very misleading index of the occurrence of tuberculosis, because duration of fatal disease may vary from a few weeks to many years and because recently available chemotheraphy has sharply curtailed fatal outcome. Mortality is most reliable when case fatality is very high, as with human rabies (100 per cent), or lung cancer (over 90 per cent within two years, even with early diagnosis and surgery). Finally, allowance must be made for relative changes in the rules governing assignment of the cause of death (see Chapter 7).

A fourth point relates to how soon disease becomes evident after first exposure to a disease agent. With most infectious diseases other than tuberculosis, the interval from effective exposure to disease onset (the incubation period) is measured in days. Single exposure to many non-infectious agents (pollens, poisons of many types) may produce disease within minutes or hours. However, when prolonged exposure is required to produce disease, the incubation period is both hard to define and quite variable. Cigarette smoking is accepted as causally related to lung cancer, but fifteen or more years, depending on level of cigarette consumption, must elapse from beginning of smoking to development of disease. Clearly, the distributions of disease onsets in time most closely parallel temporal variations in activity of the causative agents of acute conditions associated with short and uniform incubation periods.

Finally, two important words are employed in describing the occurrence of disease over time in a defined place. Diseases regularly and continuously present are referred to as *endemic,* and the usual frequency of occurrence, including possible seasonal variations, is referred to as the *endemic level.* The term *epidemic* is often misused to apply to any large clustering of cases in time and space. More correctly, an *epidemic* is defined by the fact that the number of cases, small or large, represents a significant excess over that expected on the basis of cumulated previous experience. Thus, in 1854, John Snow recognized the occurrence of an epidemic of cholera in the Golden Square area when there was a sharp increase in the number of cases per day over that which had been prevailing. The principle is well illustrated in Figure 11-1 in which weekly pneumonia and influenza deaths in United States cities are plotted.

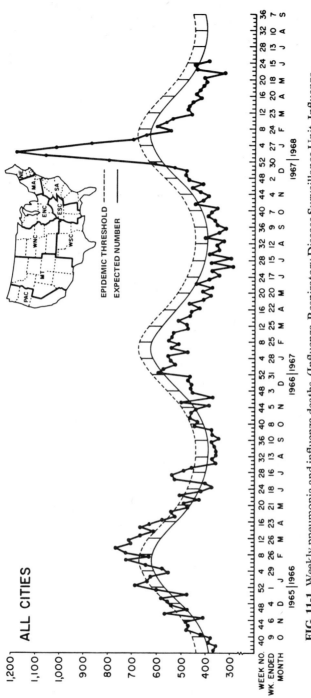

FIG. 11-1 Weekly pneumonia and influenza deaths. (Influenza-Respiratory Disease Surveillance Unit. Influenza-Respiratory Disease Surveillance Report No. 84. National Communicable Disease Center.)

Deaths from these causes have a regular seasonal pattern, described by a smooth curve, about which the weekly figures vary. The *usual* upper limit of variation (which would contain 95 per cent of the weekly plots) is shown by a dotted line. When the observed numbers of deaths exceed this line for more than two successive weeks, an *unusual* disease occurrence, or *epidemic*, is indicated, in this case of influenza. By this definition, a major epidemic occurred in the winter of 1967–1968 and a small one, two years previously. In the interest of minimizing public alarm, public health authorities employ the term *outbreak*, rather than *epidemic*, unless the number of cases is indeed very large. Epidemics often spread from place to place and the term *pandemic* has been coined to describe excess disease occurring in many countries, as with Asian influenza in 1957. Although ordinarily applied to acute diseases occurring in outbreaks of a few weeks or months duration, the concept of epidemic is equally applicable to chronic diseases if the time scale is shifted from days or weeks to years. The most notable example is lung cancer, which still is on the ascending limb of a pandemic curve which began after World War I.

11-2   Clustering in Time

The concept of incubation period implies that, given a point-in-time application of an etiologic agent, disease (if it occurs) will follow within a predictable range of time. Under natural conditions, infectious diseases are characterized by remarkably constant average incubation periods. However, the longer the average incubation period, the greater the usual range of variation. These principles presumably hold for both infectious and noninfectious agents. Their operation, when numbers of susceptible persons are exposed, results in clustering of disease onsets in time. Recognition of this phenomenon can be of major assistance in explaining disease occurrence.

The most obvious example is a sharp outbreak of noncontagious disease of known etiology. If the distribution of onsets over time does not exceed the usual range of variation of the incubation period (difference between shortest and longest usual period), it is likely that all were exposed at the same time (and probably at the same place). Further, the approximate time of exposure can be calculated by assuming that the first case represents the shortest usual incubation period and the last case the longest, thus focusing the investigation in time. This approach is particularly helpful with diseases such as typhoid or leptospirosis, in which the average incubation period is ten or more days and the range of variation fairly wide.

Another example relates to conditions of less certain etiology. Air pollution from automobile exhausts and the stacks of industrial furnaces has been an ever-increasing concern in major metropolitan areas, but, to date, it has not been possible to demonstrate that specific air pollutants or the total pollutants at their usual levels of concentration adversely affect health. However, when atmospheric inversions occur, the concentrations build up acutely. In Donora, Pennsylvania in 1948 (1), in London on many occasions, and more recently in New York City (2), acute episodes have been followed promptly by epidemics of asthmatic attacks and sharp increases in the daily number of deaths. The clustering in these instances provides fairly dramatic evidence that high levels of atmospheric pollution can adversely affect health, even though the specific responsible pollutants and their mechanisms of action remain to be identified.

Time clusters often are camouflaged because the affected persons received their exposures at different times. When this happens as a natural phenomenon as with an infectious agent passing from person to person, the resulting aggregate of disease occurrence may constitute an epidemic. To fully reveal the cluster in time, it would be necessary to determine precisely the time of exposure of each patient, set this at day zero on the time axis, and then plot the day of onset. Although the precise time of exposure typically cannot be determined in naturally occurring disease, instances where the only exposure was on a known date can be cumulated. This basic method has provided our knowledge of the natural range of variation in incubation periods for long-familiar diseases such as measles, mumps, and poliomyelitis. For many of the newly recognized viruses, proof that they actually cause disease is still lacking. One type of evidence that would support their role as disease agents would be demonstration that onsets of disease in infected persons with known times of exposure do cluster along the time axis. In practice, this approach has little applicability to the viruses in question, because the frequent occurrence of inapparent infections makes it nearly impossible for a given infected person to know with certainty the time of his effective exposure.

The foregoing basic approach, however, has been helpful in elucidating causation in some diseases. In the prevaccine era of poliomyelitis there was great interest in identifying "provoking" factors which helped determine that infection would result in paralytic disease. In this example, the approach was modified by setting disease onset at day zero and looking backward along the time axis for a clustering of possible provoking events. In this manner, recent tonsillectomy, inoculations (especially with irritant vaccines), and unusual physical exertion were singled out as suspect factors. With the advent of polio vaccines, this approach found a new and unexpected application. In the well-publicized Cutter episode some of the newly licensed Salk vaccine contained traces of live, virulent poliovirus which caused disease in a small proportion of vaccinated persons and their family contacts. As shown in Figure 11-2, cases in vaccinated persons clustered between three and twenty-five days after inoculation with

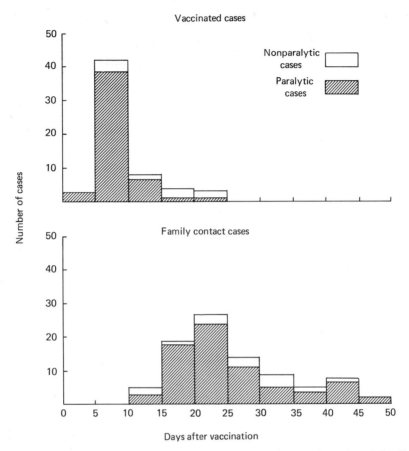

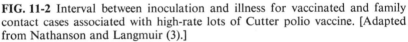

FIG. 11-2 Interval between inoculation and illness for vaccinated and family contact cases associated with high-rate lots of Cutter polio vaccine. [Adapted from Nathanson and Langmuir (3).]

a large peak in the 5–9 day interval, whereas those in family contacts of vaccinees formed a second wave with its crest about two weeks later (3). Although other aspects of association (plus demonstrating residual live virus in unused vaccine) provided stronger evidence for vaccine causation of disease, knowledge of this time distribution was utilized in subsequent continuing national surveillance of poliomyelitis instituted by the National Communicable Disease Center. All paralytic cases which had received vaccine within thirty days prior to onset were investigated to reveal possible clusters of patients receiving vaccine from a single lot.

With the introduction of Sabin live poliovirus vaccines, still another example was provided when a very small number of cases of paralytic disease occurred among the several million recipients of type 3 vaccine. The relation between Sabin vaccine and disease has been a highly controversial subject, but one strong bit of evidence supporting it was the concentration of case onsets within five to thirty days following vaccination. This is evident in Figure 11-3, in which are compared cases following vaccine feeding in epidemic areas (presumably caused by wild virus) and in nonepidemic areas (possibly caused by vaccine). Many other examples, centered chiefly about iatrogenically influenced disease, could be cited, especially in ferreting out mechanisms by which serum hepatitis has been

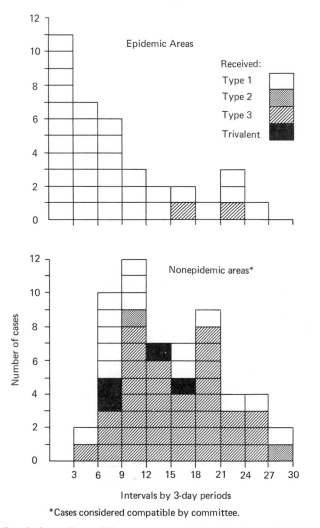

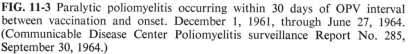

Intervals by 3-day periods

*Cases considered compatible by committee.

FIG. 11-3 Paralytic poliomyelitis occurring within 30 days of OPV interval between vaccination and onset. December 1, 1961, through June 27, 1964. (Communicable Disease Center Poliomyelitis surveillance Report No. 285, September 30, 1964.)

transmitted. Notable examples of this include serum-containing yellow fever vaccine in Brazil (4) and among United States soldiers in World War II (5), gelfoam (made from human fibrin) used to control bleeding in surgery, and inoculation procedures in which syringes and needles were reused without adequate cleaning and sterilization (the virus of serum hepatitis is notably heat resistant). In a particularly interesting example, Ellis (6) reviewed the health records of some 4,100 British military personnel who had developed nonsurgical jaundice with particular reference to inoculation with vaccinia or typhoid vaccine in the interval 11 to 340 days before disease onset. There were 379 who had received vaccinia and 576 to whom typhoid had been given. Arranging these patients so that day of onset became day zero, significant clustering in date of typhoid vaccine inoculation was observed in the intervals 11–40 and 41–70 days before onset. No such clustering was related to vaccinia, in the administration of which no reuse of needles occurs. Not only did this study further incriminate the practice of reusing injection equipment, but it provided evidence in the 11–40 day cluster that the virus of infectious heptatitis also had been transmitted by inoculation.

11-3   Short-term Variations

As short-term variations we will consider only unpredictable episodes of excess disease occurrence, that is, *epidemics* whose duration is measured in days, weeks, or perhaps months. By far the most common examples are the so-called "point" epidemics in which cases are concentrated within a few days. Their occurrence suggests that the affected persons were exposed to the same causal factor at nearly the same time, that the disease is not readily spread by contact, and that the average incubation period is short. Because of this, investigation of the outbreak can be sharply restricted in time and typically yields a satisfactory explanation, not infrequently implicating heretofore unsuspected mechanisms. Examples would include brief bacterial contaminations of water supplies (possibly because of failure to add chlorine during a holiday), and the acute air pollution episodes mentioned in the preceding section. Most often, however, they result from ingestion of chemically or microbially contaminated food. Unless large numbers of persons are affected (as in school or military groups, or at company or church picnics or banquets) or some victims suffer fatal disease (as with botulism), these episodes often escape official attention.

The brief duration of the "point" epidemics reflects the brevity of the activity of the disease source. By the same token, when outbreaks of noncontagious disease persist more than a few days, one must infer persistence of the disease source and it becomes even more important to identify and terminate it. The 1965 community-wide outbreak of salmonellosis in Madera, California was quickly traced to the water supply (7). When cases are relatively few and not clustered geographically, the problem becomes more difficult. Between December 1964 and July 1966 sixty-eight patients entered Omaha, Nebraska hospitals acutely ill with serious primary myocardial disease of uncertain etiology. Of these, thirty died. Most were residents of Omaha and they were not clustered in space or time. The common link, discovered only after many months had passed, was the habitual consumption by the victims of ten or more glasses of beer a day, almost all of brand "Z." Investigation revealed that traces of cobalt (1.1 to 1.2 parts per million) had been added to brand "Z," beginning a few months before the first appearance of what is now referred to as "beer drinkers'" disease. The outbreak terminated when the brewery was persuaded to omit the cobalt (8). On a national scale, botulism resulting from smoked fish from a particular producer or salmonellosis from contamination of one brand of powdered milk represent fairly recent similar problems.

Except for the "continuing source" type of outbreaks just described, epidemics of infectious diseases are generally self-limited. The curve of disease occurrence rises and then falls, often taking the approximate form of the familiar bell-shaped curve of the normal distribution. Evaluation of epidemic control measures is obviously complicated by the knowledge that, had no control efforts been made, the disease would have declined in any event. The question is whether or not the decline was hastened by the control measures. According to one apocryphal definition, an epidemiologist is "an expert from out of town who slides to glory on the descending limb of the epidemic curve."

The basic difference between a "point" epidemic and usual self-limited epidemics of infectious disease, other than duration, is that the rise of the epidemic reflects a progressive increase in the numbers of sources of infection and the fall mirrors a similarly progressive decline (often symmetrical). With contact-transmitted diseases, the sources are infected persons who may or may not experience overt disease. The epidemic owes its origin to the existence in the population of enough susceptibles that the infection has a high chance of spreading. As it spreads, those infected become immunes and the supply of susceptibles is depleted to the point that spread tapers off and finally ceases. The rapidity with which such an epidemic reaches its peak and its duration depend upon infectivity of the agent, length of the incubation period, initial proportion of susceptibles in the population, and intimacy of contact. An example of a school-centered outbreak of influenza resulting from group B influenza virus is provided in Figure 11-4 (9). This study illustrates the rapidity of build-up of cases in the school population when the incubation period is short (24 to 72 hours) and the slower progress among family contacts of the

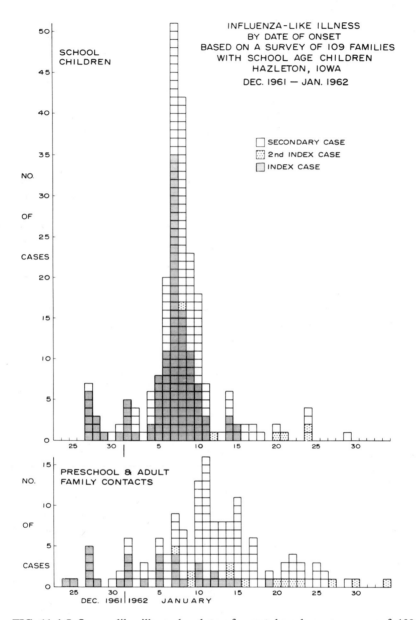

FIG. 11-4 Influenza-like illness by date of onset based on a survey of 109 families with school-age children, Hazelton, Iowa, December, 1961–January, 1962. (Tom D. Y. Chin et al. Epidemiologic studies of Type B influenza in 1961–62. *Amer. J. Public Health* **53**:1068–1074, 1963.)

infected school children. When an arthropod vector transmits the agent from man to man (the body louse in epidemic typhus, the *Aedes aegypti* mosquito in urban yellow fever), the above principles continue to operate, but a new requirement is that conditions favoring an abundance of the vector must also prevail.

With zoonoses such as St. Louis encephalitis, the primary sources of infection are lower vertebrate and the immediate sources are infected culex mosquitoes. The proportion of immunes in the human population rarely is high enough to influence the pattern of human infection. Rather, a change in the proportion of susceptibles among the lower vertebrate hosts, a seasonally determined variation in abundance of the mosquito vector, and the length of the extrinsic incubation period (in the vector) determine the onset time, slope of the curve, and duration of the epidemic. Where, as in California, St. Louis encephalitis and western equine encephalomyelitis (WEE) occur in the same areas and utilize the same host and vector species, WEE outbreaks begin earlier and progress more rapidly because the extrinsic incubation period is much shorter than that of St. Louis virus.

11-4   Periodic Variations

Frequency of disease occurrence often rises and falls with predictable regularity. Many diseases exhibit annual or seasonal peaks and some occur in cycles of several years' duration.

Seasonal variation implies a link between the activity of the underlying cause and some aspect of season, such as mean temperature, amount or type of precipitation, length of day, or some requisite sequential combination of these. The link is easy to find when the biological environment is involved. Zoonotic diseases depending on arthropod transmission vary in relation to seasonal variation in stage of development (chiefly of ticks), activity, and abundance of the vector. Tick activity is maximal in the spring and early summer, thus setting the seasonal pattern for tularemia and Rocky Mountain spotted fever. Rat flea populations closely parallel mean temperature and hence, so does the occurrence of murine typhus in the Southeastern United States. However, the curves of disease occurrence and vector abundance rarely coincide exactly, and may not even be parallel. St. Louis encephalitis and the other viral encephalitides in North America occur in late summer and early fall. Populations of the mosquito vectors become abundant several weeks in advance of human disease, but disease occurrence and vector population decline in close parallel, separated only by the incubation period in man. The initial lag in human disease reflects the time necessary for virus buildup in its mosquito-avian host reservoir before spillover to man occurs.

Respiratory illnesses and other diseases with airborne transmission are less frequent in the summer months, presumably in part because schools are closed and many play and social contacts occur out of doors, where great dilution of airborne agents occurs. Reopening of schools coincides with a general resurgence of respiratory disease, but different agents predominate as the season progresses. Influenza most often peaks in mid-winter, but measles, spread in the same manner, prefers the late winter and spring, and mumps often carries well into the summer. Although differences in incubation period no doubt constitute a partial explanation, these differences in seasonal appearance are still not fully understood.

Enteric infections tend to flourish in the warmer months, the annual increase appearing earlier in the southern than in the northern parts of the United States. With enteric bacteria, warmer temperatures favor multiplication of the agent in unrefrigerated food and milk, filth fly populations increase, and summer recreational activities may be associated with lowering of sanitary precautions. Explanations for the seasonal pattern of enteric viruses are less satisfying. The prototype disease, polio-myelitis, in the prevaccination era reached its peak in June and July in the Southern states and in August and September in the North. Although flies and other means of indirect transmission operate more often in the warmer months, the major spread of infection in the United States is believed to be by intimate play contact between young children, most of it out of doors. Conceivably, poor personal hygiene of children becomes more relevant when warm weather dictates a minimum of clothing. However, a completely opposite seasonal pattern is manifested by infectious hepatitis, another viral disease for which fecal-oral transmission is postulated. The late winter peaking of this disease suggests that season must exert a different kind of influence on enteric virus spread than has so far been conceived.

Seasonal variation is not confined to infectious diseases. For some, such as hay fever from plant pollens or accidents resulting from various seasonally dictated forms of sport or recreation, seasonal variations are widely recognized and readily explained. Well known but unexplained is the fact that daily mortality varies markedly, being lowest in late summer and highest in December and January. Perhaps more understandable, daily births also vary, being highest in March in the United States. The list of diseases manifesting seasonal variation could be extended encyclopedically. The important points, however, have already been made, namely that seasonal variation is common, that it typically is not fully explained, and that search for satisfactory explanations constitutes another potentially profitable approach to overall explanations of disease causation. A newly recognized example of seasonal variation in disease which is being explored is the relation between summer and both clinical onset and mortality in certain malignant states in children, notably, acute leukemia and neuroblastomas (10).

To examine trends over periods of several years, annual disease experience (incidence, prevalence, or mortality) is plotted. For diseases with a marked seasonal pattern, annual figures are often based on the "epidemiologic" year (demarcated by the week of lowest incidence), rather than on the calendar year. With poliomyelitis in the United States, the new year usually began some time in March. *Cyclic variation* (periodicity of longer than one year) has been described for a number of infectious diseases, all of which are also characterized by seasonal variations. Measles (rubeola) in major urban centers occurs with greater than usual frequency at intervals that average slightly less than three years. Before 1950, deaths due to meningococcal meningitis occurred on a nationwide basis in cycles of 7–9 years. The last such peak was in 1942–1944, the interruption of the cycle presumably resulting from the advent of sulfonamides and penicillin. Figure 11-5 illustrates the very similar cyclic occurrence of infectious hepatitis in the United States since 1952. These cyclic patterns are generally considered to reflect variations in herd immunity. In the interepidemic periods, the annual waves are brought to termination (presumably by the advent of season-related circumstances unfavorable to agent spread) before the annual number of infections equals the annual input of susceptibles by birth. This results in an increase in the proportion of susceptibles to the point that spread is greatly facilitated. With highly infectious agents such as measles or influenza viruses, the epidemic consists of an enlarged annual wave. With less infectious agents, such as that of infectious hepatitis, seasonal lows are elevated over three or more years, with the usual seasonal pattern imprinted on the epidemic wave. It should be emphasized that, although plausible, the mechanism outlined above remains to be fully documented.

11-5 Secular or Long-term Trends

Concern here is with changes in disease occurrence over periods measured in decades or centuries. For comparisons over long periods, disease occurrence must be expressed in terms of rates (morbidity or mortality), because changes in numerical incidence could result simply from changes in size of population. One exception is disease that is very infrequent and possibly on the verge of disappearance. Not only do rates have little meaning, but main interest centers in the actual number and distribution of cases. Examples in the United States include indigenous malaria and smallpox as they neared extinction and rabies in man, which varies annually between one and five or six cases.

Availability and comparability of data are important limiting factors

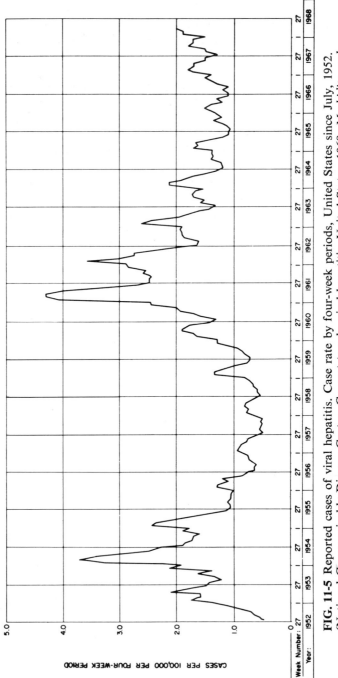

FIG. 11-5 Reported cases of viral hepatitis. Case rate by four-week periods, United States since July, 1952. (National Communicable Disease Center. Current trends, viral hepatitis, United States, 1968. *Morbidity and Mortality Weekly Rep.* **17**: No. 14, 1968.)

in the study of long-term trends. Systematically collected morbidity information exists only for notifiable diseases (chiefly infectious) and conditions such as serious mental illness for which most patients are hospitalized. As noted in Chapter 10, availability and reliability of data vary greatly between nations and the problem of comparability over long periods of time also has been discussed. Not previously mentioned is the completeness with which notifiable diseases are reported. Incompleteness of reporting is clearly important to interpreting long-term trends, unless one can establish that the degree of completeness remained reasonably constant. This is rarely possible. In the case of poliomyelitis, the inclusion of cases of nonparalytic or slightly paralytic disease, begun in the 1940s, clearly increased the completeness of record, but to an unknown degree.

Because of the frequently insoluble problems related to using morbidity data, summarized above, data for mortality have been more commonly and profitably employed in examining long-term trends in disease occurrence. Cause-specific mortality, when it satisfies the requirements previously stipulated, is a useful index in those countries where deaths are completely recorded. The basic requirements, briefly, are that disease must result in death in a significant and constant proportion of cases and within a reasonably uniform period after onset. These requirements are fulfilled for many more diseases than we can describe, and the examples employed in the following discussion have been chosen to illustrate how some of the problems in interpretation of long-term data have been approached.

Changes in crude cause-specific death rates usually progress gradually, in the same direction, upward or downward, over long periods of time. When trends are observed, the activity of possible causative factors is examined to see whether a parallel trend exists. Failure to discover such parallelism provides a forceful argument against the hypothesis of causal relation. Demonstration of parallelism, however, ordinarily is of limited value in proof of a causal relation. The rise in the death rate for lung cancer since World War I parallels not just an increase in per capita consumption of cigarettes, but also increases of many other types from sales of nylon stockings to utilization of combustible petroleum products. In rare instances the trend in mortality rates differs between countries and is not constant within one country. In such cases, discovery that activity of a suspect causative factor parallels these changes in disease occurrence provides much stronger evidence for a causal relation. The parallelism between death rates for cirrhosis of the liver and per capita consumption of alcohol in the form of distilled spirits and wine is an example. In the United States, prohibition between 1920 and 1933 resulted in a marked decrease in consumption of alcohol which, as seen in Figure 11-6, coincided approximately with a major decline in cirrhosis mortality. Both trends were reversed following repeal of prohibition. During 1900–

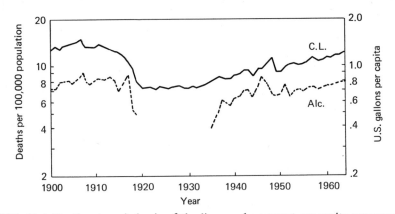

FIG. 11-6 Death rates, cirrhosis of the liver, and apparent per capita consumption of absolute alcohol from spirits and wine, United States, 1900–1964. (Milton Terris. *Amer. J. Public Health* **57**:2076–2088, 1967.)

1963 in the British Isles, very different but still parallel patterns were observed (Figure 11-7). Heavy taxation of distilled spirits, introduced during World War I and greatly augmented in World War II, resulted in sharp declines in consumption of alcohol in the form of distilled spirits which were paralleled by decreases in mortality from cirrhosis. Since 1945, use of distilled spirits has increased (presumably because of overall improvement in the economic status of British citizens) and so has mortality from cirrhosis (11). These parallelisms are most difficult to explain by chance, and provide strong support for the prevailing opinion that

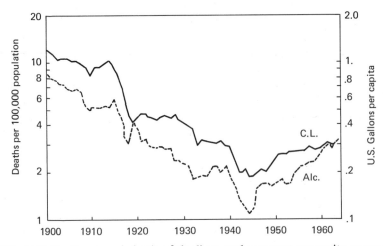

FIG. 11-7 Death rates, cirrhosis of the liver, and apparent per capita consumption of absolute alcohol from spirits and wine, United Kingdom, 1900–1963. (Milton Terris. *Amer. J. Public Health* **57**:2076–2088, 1967.)

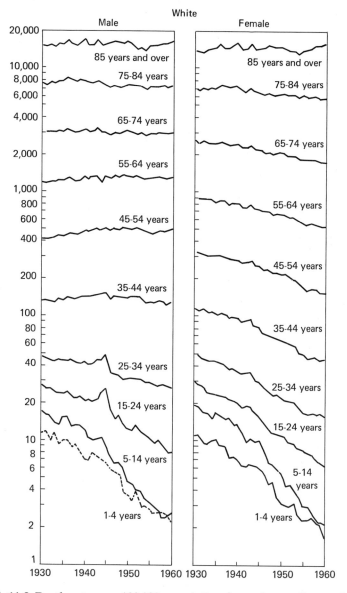

FIG. 11-8 Death rates per 100,000 population for major cardiovascular-renal diseases, by age and sex for the white population: United States, 1930–1960. (Vital and Health Statistics. National Center for Health Statistics, Series 3, No. 1.)

alcoholism contributes greatly to the occurrence of fatal cirrhoses of the liver.

When disease occurrence is strongly associated with age (a usual situation), allowance must be made for changes in age composition of the population before comparisons of death rates over long time spans are made. For the United States, the death rate in 1950 for major cardio-vascular-renal (CVR) diseases was 511 per 100,000 population, as compared with 345 in 1900. Following age-adjustment (based on the 1940

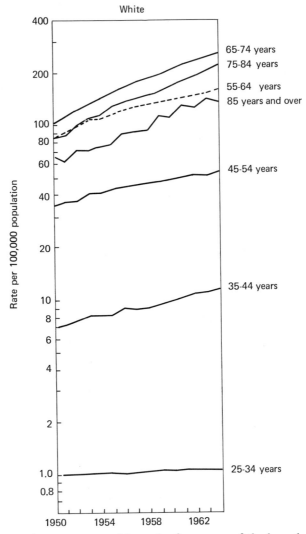

FIG. 11-9 Death rates among white males for cancer of the lung, by specified age groups: 1950–1964. (Vital and Health Statistics, Series 20, Number 4.)

United States population), the corresponding figures were 429 and 422. The detailed trend for CVR diseases over three decades, 1930–1960, is shown in Figure 11-8. Age-sex-specific rates for the white population in no instance increased perceptibly, and, excepting chiefly males of thirty-five years and older, usually declined appreciably. A very different picture is seen for lung cancer, the death rates for which doubled between 1950 and 1964 (12.2 versus 24.0 per 100,000 population). Among white males death rates increased continuously during this period for each age group above thirty-four years (Figure 11-9). In view of this finding, it is not surprising that the nearly twofold difference in United States death rates was little reduced by age adjustment (11.8 versus 20.7 deaths per 100,000).

Although changes in age composition of the population can be easily dealt with, as illustrated above, the problem of comparability over time in standards of diagnosis is more difficult. One approach is to collect series of cases in which autopsies were performed and determine the proportion in which clinical diagnosis was confirmed. Not only does this represent a very laborious procedure, but one can hardly generalize from the experience of an autopsied population (which will have received better than average medical care) to that of the entire population of deaths. Two other, more readily applied, approaches are commonly used. One is to compare the trend in the disease under study with trends in other diseases which present diagnostic problems of similar difficulty. In Table 11-1 death rates for lung cancer in United States white males, ages 45–54 and 55–64, over the period 1930–1960 are compared with similar figures for cancers of the stomach, urinary bladder, and prostate, and for leukemia. The downward trend in gastric cancer and the disproportionate overall increase in lung cancer gives support to the belief that the rise in lung cancer is not an artifact of diagnosis.

TABLE 11-1

Mortality rates (per 100,000 population) for malignant neoplasms of the lung, stomach, urinary bladder and prostate, and for leukemia, United States white males, ages 45–54 and 55–64, 1930 to 1960.

	LUNG CANCER		GASTRIC CANCER		URINARY BLADDER		PROSTATE		LEUKEMIA	
	45–54	55–64	45–54	55–64	45–54	55–64	45–54	55–64	45–54	55–64
1930	7.8	13.0	34.2	99.3	5.1	15.9	2.8	23.0	3.3	6.2
1940	20.4	40.6	26.0	78.1	5.2	15.8	3.6	27.8	5.8	10.9
1950	35.1	85.3	16.6	54.2	4.1	16.9	2.6	21.9	6.7	14.4
1960	49.2	139.2	11.03	34.4	3.3	14.1	2.1	16.1	7.3	16.6

Sources: National Cancer Institute Monograph No. 6, 1961; P.H.S. Pub. No. 113, 1963.

The other approach is to compare the experience of the two sexes. This comparison is meaningful only for diseases common to both sexes and when the trends are not parallel. As one example, we may refer back to Figure 11-8, which reveals appreciable declines between 1930 and 1960 in CVR disease deaths among females in all age groups below seventy-five years. The reality of these trends is supported by the fact that males in corresponding age groups over thirty-four years did not experience similar declines, even though they presumably benefited from comparable medical care. More dramatic is the contrasting experience of older males and females (ages 55–64) with respect to malignant neoplasms as a group, shown in Figure 11-10. In 1930, rates for females exceeded those for males in both whites and nonwhites. However, rates for males rose (sharply in the case of nonwhites), whereas those for females declined (whites) or rose only slightly (nonwhites), with the result that male rates had substantially surpassed female rates by 1960.

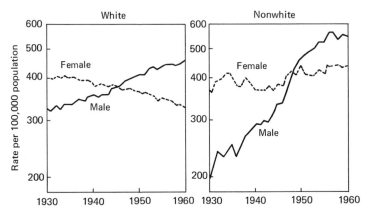

FIG. 11-10 Death rates for malignant neoplasms, 55-to-64-year age group, by color and sex: United States, 1930–1960. (Vital and Health Statistics, Series 3, Number 1.)

A final problem relates to diseases in which the "incubation period" is very long and there is a strong association with age. In this context, "incubation period" is defined as the interval between infection (as in tuberculosis) or initial exposure (as with cigarette smoking) and death from resulting disease. The problem is to discover the trend in activity of the underlying cause(s). One might, for example, examine the age-mortality curves for tuberculosis in the United States for selected years from 1900 to 1960, as is done for white males in Figure 11-11 (12). The several curves are similar in reflecting high rates in early childhood which drop sharply and then increase progressively with age in adult life. However, each age-specific rate declines with time (more evident in the younger

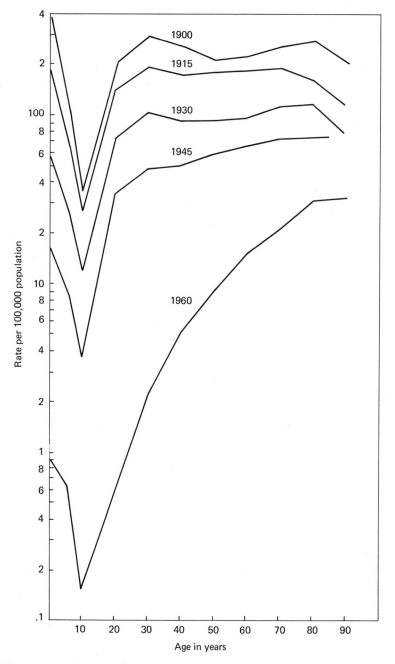

FIG. 11-11 Death rates from tuberculosis by age group for selected years. (Doege, Theodore C. Tuberculosis mortality in the United States, 1900 to 1960. *J. Amer. Med. Assn.* **192**:1045–1048, 1965.)

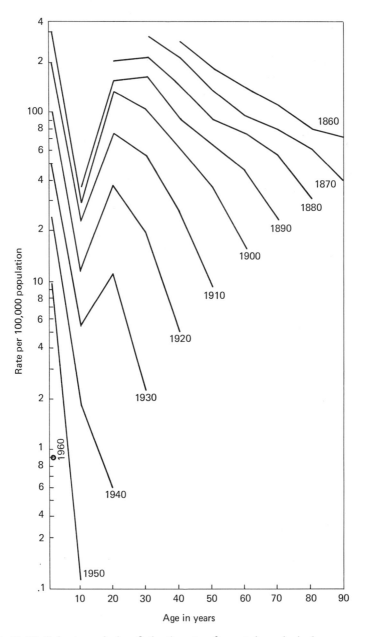

FIG. 11-12 Cohort analysis of death rates from tuberculosis by age group, 1860–1960. The line associated with each year indicates death rates by age group for persons born in that year. (Doege, Theodore C. Tuberculosis mortality in the United States, 1900 to 1960. *J. Amer. Med. Assn.* **192**:1045–1048, 1965.)

ages). This could suggest a progressive decrease in activity of the tubercle bacillus, which affected younger age groups somewhat more than the older. A different picture is seen if one rearranges the data so that the curves connect points representing the age-specific death rates for population segments born at the same time (*cohorts*) as in Figure 11-12. These curves, representing changes in death rates with age during the life experience of each cohort, show that, in actual fact, the risk of dying from tuberculosis among adults does not rise progressively with age, but declines for all cohorts after age twenty-five to thirty. Also, for any age group, the risk of death decreases for successively born cohorts. This approach, called *cohort analysis*, provides strong support for the prevalent hypothesis that tuberculosis disease and mortality in adults ordinarily results, not from newly acquired infection or reinfection, but from reactivation of infection acquired early in life. Thus, in any given year, the rise in death rates with age during adult life is determined more by the progressively decreasing prevalence of infection during childhood than by age itself.

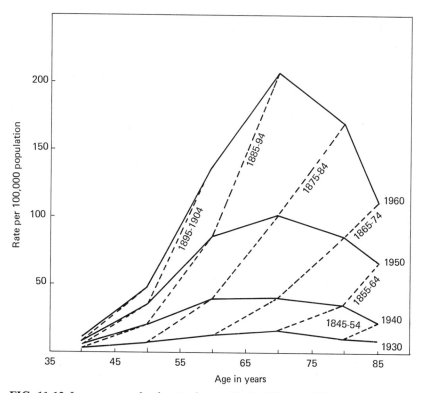

FIG. 11-13 Lung cancer death rates by age. United States white males, 40 years of age and older, for selected years (solid lines) and for certain cohorts (broken lines). (National Cancer Institute Monograph No. 6, 1961, P.H.S. Pub. No. 113, 1963.)

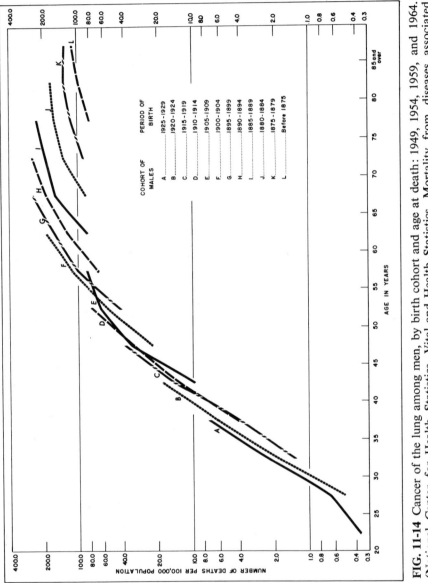

FIG. 11-14 Cancer of the lung among men, by birth cohort and age at death: 1949, 1954, 1959, and 1964. (National Center for Health Statistics, Vital and Health Statistics. Mortality from diseases associated with smoking: United States 1590–64. U.S. Department of Health, Education and Welfare.)

A final and less cheerful example is afforded by lung cancer. The curves for age-specific death rates among United States males in the census years 1930 to 1960, are shown in Figure 11-13 (solid lines). The curves are similar in shape, the risk increasing until age 65–74 years, and then declining slightly. However, for each age group, the rates observed at successive ten-year intervals increase progressively. The full import of this trend is better seen when *cohort analysis* is employed. The broken lines in Figure 11-13 show the application of this method to the same data. Not only is there no age range over which death rates decline, but, for each of six successive ten-year cohorts born since 1845, the rise has begun earlier and its slope has been steeper. As seen in Figure 11-14 (based on five-year cohorts), the same statement can be extended to include cohorts born as recently as 1925–1929. Clearly, the activity of the causative factor(s) appears to be still increasing and, unless something drastic is done (presumably, curtailment of consumption of cigarettes), the risk of lung cancer will continue to rise.

11-6   Summary

Disease variation with time reflects temporal variation in activity of the causes. This parallelism is greatest for diseases associated with short and uniform incubation periods. Study of disease trends over decades is complicated by changes in quality and completeness of data. Use of disease-specific mortality as an index requires that the disease must cause death with uniform and significant frequency within a reasonably constant period after onset.

Endemic refers to diseases continuously present in a place and *endemic level* describes their usual frequency of occurrence; significantly greater frequency is called *epidemic*.

The relative uniformity of incubation period for specific diseases results in obvious clustering of disease in time when many persons are exposed simultaneously. Such time clusters are camouflaged when persons are exposed at different times, but their demonstration, by setting at zero the day of possible exposure and looking forward or by taking the day of disease onset and looking backward, provides strong evidence for causal relations.

Short-term increases in disease other than seasonal are epidemics. The most common are "point epidemics" of noncontagious diseases resulting from simultaneous exposure of groups of persons and characterized by brief duration. Outbreaks of noncontagious disease lasting more than a few days indicate a continuing source. Epidemics of contagious diseases are self-limited; incidence rises as numbers of sources (infected persons) increase and declines when the proportion nonimmune become too small to support agent spread. Epidemics of zoonoses are also self-limited, because of depletion of nonimmunes in the reservoir host and season-determined decline in vector abundance.

Seasonal variation characterizes many diseases, infectious and non-infectious, and implies a link between some aspect of season and an important cause. This link is usually obvious for zoonoses and is at least partially understood for most other infectious diseases. Especially for certain chronic conditions, elucidation of the link with season may contribute importantly to understanding causation. A number of infectious diseases exhibit an additional variation, with a periodicity of two or more years (cyclic variation), believed to reflect the influence of herd immunity.

Changes in disease occurrence over periods measured in decades or centuries are called secular trends, description of which requires the use of rates rather than numbers of cases. Because of lack of availability of systematically collected morbidity data for many diseases and varying completeness of that which is available, profitable study of long-term trends has been largely restricted to diseases for which cause-specific mortality provides a satisfactory index.

When trends in disease are observed, the activity of possible causative factors is examined. Demonstration of parallelism is essential to proof of causal relation, but is of only limited positive value unless found in countries with very different trends or shown to persist within a country despite the occurrence of marked changes in trend.

When disease is strongly associated with age, comparison of death rates over long periods of time requires that they be adjusted for age. To establish comparability of diagnostic criteria over time is difficult, but can be approached by comparing age-specific rates for diseases posing equivalent diagnostic problems or sex-specific rates for the disease under study (valuable only when the trends for the two sexes diverge).

Interpretation of trends for diseases with long and ill-defined incubation periods may be misleading, unless the lifetime experiences (sequential age-specific death rates) of successive population cohorts (born in the same period) are compared. This method (known as cohort analysis) is widely applicable and has been illustrated for tuberculosis and lung cancer. It revealed that risk of tuberculosis declines, rather than increases, with age in adult life, whereas risk for lung cancer increases more sharply than suggested by current-year age profiles.

GLOSSARY

Iatrogenic(ally)   Physician-induced.

Leptospirosis   A zoonotic disease caused by a member of the bacterial group known as leptospira and harbored by many species of lower animals (rats, dogs, cattle, in particular).

Leukemia Malignant disease of the tissues producing lymphocytes (lymphatic leukemia) or polymorphonuclear cells of the blood (myelogenous leukemia), typically characterized by great increases in the blood of abnormal forms of the respective types of cells.

Neoplasm (malignant) Abnormal growth or tumor (cancer).

Serum hepatitis Disease caused by a virus of still unknown nature which persists indefinitely in blood and tissues of healthy carriers; clinically similar to infectious hepatitis but characterized by a much longer incubation period.

REFERENCES

1. Schrenk, H. H., Heimann, H., Clayton, G. D., Gafafer, W. M., and Wexler, H. Air Pollution in Donora, Pa.: Epidemiology of the Unusual Smog Episode of October, 1948. Public Health Bull. No. 306. Washington, D.C.: Federal Security Agency, 1949.

2. McCarroll, James, and Bradley, William. Excess mortality as an indicator of health effects of air pollution. *Amer. J. Public Health* **56**:1933–1942, 1966.

3. Nathanson, Neal, and Langmuir, Alexander D. The Cutter incident. Poliomyelitis following formaldehyde-inactivated poliovirus vaccination in the United States during the spring of 1955. *Amer. J. Hyg.* **78**:16–81, 1963.

4. Fox, John P., Manso, C., Penna, H. A., and Para, M. Observations on the occurrence of icterus in Brazil following vaccination against yellow fever. *Amer. J. Hyg.* **36**:68–116, 1942.

5. Sawyer, W. A., *et al.* Jaundice in army personnel in the western region of the United States and its relation to vaccination against yellow fever. *Amer. J. Hyg.* **39**:337–430; **40**:35–107, 1944.

6. Ellis, F. P. The transmission of hepatitis virus by routine immunization procedures. *J. Hyg.* (*Camb.*) **53**:124–128, 1955.

7. Renteln, Henry A., and Hinman, Alan R. A waterborne epidemic of gastroenteritis in Madera, California. *Amer. J. Epidem.* **86**:1–10, 1967.

8. McDermott, Paul H., Delancy, Robert L., Egan, John D., and Sullivan, James F. Myocardosis and cardiac failure in men. *J. Amer. Med. Ass.* **198**:253–256, 1966.

9. Chin, Tom D. Y., Mosley, W. H., Poland, J. D., Rush, D., Belden, E. A., and Johnson, O. Epidemiologic studies of type B influenza in 1961–62. *Amer. J. Public Health* **53**:1068–1074, 1963.

10. Lee, John A. H. Summer and death from neuroblastoma. *Brit. Med. J.* **2**:404–407, 1967.

11. Terris, Milton. Epidemiology of cirrhosis of the liver. National mortality data. *Amer. J. Public Health* **57**:2076–2088, 1967.

12. Doege, Theodore C. Tuberculosis mortality in the United States, 1900 to 1960. *J. Amer. Med. Ass.* **192**:1045–1048, 1965.

12

The Nature of
Epidemiologic Research

The preoccupation of epidemiology with understanding the occurrence of disease in populations and with exploiting insights gained for the prevention and control of disease has been stressed in this book. Full understanding means full knowledge of disease causation, the inherent complexity of which was outlined in Chapter 3. The present chapter is concerned with how we obtain this knowledge.

12-1 Goals of Epidemiologic Research

It is a truism to say that our understanding of causation of diseases is satisfactory for only a few. Our state of knowledge ranges from little more than the pattern of occurrence of diseases such as infectious hepatitis to very effective understanding of such diseases as diphtheria or measles. For measles, adequate characterization of the causative virus is a still new achievement, and effective vaccines have only recently become available. Traditionally, in addition to describing disease occurrence and characterizing the primary agent, epidemiologic research has sought increased specificity in diagnosis, understanding of pathogenesis with special interest in portals of invasion and avenues of shedding of the agent, determination of transmission and reservoir mechanisms, discovery and evaluation of contributing factors, and development and evaluation of measures for prevention and control.

Etiologically specific diagnosis of disease is particularly important. As noted in Chapter 9, the clinical picture of disease is an unreliable guide to etiology. Clinically similar syndromes may be caused by several agents, and a given agent may elicit a wide spectrum of clinical response. "Atypical pneumonia" is a case in point. This syndrome emerged as a presumed etiologic entity of importance with the advent of effective therapeutic agents to combat the common bacterial pneumonias. Presently, we know that this syndrome may be caused by Q fever rickettsiae, ornithosis, adeno and influenza viruses, but the most important cause is what Monroe Eaton described as the virus of primary atypical pneumonia (the Eaton agent), now recognized as *Mycoplasma pneumoniae* (1). As methods for recognizing present or past infection evolved, it also became clear that atypical pneumonia constitutes just one end of the spectrum of clinical response to infection with the Eaton agent (2). Further, when methods for preventing disease from Eaton agent are developed, evaluation of their effectiveness will similarly require the ability to specifically recognize infection with *M. pneumoniae*.

A major contemporary goal of epidemiologic research is to assess the disease potential of agents not yet associated with disease. This is a reversal of the classical approach in which the epidemiologist seeks to discover the cause of a presumed disease entity. Presently, he is confronted with a host of agents whose relation to disease remains to be determined. One important class of such "agents in search of a disease" includes the many viruses which have been recovered from man (chiefly in respiratory or fecal specimens), from arthropods, and from lower animals. Another class, posing more difficult problems of evaluation, is made up of the host of potentially noxious noninfectious agents to which man is exposed in his increasingly complex environment. These include emissions from automobiles and industry which pollute the air; food additives; an awesome array of new drugs; natural and man-made irradiation; and the spillover of our chemical warfare against insects, to which Rachel Carson has so dramatically drawn our attention (3).

12-2   The Nature of Epidemiologic Research

By definition, epidemiologic research is that relevant to understanding of disease occurrence. As in other disciplines, recognition of significant problems and formulation of methods for their solution demand imagination, curiosity, and ingenuity in the application of scientific discipline. However, investigations of widely different types may be relevant even when concern is with causation and prevention of a single disease. For purposes of further discussion, these are conveniently classified according to their setting (laboratory or field) and the basic method employed (experimental or observational).

Laboratory studies are inherently experimental and may take many forms. One relevant example is the Nobel Prize-winning work of Enders and his colleagues. By showing that polioviruses multiply in tissue culture with readily visible destructive effects, these workers provided a major tool for detecting polioviruses in man and suspected environmental sources (sewage, flies), for demonstrating seroimmunity and for producing the large amounts of virus required in the production of vaccines (4).

Experimental epidemiology involves manipulation of animal or human populations (including, in recent times, populations simulated on computers). The earliest studies so designated utilized herds of laboratory animals and a natural pathogen as models to study the influence on disease occurrence of such factors as agent virulence, host nutritional state, and proportion of hosts susceptible. The distinguishing features of experimental epidemiologic studies are: (1) that the investigator assigns the experimental subjects to treatment or control groups by some formal method of randomization (to exclude possible investigator bias and to entitle him to use statistical tests in interpreting results); and (2) that the factor under study is imposed or withheld by the investigator. Vaccine trials represent the most common type of experimental study in man.

Observational studies in a field setting (clinic or community) comprise the bulk of epidemiologic research. Observation is focused on events, chiefly possible "exposures" and disease occurrence, which have occurred or are occurring in the study population in the course of normal living. Thus, unlike experimental epidemiology, grouping of population members for analysis is on the basis of characteristics (age, race, sex, occupation, smoking, diet, family size, and so on) which were not and could not have been assigned by the investigator. Surveys constitute the simplest form of observational study and are undertaken to describe the distribution of disease, of disease sequellae, or of various factors possibly contributing to disease.

More sophisticated in concept and design are analytic studies undertaken to test hypotheses as to disease occurrence that have been developed on the basis of descriptive data, including that yielded by surveys. The type hypothesis to be explored is that a specified factor is causally related to the occurrence of a particular disease. The statistical association which would support the hypothesis can be sought in two ways. A common first approach is to compare groups of patients (for example, those with lung cancer) and of nonpatients with respect to prior exposure (for example, to cigarette smoking). This retrospective* ("looking backward") approach is relatively quick and inexpensive. However, although it may reveal association (e.g., smoking is more common among lung cancer patients than among nonpatients), it provides no direct measure of the risk related to exposure (i.e., how much greater is the incidence of lung cancer in smokers than in nonsmokers). This can be obtained only by prospective* studies in which the development of disease is observed in exposed and unexposed groups.

*The terms *retrospective* and *prospective* refer to how data are analyzed and not to how or when they are collected. To avoid the confusion engendered by the quite different everyday meanings of these words, McMahon and co-authors (*Epidemiologic Methods*, Boston: Little, Brown, 1960) chose to employ new terms, i,e, *case-history* for retrospective and *cohort* for prospective. We have retained the old terminology, but readers should know that these synonyms exist and are being used with increasing frequency.

12-3   Laboratory Studies

Because of the broad scope of epidemiology and the frequently important implications of many types of biological knowledge to health and disease, there is no sharp criterion by which laboratory studies can be identified as relevant to epidemiology. Thus, within the field of virology, the search for ways to propagate viruses and to reproduce disease, the study of host range, antigenic character and viability in the free state, and the development of methods for specific recognition of infections are clearly relevant to epidemiology. However, modern virology also embraces the important and basic field of molecular biology. This deals with the ultrastructure and function of viral particles, and the processes of cell invasion and viral replication which, controlled by the viral genetic material (nucleic acid), involves diversion of normal cell processes to synthesis of viral components and their assembly into mature particles. Although the resulting basic knowledge ultimately will be significant to human health, it is not currently relevant to epidemiology.

Of particular importance are studies centered about the experimental reproduction of disease. When successful, as with yellow fever virus in rhesus monkeys or with chemicals (carcinogens) which induce cancers in experimental animals, such studies provide crucial evidence for the etiologic role of suspect agents and an experimental model of disease. Such a model permits studies of agent–host relations and of factors related to host resistance and susceptibility. In monkeys with experimental yellow fever detailed studies were made of the sites of virus multiplication, the related tissue changes, the time sequence of virus circulation in the blood, and the appearance of serum antibody. The monkey model also was used to test mechanisms of transmission of infection, and in crucial pilot studies of the safety and effectiveness of the 17D strain of yellow fever virus as a live virus vaccine (5).

Once a primary etiologic agent has been identified, its characterization with respect to epidemiologically relevant properties becomes an important objective. A first step is classification, because the agent may share properties with previously known agents of the same class. Demonstration that the Eaton agent (of primary atypical pneumonia) is a tiny bacterium of the mycoplasma group, rather than a virus, led to improved methods for agent detection and identification, further encouraged antibiotic therapy, and stimulated efforts to develop a specific vaccine (6). The crucial laboratory studies of poliomyelitis have already been discussed. In addition to providing a tool for virus detection, antibody tests, and vaccine production, the ready cultivability of polioviruses facilitated their antigenic characterization and important studies of host range and viability in the free state. Indeed, the tremendous strides made since 1950 in understanding and controlling poliomyelitis stem almost entirely from the key laboratory observations of Enders and his colleagues.

The laboratory also can aid in the study of the natural history of diseases, as can be abundantly illustrated for arboviruses. Whether we consider such long-known diseases as yellow fever, Russian Far East encephalitis, or Eastern equine encephalomyelitis, or relative newcomers such as Kyasanur Forest disease or Bolivian hemorrhagic fever, the central problem is to define the various components of the sylvatic cycle of the agent. Resolution of this problem must of course begin with field studies of the relative seasonal abundance of the vertebrate and invertebrate species present in areas of known viral activity. In the laboratory, blood and tissues of vertebrates and pools of arthropods collected in the field are studied for evidence, specific antibody or infective virus, that may implicate particular species in the reservoir mechanism.

Potentially even more meaningful is the study of live-caught vertebrates and arthropods. Vertebrates are tested for susceptibility to infection as measured by the development of viremia (appearance of virus in the blood). Unless viremia is sufficient in amount and duration that a blood-sucking arthropod could ingest an infective blood meal, the species under study can be excluded forthwith as a participant in the reservoir mechanism. Also, information as to antibody response and persistence after experimental infection is important to interpretation of sero-survey data. Arthropods are studied for their susceptibility to infection, the time required for them to become infectious ("extrinsic incubation period"), their efficiency in transmitting infection to susceptible vertebrates, and the time during which they remain infectious. Finally, when candidate vertebrate and invertebrate species have been identified, the laboratory is the site of the crucial tests that will prove beyond question that consecutive cycles of transmission in the candidate species are possible.

Although the story of sylvatic yellow fever in the Americas and in Africa is reasonably complete, important unresolved problems remain concerning other long-studied diseases, including St. Louis encephalitis and Eastern or Western equine encephalomyelitis. These problems include determining which mosquito and vertebrate species are maintaining the virus in each infected area and discovering the mechanism responsible for the annual reappearance of the virus. Postulated mechanisms include introduction by migrating birds, persistence of virus in hibernating mosquitoes or vertebrates (reptiles or bats), and recrudescent viremia in latently infected vertebrate hosts. Both of these latter possibilities may be best explored in the laboratory.

Another role of the laboratory is in development of methods for preventing or controlling disease, either by interfering with transmission or by enhancing host defenses. Allusion has already been made to the development of the 17D vaccine against yellow fever. During World War

II, epidemic typhus again became a disease of major importance, a situation which stimulated efforts to control the arthropod vector, the human body louse, and to develop a vaccine. A long series of laboratory studies, utilizing laboratory-reared louse colonies, culminated in a dusting powder containing long-acting DDT which could be applied simply, cheaply, and with ready acceptance to large population segments. This remedy passed its crucial field test in the historic epidemic in Naples in 1943 (7). Previous efforts to control civilian outbreaks had depended upon hot soapy showers for people and concurrent autoclaving of their clothing. Because the clothing usually underwent severe shrinkage, popular resistance to this form of louse control was great. In marked contrast, the DDT powder did not damage clothing and, since it gave immediate relief from louse biting, was eagerly sought and popularly referred to as "sleeping powder."

The demonstration by Herald Cox that *Rickettsia prowazekii* could be readily grown in chick embryo yolk sacs provided an abundant source of antigen which, after partial purification and formol inactivation, constituted an effective typhus vaccine (8). After preliminary trials in man to measure antibody response, the vaccine was employed routinely for the protection of military personnel. Passage in the chick embryo also resulted in a variant strain of *R. prowazekii* (strain E) which was shown to have reduced pathogenicity and virulence for laboratory animals and to induce specific resistance to experimental disease. These basic laboratory observations justified exploration of the safety and effectiveness of strain E as a live-rickettsia vaccine to protect man against typhus (9). The studies in man are described in a later section.

Occasionally, approaches to control and natural history are made simultaneously. Such might be the case when, as with elevated serum cholesterol, the relationship of a factor to a specific entity such as coronary artery disease is not clearly established. In this instance, laboratory studies have indicated that diets containing relatively high proportions of polyunsaturated fats may lead to reduction in serum cholesterol levels. Pilot tests of this as a possible preventive step have been under way for some time, and major field trials are in prospect (10). Resulting reduction in disease incidence would testify to the contribution by elevated serum cholesterol to the occurrence of coronary heart disease.

12-4   Experimental Epidemiology

General considerations   Experimental manipulation of populations, animal or human, has contributed significantly to understanding of disease occurrence. When applicable, this approach can provide a degree of support for causal relations greatly exceeding that afforded by associations demonstrated in observational studies. This advantage stems chiefly from the fact that subjects are assigned to experimental and control groups by some formal method of randomization. When the population to be sampled is fairly homogeneous (for example, of the same sex and within a specified age group), assignment to treatment groups can easily be made by using a table of random numbers. If the population is not homogeneous, an alternate design can be used to insure that the treatment groups are comparable with respect to such attributes as age, sex, or race. This involves dividing the population into subgroups homogeneous for the above attributes and sampling at random within each subgroup to determine individual assignments to the treatment groups.

The use of a formal method of randomization in forming experimental or treatment groups has three main advantages. Least important, it increases the likelihood that the groups will be comparable with respect to possibly important variables not taken into account in forming the groups. More important, it precludes possible prejudicial selection or assignment to treatment groups by the investigator. Of greatest importance, it allows the investigator to take full advantage of statistical tests of hypotheses and confidence intervals. He can make use of probability theory to arrive at statements of the IF . . . THEN type:

> IF *we take repeated pairs of samples from identical populations,* THEN *a difference this large or larger would result with a probability (or relative frequency) equal to P per cent.*

Such statements have maximum usefulness when groups are similar with respect to all factors (variables) except that under study. The likelihood of a false claim of significance can be controlled by our choice of level of significance, or P (let us say 1 per cent or $p < .01$). Our basic conclusion, then, is that the difference observed requires some explanation other than sampling error. The conclusion that it was causally related to the experimentally imposed factor is a matter of judgment, based in large part on factual knowledge of the problem under study, but also on whether the experiment was well designed and extraneous factors were adequately controlled. This aspect was discussed more fully in Chapter 8.

Use of animal models   Experimental epidemiology began with studies in populations of laboratory animals, using as models diseases of animals analogous to important diseases of man. These evolved first in Britain, where Topley and his colleagues were the principal exponents (11), and soon after in the United States with the work of L. T. Webster and associates at the Rockefeller Institute (12). In both countries the early work was done chiefly with mouse typhoid in mice and interest centered on the relative importance of certain environmental, host, and agent factors to the occurrence of infection and disease. Introduction of the agent into fully susceptible herds consistently resulted in epidemics which terminated with a small number of survivors. If new susceptibles were added at some regular rate (as would be the case in human populations), epidemics could be kept going or an endemic pattern established. The concept of herd immunity evolved when it became apparent that spread of the agent ceased when something less than 100 per cent of the herd had become immune. A point of difference between British and American workers, still unresolved, had to do with change in agent virulence as a factor in the evolution of epidemics. Webster's group utilized the possibility of selective inbreeding of mice to demonstrate that genetically determined resistance was directed against specific diseases or types of diseases (for example, viral encephalitis) rather than being general.

In more recent times airborne spread of infection has been studied. C. H. Andrewes of Britain, using young chicks and Newcastle disease virus, showed that spread of a respiratory infection requires very intimate contact between infected and susceptible individuals (13). Additional factors affecting airborne spread were studied by Schulman and Kilbourne, using mice and several strains of influenza A viruses (14). These included age (not important for infector mice, but older mice were more susceptible), postinfection immunity (solidly effective), immunity induced by killed vaccine (vaccinated mice were less susceptible to contact infection but, when infected, were good infectors), relative humidity (humidity under 50 per cent favors transmission), season, and virus strain. Table 12-1 presents data showing that transmission is reduced in the summer,

TABLE 12-1

Seasonal differences in contact transmission of influenza A2 virus infection in mice

ENVIRONMENTAL CONTROL	NO. MICE INFECTED/NO. EXPOSED	
	SUMMER	WINTER
Steam heat and room air air conditioner	1/120 (0.8%)	48/216 (22.2%)
Constant temperature (72°F) and relative humidity (50%)	109/320 (34.1%)	192/330 (58.2%)

Source: Adapted from *J. Exp. Med.* **118**:267, 1963.

even when temperature and humidity were kept constant. Of special interest, even though virus strains were equally infective and pathogenic for mice, they differed greatly in transmissibility by contact (see Table 12-2). Possibly because of their greater content of neuraminidase (enzyme

TABLE 12-2

Comparison of transmissibility of different strains of influenza virus

| VIRUS | INFECTOR MICE | | CONTACT MICE |
	PULMONARY VIRUS TITER, 48 HR*	LUNG LESIONS DAY 7†	NO. INFECTED (PER CENT)
Swine (S-15)	7.8	45	2/20 (10)
A_o(PR8)	7.5	42.5	1/20 (5)
A_o(NWS)	7.6	65	3/40 (7.5)
A_2(RI/5⁻)	6.8	2.5‡	6/20 (30)
A_2(Jap.305)	7.6	60	25/40 (62.5)
B (Lee)	6.9	20	1/20 (5)

*Mean of individual titrations, five animals in each group $\log_{10}$, EID_{50}.
†Extent of lung lesions (per cent), five animals in each group.
‡Lesion ($<25\%$ of lung) in one of five animals.
Source: Schulman, Jerome L. *J. Exp. Med.* **125**:481, 1967.

attacking mucoprotein), A2 strains were more abundantly shed (and more readily transmitted) by infected mice than were other strains.

A major problem of classical experimental epidemiology is in translating laboratory findings to natural disease occurrence, even in the same animal species. This problem was encountered by Howard Schneider, in extending observations made jointly with Webster, which suggest the existence of a dietary factor important to mouse resistance to mouse typhoid. Using genetically selected strains of mice (resistant, susceptible, and heterogeneous) and of the mouse typhoid organism (virulent, avirulent, and heterogeneous) in all nine possible combinations (see Figure 12-1), Schneider showed that the dietary factor contributed to resistance only when heterogeneous mice were challenged with heterogeneous organisms (15). Reasoning that both naturally occurring organisms and wild mice would be genetically heterogeneous, he inferred that the dietary factor would be of substantial importance in naturally occurring disease. When he put this to direct test (after a frustrating year spent in persuading wild mice to breed in captivity), he found that natural selection already had rendered all wild mice highly resistant.

Experiments with human populations Because translating observations made in animals to man poses an even more difficult problem, experiments involving human populations are of particular interest. When any significant risk to health exists, such experiments can be justified morally only after all possible tests in lower animals have been conducted, when the subjects involved are true volunteers who have been fully apprised of the risk, and when the importance of the problem and the promise

		HOST-GENOTYPE		
		Inbred, selected resistant	Random-bred, (outbred) nonselected	Inbred, selected susceptible
Pathogen-Genotype	Uniformly virulent	None	None	None
	Mixed virulent and avirulent	None	Demonstrable effect	None
	Uniformly avirulent	None	None	None

FIG. 12-1 The biological dimensions of the dietary effect in natural resistance to infection. (Howard A. Schneider. *J. Exper. Med.* **84**:320, 1946.)

of the anticipated results clearly outweigh the anticipated risk. When, as with infectious hepatitis, man is the only known susceptible host and no effective therapy exists, only limited and crucial experiments are justified. Working in a large institution for mentally retarded children where a particularly benign form of the disease was endemic, Krugman and co-workers (16) described the pattern of viremia and fecal excretion of virus in relation to the clinical manifestations of infectious hepatitis, as depicted in Figure 12-2. They also found that gamma globulin in appropriate

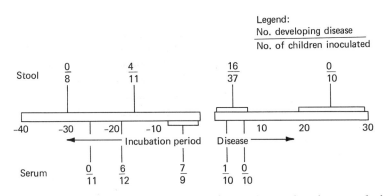

FIG. 12-2 Infectious hepatitis. Detection of virus in stool and serum during incubation period and disease. (Adapted from S. Krugman *et al. New Eng. J. Med.* **261**:729–734, 1959.)

dosage (0.02 ml/kg of body weight) protects against disease for about six weeks but does not prevent subclinical, immunizing infection, as shown in Figure 12-3 (17). Working with a much more benign disease, Andrewes and coworkers (18) used human volunteers to establish certain characteristics of the agents of the common cold, to study their transmission and also to test the importance of factors presumed to lower host resistance. One example of their findings apparently refuted a widely held belief; severe chilling (induced by sitting in a draft, wrapped in a wet sheet, and with feet in an ice water bath) failed to increase susceptibility to disease.

The testing and evaluation of vaccines or other preventive measures is the most common type of experimental study in man. Experience with the attenuated strain E of *Rickettsia prowazekii* as a vaccine to protect man against epidemic typhus illustrates the important phases of this problem. When the basic work in laboratory animals (described in a preceding section) had been completed, trials in man began with small pilot studies in laboratory personnel. These and later tests on prisoner volunteers, including placebo-inoculated controls, suggested the primary safety of

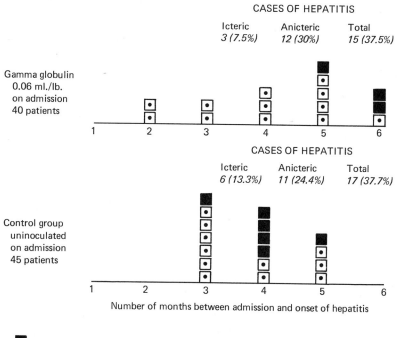

FIG. 12-3 Effect of gamma globulin on the incidence of icteric and anicteric hepatitis. Gamma globulin suppressed jaundice but did not prevent hepatitis infection. (From S. Krugman and R. Ward. *Yale J. Biol. Med.* **34**:329, 1961/2.)

TABLE 12-3

Persistence of complement fixing and neutralizing antibodies after immunization with strain E

NUMBER OF SERA WITH ANTIBODY TITERS OF 1:x FOR

INTERVAL POST-INOCULATION MONTHS	CF ANTIBODY*						NEUTRALIZING ANTIBODY						
	Total tested†	<2	2-4	8-16	32	64+	Total tested†	0	1-2	3-5	6-11	12-23	24+
2	114	21	8	36	28	21	28	1			6	7	15
6	108	11	13	53	16	15	27	1	3		12	6	5
12	83	64	4	13	1	1	44	1	1	8	17	10	7
24	44	26	13	2	3		40	1	6	13	6	7	7
36	25	18	6	1			24		1	3	12	5	3
48	22	18	4				22		2	2	8	9	1
60-66	13	8	2	3			13	1		1	3	8	

*Titers as measured with 2 units of antigen.
†Because a few volunteers were intermittently willing to be bled, because another few men were freed and later returned, and because the three New Orleans volunteers are included in the 60–66 month group, the volunteers observed differ slightly from interval to interval beyond the differences resulting from simple subtraction.

Source: Fox, J. P., Jordan, M. E., and Gelfand, H. M. J. Immun. 79:349, 1957.

TABLE 12-4

Summary of results observed after challenge infections with virulent *Rickettsia prowazekii* given to persons immunized with strain E or Cox-type vaccines and to normal controls

INTERVAL MONTHS	IMMUNI-ZATION	NUMBER OF VOLUNTEERS		NUMBER WITH CF TITERS* OF 1:x							
				PRE-CHALLENGE				MAXIMUM POST-CHALLENGE			
		TOTAL	FEBRILE	2	2–4	8–16	32+	2–4	8–16	32–64	128+
2–36	Strain E	28	(1)†	6	10	7	5	1	12	10	5
	Cox	6	3 (5)†	6						1	5
	control	10	10	10						4	6
48	Strain E	4	1‡	3	1				1	2	1‡
	control	2	2	2						1	1
60	Strain E	1	1‡	1							1‡
	control	3	2 (3)†	3						2	1
66	Strain E	3	(1)§	1		2					3
	control	3	3	3						1	2

*CF titers as measured with 2 units of antigen.
†Figures in parentheses include abortive febrile response, probably the result of challenge, but which did not require treatment.
‡Indicates men given strain E who failed to develop any detectable antibody after vaccination.
§Figure in parentheses is abortive febrile response, associated with respiratory infection on day 5.
Source: Fox, J. P., Jordan, M. E., and Gelfand, H. M. *J. Immun.* **79**:350, 1957.

strain E infection for man and demonstrated the effectiveness of infection in stimulating antibody response (19). As shown in Tables 12-3 and 12-4, continued observation of these volunteers for nearly six years with periodic challenge with virulent rickettsiae of small groups of vaccinated and control volunteers, testified to the persistence of both seroimmunity and resistance to challenge-induced disease. In these studies the availability of an effective antibiotic (tetracycline) for treatment made very small the risks associated with both primary safety testing and the later virulent challenges. The final step in this story was a study of much larger scale on primary safety and antibody response in the altiplano of Peru where typhus persists as a real disease threat (20). As shown in Table 12-5, larger doses of vaccine induced undesirable immediate reactions in all recipients and delayed reactions of unacceptable severity in some non-immunes. Fortunately, smaller doses (0.25 or 0.1 per cent yolk sac) were shown to be acceptably safe and (not shown) 95 per cent effective in inducing antibody response. As with the pilot studies, these more extended studies in the civilian population included the use of placebo-inoculated controls to measure the frequency of background illness that might be confused with reactions to the vaccine. A much larger and better-known example of a vaccine trial, that conducted by Francis to test the Salk polio vaccine, was described in Chapter 1.

Experiments with computer-simulated populations using stochastic models
Experimental epidemiologic studies also can be carried out by computer simulation of the spread of infection in arbitrarily designed populations. Many years ago, Reed and Frost developed a simple probability model for the study of epidemics of contact-transmitted disease. Parameters which could be varied included average number of effective contacts per case and proportion of susceptibles in the simulated population. Using a simple apparatus involving serial drawing of color-coded marbles (the population), a series of epidemics could be observed in order to determine the variation in epidemic sizes with various contact rates and original proportions of susceptibles (21). The advent of the computer, coupled with skillful programming, has tremendously facilitated the observation of such simulated epidemics.

In a recent series of studies, using appropriately modified extensions of the Reed–Frost model, Elveback and coworkers (22) have explored the effect of interference (transitory state induced by a viral infection in which the host is refractory to infection with heterologous viruses) when two competing viral agents are introduced into a population. The model can take account of differences in infectivity between the two agents and at various stages of infection with either virus (by adjusting contact rates), the duration of the refractory period as a result of interference can be adjusted and the proportions susceptible to either agent in the original population can be varied. Data based on several hundred simulated epidemics per change in variable suggest that in randomly mixing populations interference would have little influence on the size and course of epidemics under natural conditions, but that appropriate large-scale use of a live virus vaccine, for example, live poliovirus, would significantly curtail an outbreak from a heterologous enterovirus (of the coxsackie group, for example). Figure 12-4 presents the supporting data.

A more complex model has been developed to simulate the spread of infection in a community of families. The contact rate within households is taken to be high. Spread among small children is represented by exposure of preschoolers in the playgroup, and family clusters correspond

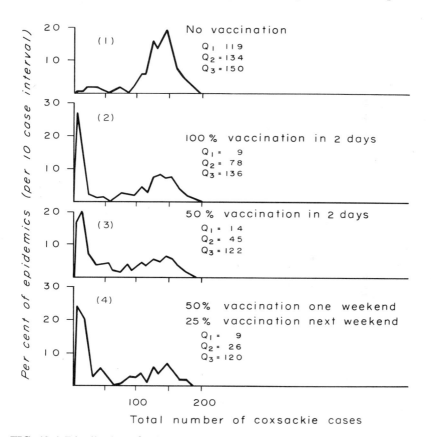

FIG. 12-4 Distribution of epidemic size for four vaccination schedules (population 400). Q_1, Q_2, Q_3 = first, second and third quartiles, respectively; in the trials with no vaccination, for example, 25 per cent of epidemics terminated with less than 119 cases, 50 per cent with less than 134 cases, and 75 per cent resulted in no more than 150 cases. (L. R. Elveback *et al.* A stochastic model for competition between viral agents in the presence of interference. 1. Live virus vaccine in a randomly mixing population, Model III. *Amer. J. Epidem.* **87**:373–384, 1968.)

TABLE 12-5

Summary of reactions in groups vaccinated with strain E in Peru

A. Immediate reactions

% CONCENTRATION OF STRAIN E YOLK SAC	No. OF PERSONS VACCINATED	PERCENTAGE OF VACCINATED PERSONS WITH REACTIONS							
		FEVER*	HEADACHE	NAUSEA	VOMITING	MALAISE	IN BED†	LOCAL REACTION 1+‡	LYMPH ADENITIS
10.0	101	64	71	17	7	61	7	54	42
1.0	951	30	49	9	3	29	2	30	21
0.25	252	5	23	1	1	14	1	29	14
0.1	955	5	17	2	1	8		7	7
Placebo	885	2	7	1	1	2		1	1

B. Delayed reactions (9–14 days after vaccination)

% Concentration of Strain E Yolk Sac	No. of Persons Vaccinated§	Percentage of vaccinated persons with reactions										
		Of all grades	Of grade‖			Of days duration			Fever	Head-ache	N or V**	In bed
			1	2	3	1–3	4–6	7 Plus				
10.0	83	20	7	10	4	8	2	10	7	19	4	4
1.0	754	29	21	8	1	15	10	4	10	29	3	1
0.25	121	19	12	6	1	12	6	1	3	18	1	1
0.1	724	26	19	6	1	12	11	3	5	25	3	1
Placebo	885	11	9	2		7	3	1	2	11	1	0

*Fever based on temperature readings in excess of 38°C or on history of "fever and chilliness."

†Confined to bed for at least one day.

‡Local reactions were graded on the size of the area of redness and swelling, an area of about 3 centimeters in diameter being graded as 1+. Persons immune prior to vaccination have been excluded except in the placebo controls, because virtually no delayed reactions occurred in such persons.

§Persons immune prior to vaccination have been excluded except in the placebo controls, because virtually no delayed reactions occurred in such persons.

‖Reactions roughly graded as follows: grade 1, headache alone for any duration (unless very intense) or fever and headache or other symptoms for less than 4 days; grade 2, intense headache alone, or other combinations of manifestations for 4 days or more; grade 3, more seriously ill, i.e., confined to bed for several days at home or in hospital.

**N or V = nausea or vomiting.

Source: Adapted from Fox, J. P., *et al.*, *Amer. J. Hyg.* **61**:191 and 193, 1955.

to contact between close neighbors. Older children are exposed in the grade school, which can be opened or closed at any point in the epidemic. This model was designed to study spread of infection in a suburban community of the United States. Still another model deals with the spread of infection through environmental contamination, as well as person-to-person contact, and is appropriate for studying the effectiveness of mass use of live poliovirus vaccine to combat a poliomyelitis epidemic in a population in which endemic infection with other interfering enteroviruses is widespread.

Natural experiments Finally, one cannot leave the realm of experimental epidemiology without noting that nature herself on occasion conducts fortuitous experiments which, if recognized as such, can provide invaluable information. The prototype of natural experiments, already described briefly in Chapter 2, was Snow's "Grand Experiment" conducted in London in 1854 in which he recognized that two randomly mixed populations, alike in other important repects, could be differentiated by the source of the water running from the taps in their individual

TABLE 12-6

Deaths from cholera per 10,000 houses and source of water supply of these houses, London 1853

SOURCE OF WATER SUPPLY	NUMBER OF HOUSES	DEATHS FROM CHOLERA	DEATHS IN EACH 10,000 HOUSES
Southwark and Vauxhall Company	40,046	1,263	315
Lambeth Company	26,107	98	37
Rest of London	256,423	1,422	59

Source: Snow on Cholera. New York: Commonwealth Fund, 1936, p. 86.

households (23). Snow's data are presented again in Table 12-6. The Lambeth water came from an intake on the Thames River well above London, whereas that of the Southwark and Vauxhall Company was from the sewage-polluted river basin. The great difference in the occurrence of cholera among these two populations afforded clear demonstration of the importance of water supply, even though the nature of the disease agent had not then been established.

In a less spectacular, but more recent, instance evidence for the value of BCG vaccine in combating tuberculosis was obtained in a Danish girls' school during World War II (24). A teacher with undetected open tuberculosis provided an unsuspected challenge exposure to more than 300 students who were nearly equally divided among three categories, tuberculin-negative, tuberculin-positive because of BCG, and tuberculin-positive because of prior natural infection. Examination of these children after the exposure was recognized revealed more than forty cases of tuberculosis among the tuberculin-negative children as compared with two and four cases, respectively, in the BCG and naturally tuberculin-positive groups (see Table 12-7).

TABLE 12-7

Efficacy of BCG vaccine in an epidemic of tuberculosis in a state school, Denmark 1943

PRE-EXPOSURE STATUS	NO. EXPOSED	NO. CASES TUBERCULOSIS	PER CENT
BCG Vaccine	106	2	1.9
Naturally tuberculin positive	105	4	3.8
Tuberculin negative	94	41	58.6

Source: Adapted from Tage V. Hyge. The efficacy of BCG vaccine. *Acta Tuberc. Scand.* **32**:106, 1956.

12-5   Epidemiologic Surveys and Surveillance

Underlying concepts   In this politically oriented age, the word "survey" calls to many minds Gallup or Roper and their public opinion polls. Although undertaken with rather different objectives, such polls do share one important aspect with many epidemiologic surveys. Just as it rarely is possible to query every member of a population regarding his political preference, so it is even more rarely possible to determine for every member of a population his status with respect to any particular disease or suspect determinant of disease. Instead, we must be satisfied with information concerning some sample of the population selected by known and appropriate methods. Our ability to generalize from the sample surveyed to the population under study depends on the care taken to insure that all members of the general population had a known and nonzero chance of being included in the sample. The untimely demise of the once widely circulated magazine, the *Literary Digest*, was directly attributable to its failure to observe the foregoing rule in attempting to predict the outcome of the 1932 presidential election. Opinions were sought from a randomly selected sample of telephone subscribers. At the depths of the Depression, nonsubscribers to telephone service constituted a large proportion of the population whose opinion, not sampled by the *Literary Digest*, determined the election of Franklin D. Roosevelt. Although the survey concept is very simple, its proper implementation, as indicated already in Chapter 8, requires familiarity with the theory and practice of sampling. Indeed, as will be emphasized again in subsequent sections, well-conceived sampling is important to all epidemiologic studies.

Epidemiologic surveys are undertaken when existing information concerning the interrelation between man and a disease agent or a suspected disease determinant is inadequate. The reasons for such inadequacy include previous lack of sensitive or specific diagnostic methods, the fact that the disease rarely requires medical attention (for example, the common cold), lack of official requirement for disease reporting, and incomplete compliance when such a requirement exists. Although surveys of factors indirectly determining disease occurrence are important, for example, type of housing, diet, smoking, distribution of suspect host and vector species, or extent of immunization, the following examples are limited to surveys of the impact of disease agents on man. Such impact may be reflected by evidence for current activity of the agent (disease or the presence of the agent) or for prior activity such as persisting specific antibody or dermal sensitivity (e.g., positive reaction to tuberculin) or the presence of characteristic disability (e.g., paralysis of poliomyelitis). Most such surveys fall into one or another of a few basic types. One special, continuing type, the National Health Survey of general morbidity in the United States, was described in Chapter 7.

Sero-surveys Surveys of seroimmunity (serologic epidemiology) are basic to the study of infectious diseases (25). Poliomyelitis provides an important example. Because of the great frequency with which poliovirus infection leads to inapparent or atypical disease, the occurrence of "characteristic" paralytic disease provides a highly misleading picture of the extent and pattern of human infection with polioviruses. A far different picture is revealed by the method of sero-survey which, in essence, consists of seeking the presence of poliovirus antibodies in the sera of an appropriately selected sample of the population. The most important outcome of sero-surveys of poliomyelitis was the demonstration of an apparent paradox in that paralytic disease is least frequent in populations which, on the basis of antibody prevalence, have experienced the most poliovirus infection. This problem was resolved when it was realized that early acquisition of infection (favored by abundant presence of virus) resulted in paralytic disease only infrequently. Thus infection was far more prevalent in areas with inadequate environmental sanitation, whereas disease was much more common and occurred at older ages in areas with good sanitation. Surveys of isolated population groups such as remote Eskimo communities in Alaska or the natives of Tahiti have revealed when particular polioviruses were last present and have provided strong evidence that poliovirus antibodies (and presumably immunity) are long enduring in the absence of reinfection. The age patterns of seroimmunity, in two Alaskan communities shown in Figure 12-5, make it clear that types 2, 1, and 3 polioviruses had been absent for about 20, 30, and 40 years, respectively, before the survey and that the antibodies detected had persisted over these periods without stimulation by reinfection (26).

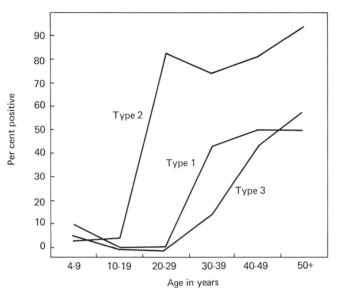

FIG. 12-5 Comparative age distributional rates at which neutralizing antibodies (as determined qualitatively) for three strains of poliomyelitis virus (types 1, 2 and 3) appeared in the population of two Eskimo villages (Barrow and Wainwright). (John R. Paul, John T. Riordan, and Joseph L. Melnick. *Amer. J. Hyg.* **54**:282, 1951.)

Sero-surveys also have contributed greatly to understanding the epidemiology of yellow fever. Examination of human sera collected in many parts of the world served to define the geographic distribution of yellow fever virus (restricted to Africa and South and Central America). Even more importantly, such studies revealed antibody to yellow fever virus in residents of large areas (the interior of Brazil and of central Africa) where the disease had not been recognized clinically and where the only vector then known, the *Aedes aegypti* mosquito, did not exist. These observations led to the recognition that yellow fever has a sylvatic cycle, the elucidation of which required further sero-surveys (this time of lower animals) to determine the important reservoir hosts.

Another use of the sero-survey relates to newly encountered agents potentially pathogenic for man. During intensive field studies of yellow fever and other arthropod-transmitted virus diseases more than 200 new arboviruses have been recovered and identified as distinct entities. For each new virus, the key questions are "Has it made contact with man?"

and, if so, "Does it cause disease?" Although systematic study of patients with undiagnosed infectious illness is the only way to answer the latter question, simple sero-surveys for antibody to a newly identified agent provide a direct way for discovering whether the agent has made contact with man. For many new arboviruses, no evidence for human contact exists. For others, such as the Ilheus virus, human infection has been established, but disease potential remains unknown. For still others, such as West Nile virus, widespread human infection has been documented and a variety of associated disease syndromes have been described (27).

Surveys of disease   Such degenerative diseases as diabetes or cancer of the cervix are well known in their advanced stages. However, more knowledge concerning their early stages is both desirable and now attainable, because of the recent availability of relatively simple and rapid screening methods for the detection of incipient disease. Heretofore, detection of incipient diabetes has required determining blood sugar levels before and at several intervals following a test meal taken after overnight fasting. Currently, early detection can be achieved by a rapid two-stage procedure amenable to mass application. A measured amount of a special corn syrup in a carbonated diluent is fed and two hours later a finger blood specimen is checked by an Auto Analyzer. One study using this method suggests that the prevalence of diabetes may be at least 3.9 per cent, rather than 1 per cent, in the United States population (28). In the case of cervical cancer, skilled microscopic examination of a properly stained smear from the cervix, as described by Papanicolaou, reliably detects disease in its earliest stages (29). Wide application of these methods is giving a far better picture of the pattern of occurrence of these two important diseases and thereby greatly increases the possibility for identifying and evaluating potential causative factors.

Another situation is exemplified by the emergence of previously known disease in unexpected circumstances or the emergence of heretofore unknown diseases. Although either situation calls for studies of many types, the first step is a survey of proven or presumed cases. Sero-surveys had revealed the past occurrence of infection with yellow fever in the absence of stegomyia mosquitoes, but they did not provide a reliable guide to current virus activity. To obtain this necessary information in Brazil, a unique form of disease survey (the viscerotomy program) was instituted. By means of a specially designed instrument, the viscerotome (see Figure 12-6), small pieces of liver were collected for histopathologic examination in all instances of death within ten days of onset of a febrile illness. This revealed the place and time of occurrence of fatal cases of yellow fever, most of which had not been diagnosed antemortem because of unavailability of medical care (30). In the more novel situation of the eruption of heretofore unknown diseases, for example, the several new hemorrhagic diseases in the Far East, Argentina, and Bolivia, search for the presumed

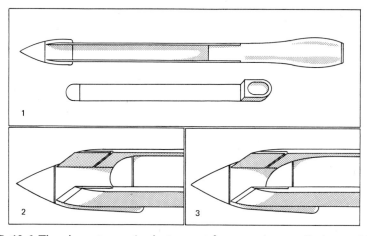

FIG. 12-6 The viscerotome. An instrument for removing small pieces of liver after death to search for fatal cases of yellow fever. (George K. Strode, ed., *Yellow Fever.* New York: McGraw-Hill, 1951.)

microbial agent has excited the greatest interest, but surveys to discover the extent and pattern of disease occurrence constituted the important first attacks on these problems.

Surveillance   As so far illustrated, surveys have been based on single observations of individuals and, with some exceptions (the National Health Survey and the yellow fever viscerotomy program), have been oriented to provide a cross-sectional, point-in-time look at the situation. Important additional information may be gained when population groups are subjected to continuing, or longitudinal, survey (surveillance). Such surveillance of family units has been particularly rewarding in the study of common infectious diseases. Early family studies in Great Britain (31) and in Cleveland (32) focused on common respiratory illness of undefined etiology (presumably largely caused by rhinoviruses) and measured the differences related to age or family status in the frequency of introduction of disease (highest for young school children) and in spread following introduction (young children also were the best spreaders). Later family studies have focused on detecting specific infections and possibly related disease. Observation of Louisiana families with newborn infants revealed the cyclic occurrence of infection with each poliovirus type (a periodicity of three to four years was suggested), the usual infection of all susceptible family members, and the frequent reinfection of those already immune when virus invaded the family; the study also permitted direct estimates of the pathogenicity of polioviruses (33). A more ambitious effort, the Virus Watch Program, was patterned after the Louisiana poliomyelitis study, but embraced all viruses infecting the respiratory or intestinal tracts (34). Analysis of the Virus Watch data for adenoviruses, as an example, provided a direct measure of pathogenicity (44 per cent of infections result in illness) and a description of the spectrum of clinical response, and also revealed the apparent existence of two classes of infection, one abortive and the other persistent and associated with prolonged intermittent virus excretion (35).

Since family studies of the types described above demand an unusual degree of cooperation from the family, the study group is formed by active recruitment of volunteer families and the extent to which it is representative of the population from which it was recruited must remain unknown. The Stuyvesant Town and Shelter Island populations in which the Virus Watch study was carried out were fairly homogeneous from an economic point of view, and nutritional deprivation and lack of medical care were not suspected to exist in any of the families. Differences in parental educational levels did undoubtedly exist, and this, as well as past occurrence of illness in the family, may have influenced the decision to participate in the study. It could be argued that the incidence rate of infection in the study group cannot be taken as an adequate estimate for that in the community as a whole or even in all families with young children. It is more difficult to advance reasons why response to infection, when it does occur in the volunteer families, should be unrepresentative of the response of infected persons of similar age and sex in general. For example, in the Virus Watch study families it was observed that the spectrum of disease response to adenovirus type 2 infections ranged from no detectable symptoms to full-blown acute respiratory disease. It is difficult to support an argument that the range of disease response might be more narrow in the total population. In the Louisiana study of poliomyelitis, the families were purposely recruited from three economic segments of the population for purposes of comparison. In general, in studies such as these the importance of the nonrandom selection of families must be assessed point by point in terms of the nature of the information in question, and it must be remembered that there is no other way of obtaining information on the general population. In terms of the conclusions from such studies stated above, the volunteer nature of the study groups does not detract from the importance of the information.

Chronic diseases also can be studied profitably by continuing surveillance, although extended periods of observation are required. The fact that the study population usually includes volunteers continues as a limiting factor but its importance is diminished when the population observed constitutes a large proportion of the total community. One notable example is the Tecumseh (Michigan) study, begun in 1959–1960, which succeeded in enrolling 8,641 residents (88 per cent of the community) in a long, continuing effort to describe the contribution of environmental and constitutional factors to the maintenance of health and origins of illness under natural circumstances of living. Variables so far explored have included smoking, blood pressure, serum levels of cholesterol and uric acid, age, sex, and family relationship as related to such disease states as cardiovascular disease, diabetes, gout and rheumatoid arthritis (36).

Another well-known, and older, study, focused on coronary heart disease (CHD), was begun in 1950 in Framingham, Massachusetts, then a town of 28,000 population containing 10,000 persons in the 30–59-year age range from which the study population was recruited. The study design called for taking a random sample of 6,500 within the desired age range which, it was hoped, would contain 5,000 persons free of CHD who could be followed for twenty years, during which time the disease would be expected to develop in about 1,500. As shown in Table 12-8, incomplete

TABLE 12-8
Derivation of Framingham study group

	TOTAL	MEN	WOMEN
Random sample	6,507	3,074	3,433
Respondents	4,469	2,024	2,445
Volunteers	740	312	428
Respondents free of CHD	4,393	1,975	2,418
Volunteers free of CHD	734	307	427
Total free of CHD	5,127	2,282	2,845

Source: Dawber, Thomas R., Kannel, William B., and Lyell, Lorna P. An approach to longitudinal studies in the community: The Framingham Study. *Ann. N.Y. Acad. Sci.* **107**:548, 1963. Copyright The New York Academy of Sciences 1963. Reprinted by permission.

response within the randomly selected sample forced the investigators to use volunteers to complete their study group. In retrospect, the investigators commented: "Since the major effort of the Framingham study involved within-group comparisons, it would appear that a great deal of unnecessary effort may have been expended in attempting to get a random sample of the Framingham population" (37). This study has contributed both to methodology (especially of data analysis) and to definition of important disease determinants or risk factors (elevated serum cholesterol, smoking, electrocardiogram abnormalities, and high blood pressure).

In the family and community surveillance studies just described, much effort and money were expended in forming and observing the study populations. It should be noted here that, in the normal course of rendering medical care to individuals on a continuing basis, much potentially useful information is recorded. Thus, examination of the medical records of a defined population would make possible surveillance of that population for many types of nonnotifiable but medically attended diseases. As noted in Chapter 7, in the section on morbidity statistics, the use of such records for surveillance is usually precluded because of their lack of centralization, that is, members of readily definable large populations such as communities customarily make use of many sources of medical care. It also was pointed out in Chapter 7 that, in important special situations, medical records for definable populations are centralized and constitute valuable resources for epidemiologic studies. One example cited is the population of Olmsted County, Minnesota, 95 per cent of which receives its medical care from either the Mayo Clinic or the Olmsted County Medical Group. Other examples are the large definable populations served by prepaid comprehensive medical care plans in larger metropolitan areas in the United States which, as with Group Health Cooperative of Puget Sound in Seattle, may constitute 10 per cent of the population of the metropolitan area.

12-6   Underlying Concepts in Analytic Studies

Latin scholars will remember the opening sentence of Caesar's *Gallic Wars*: "All Gaul is divided into three parts." Unlike Caesar, we must view our Gaul (our population) as divided into four, rather than three, parts as we examine the relation between a suspect disease determinant such as smoking and a disease such as lung cancer or coronary heart disease. This division results from classifying each member of the population on both variables, that is, smoker or nonsmoker and diseased or not diseased. If smoking does in fact contribute to the disease, we should find significantly more disease among smokers than nonsmokers. Such a cross-sectional study of a whole population is rarely feasible or efficient and, in practice, we select samples of the population for comparative study. The basis of sampling and the nature of the resulting evidence for association between determinant and disease depend on whether we wish to look backward or forward. In the backward-looking (retrospective or "case-history") approach, we sample on the basis of the presence or absence of disease and association is indicated if we find that a significantly greater proportion of diseased persons are exposed (for example, smokers) than of persons free from disease. In the forward-looking (prospective or "cohort") approach, our sampling is based on exposure to the determinant and association is indicated if we observe that disease develops with significantly greater frequency among those exposed (for example, smokers) than among those unexposed. However, in both types of study the purpose is to answer the question, "Does exposure to factor X increase the risk of development of disease D?"

The prospective study seeks to answer this question by providing direct estimates of the risk of developing disease in an exposed group and in an unexposed group with otherwise similar characteristics. Both groups are followed through time (weeks, months, or years) and the development of the disease is noted. The final comparison is made in terms of the observed incidence rates of disease D in the two groups. Three basic difficulties tend to limit the use of the prospective approach. First, it may be difficult to identify the two populations to be sampled. How, for example, does one identify all smokers and nonsmokers in a large population? One approach that has been used is to select a single population sample within desired age and sex limits (the method of sampling is crucial) and establish eligibility for either group by interrogation (interview or questionnaire), hopefully with few misclassifications. This approach is not efficient, however, if the proportion eligible for either group is very small, for example, adults who have never had measles. Second, the time required for follow-up may be very long when the study concerns a chronic disease. Not only may the investigator who initiates the study fail to answer his question within his lifetime, but study members may move away from easy observation. Thus, institutions with long life expectancy must sponsor long-term studies and strenuous efforts to track down mobile study members may be necessary. Finally, both the original sampling effort and the long period of follow-up mean that prospective studies may be very expensive.

In retrospective studies the original question is transformed to the indirect form: "Is the frequency of prior exposure to factor X greater in the diseased than in the nondiseased?" Despite its indirectness, and because it avoids some of the difficulties described above, the retrospective study is often the method of choice, particularly as a first step. It requires identification of a population with disease and an appropriate control group free of disease. Often the disease group is selected without sampling, for example, all cases of the disease seen during a specified period in a given clinic or hospital. Selection of a proper control group, however, is a common source of difficulty. The commonly stated requirement that the control group be similar to the disease group "with respect to all factors other than that under study" is nearly impossible to fulfill. A more realistic requirement would read "with respect to those factors other than that under study which are known or may reasonably be expected to influence occurrence of the disease." The final list of matching factors might include age, sex, race, residence, income level, presence or absence of some other disease, and some aspect of family history. The next step is to identify and sample an appropriate group by use of a clearly stated rule. If the disease group is from a given hospital, matching control(s) for each case can be chosen from the admission list as the next person(s) free of the disease and resembling the case with respect to age, sex, and the other specified matching factors. It must be emphasized that matching variables are eliminated from study and that only a relatively few matching variables can be used successfully, unless the supply of eligible controls is unusually large.

Retrospective studies have been discussed after prospective studies in order to stress the indirectness of the retrospective method. However, in practice the initial approach is usually retrospective. Only after it becomes fairly evident that there is a higher exposure rate in the diseased group is the more difficult prospective study undertaken to establish beyond reasonable doubt that the incidence rate of disease is higher in the exposed group.

12-7   Looking Backward—the Retrospective (Case-History) Approach

Clinical impressions   Any epidemiologic study begins with the realization that knowledge concerning causation is incomplete. Having checked off the most obvious gaps in knowledge by reviewing the available literature, the scientist's common early step is to collect a group of reliably diagnosed patients and review their histories in search of commonly shared exposures or characteristics. In practice, this review may be motivated by little more than a "clinical impression." As the pioneer chest surgeons in St. Louis (Evarts Graham, and colleagues) grew bold enough to remove a whole lung or a segment thereof from patients with lung cancer, their services were increasingly sought and they were soon struck by the great frequency of heavy cigarette smoking among victims of that disease (38). In a similar way, as noted in Chapter 1, the Australian ophthalmologist Gregg became aware of an unusual frequency of congenital cataracts in children born during a particular period whose mothers had in common experiencing of German measles (rubella) during the period of gestation of the affected child (39). A necessary but unstated part of such "clinical impressions" is the assumption that the factor suspected, heavy smoking or rubella during pregnancy, has operated with greater frequency or greater intensity within the patient group than within their peers among the general population.

Formal retrospective studies   Design of a formal retrospective study involves defining a patient group with the disease and a comparison group free from the disease, but coming from the same general population segment as the patient group. In lung cancer studies, in which matching was employed in selecting the control group, the matching variables have included age, sex, and urban or rural residence. Sex and residence are of particular importance, because smoking patterns are known to vary with them; smoking is more common among males than females and among urban than rural residents. Hence, unless comparability with respect to these factors is assured, differences in sex and residence, rather than the presence or absence of disease, might explain differences observed in smoking pattern.

More than twenty groups of investigators in eight different countries have conducted retrospective studies of the relation between smoking and lung cancer. One of the best was conducted by Doll and Hill in Great Britain (40). For each of more than 1,400 hospitalized lung cancer patients studied, these workers selected as a matching control the first patient on the ward lists of the same sex, in the same five-year age group, and with a diagnosis other than cancer. One analysis of their data is presented in Table 12-9 in which, for both men and women, the distribution of cancer patients by daily cigarette consumption differs markedly from that of the controls. The basic observation of this and the other studies, now widely publicized, was that lung cancer patients included a much higher proportion of heavy cigarette smokers than did the control groups studied.

TABLE 12-9

Most recent amount of tobacco* smoked regularly before onset of the admitting illness, by lung cancer patients and matched control patients with other diseases

Sex	Disease Group	No. of Patients	Per cent of patients smoking indicated number of cigarettes daily					
			0	1–4	5–14	15–24	25–49	50+
Male	Cancer	1,357	0.5	3.6	38.0	32.8	22.0	3.0
	control	1,357	4.5	6.7	45.0	30.1	11.9	1.5
Female	Cancer	108	37.0	13.0	27.8	11.1	11.1	0
	control	108	54.6	16.7	20.4	7.4	0.9	0

*Includes pipes and cigars converted to "cigarette equivalents."
Source: Adapted from Richard Doll and A. Bradford Hill, A study of the aetiology of carcinoma of the lung. *Brit. Med. J.* **2**:1271–1286, 1952.

The backward look in studies of congenital cataracts and lung cancer revealed rubella virus and some component(s) of cigarette smoke as presumptive primary causal agents. With paralytic poliomyelitis, the agent was described by Landsteiner in 1909 but, with the realization that paralytic disease was an extremely infrequent outcome of infection, the search began for other factors which helped determine that a particular infection would cause paralysis. Numerous retrospective studies served to identify recent tonsillectomy, various inoculation procedures, and pregnancy as important factors predisposing to paralytic disease. In a particularly well-designed study by Hill and Knowlden (41), careful histories of all inoculation procedures were obtained for the thirty-day period preceding disease onset in patients with paralytic polio and in a carefully matched group of nonpatients. Matching was based on age, sex, and proximity of residence to the corresponding patient. This study confirmed a previous clinical impression that inoculation provoked paralytic disease and also drew attention to the greater importance of more irritating inocula and to the common correspondence between site of inoculation and the limb first paralyzed.

Estimation of risk   Although the retrospective approach permits direct estimation only of the frequency of exposure (exposure rate) to suspect disease determinants in diseased and nondiseased groups, these exposure rates may be used in some instances to estimate approximately the relative risk associated with exposure. One example is provided by Doll and Hill (40) who used the data obtained for residents of Greater London to estimate the death rates from lung cancer associated with different levels of smoking. Their estimates were based on three assumptions: (1) that the smoking habits of the control group were, for each age and sex, typical for all residents (because the controls were hospitalized patients with other disease to which smoking may have contributed, this is a

TABLE 12-10

Estimated annual death rates from lung cancer per 1,000 men and per 1,000 women living in Greater London: by age-group and average amount of tobacco smoked daily in preceding ten years

		ANNUAL DEATH RATE PER 1,000 PERSONS					
SEX AND AGE	NON SMOKERS	AVERAGE AMOUNT SMOKED DAILY IN PRECEDING TEN YEARS					NO. OF LUNG CARCINOMA PATIENTS INTERVIEWED
		Less than 5 cigs.	*5 cigs.—*	*15 cigs.—*	*25 cigs.—*	*50 cigs.+*	
Men							
25–	*0.00**	*0.03*	0.13	0.12	0.17	*0.52*	61
45–	*0.14*	0.59	1.35	1.67	2.95	4.74	539
65–74	0.00	2.38	2.66	3.88	6.95	*10.24*	130
Women							
25–	*0.006*	*0.04*	*0.03*	*0.13*		—	9
45–	0.09	*0.06*	0.34	1.19		—	39
65–74	0.32	*0.70*	0.59	2.37		—	13

*Rates based on observation of fewer than five cases of carcinoma of the lung are given in italics.

Source: Richard Doll, and A. Bradford Hill. A study of the aetiology of carcinoma of the lung. *Brit. Med. J.* 2:1271–1286, 1952. Reprinted from the *British Medical Journal*, 1952, **2**, 1271–1286, by permission of the authors and editor.

particularly questionable assumption); (2) that the smoking habits of the lung cancer patients interviewed were typical for all residents dying of the disease during the survey period; and (3) that the deaths attributed by the Registrar-General to lung cancer provided a reasonable estimate of the true number of such deaths (this assumes high average accuracy of diagnosis). Table 12-10 shows their estimates of annual death rates from lung cancer per 1,000 population by age, sex, and level of smoking, using the population of Greater London given by the Registrar-General for June 30, 1950. The numerators for these rates were obtained by distributing the lung cancer deaths reported in a given age–sex group by smoking level according to the proportions observed in the corresponding age–sex group of interviewed lung cancer patients; the denominators were formed from the corresponding age–sex groups of the general population in the same way, but using the proportions in each smoking level observed in the controls. The data for the 45–64 year age group were regarded as the most reliable, since this group contained the greatest number of lung cancer patients. As plotted in Figure 12-7, these data suggest that the death rate for men increases in direct proportion to the number of cigarettes smoked (the estimates for women, based on a smaller number of deaths, were regarded as less reliable).

Frequently it is not possible to estimate the two risks themselves (that

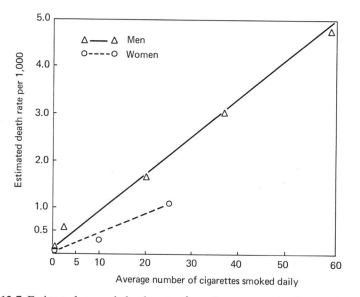

FIG. 12-7 Estimated annual death rates from lung cancer in Greater London for men and for women aged 45 to 64, in relation to the average amount of tobacco smoked daily (measured in terms of cigarettes) in the preceding ten years. (Richard Doll and A. Bradford Hill. *Brit. Med. J.* **2**:1278, 1952.) Reprinted by permission of the authors and editor.

is, for the exposed and unexposed populations) by applying exposure rates to a defined population, as was done in the foregoing example. However, given certain circumstances, one may still obtain an approximation of their ratio or the *relative risk* (ratio of disease prevalence rates in the exposed and unexposed portions of the population) by calculating the *odds ratio* estimate, as shown below. The general distribution of the study populations is summarized in a fourfold table with respect to disease (D), nondisease (d), exposure to the suspect factor (F) and no exposure (f).

	EXPOSED	UNEXPOSED
Disease group	n_{FD}	n_{fD}
Control group	n_{Fd}	n_{fd}

$$\text{The } odds\ ratio = \frac{n_{FD} \times n_{fd.}}{n_{fD} \times n_{Fd}}$$

If the disease is rare (e.g., lung cancer) and the exposure is common (e.g., smoking), if the bias introduced by using only those alive in the disease group is negligible, and if the exposure rate in the disease group reflects that of all cases in the population (the process of selection might have resulted in an unrepresentative group of patients), the odds ratio will be an adequate approximation of the relative risk. Woolf (42), in discussing a study of the relationship of peptic ulcer to blood group, gives the following data for London.

	GROUP O	GROUP A
Peptic ulcer patients	911	579
Control group	4578	4219

He estimated the ratio of risks as $911 \times 4219/579 \times 4578 = 1.45$, that is, of ulcer prevalence in Group O persons to that in Group A. In most applications of the odds ratio estimate the problem is complicated by the need to adjust for differences between the disease and control groups in age, sex, and other variables. For this more complicated procedure, the reader is referred to a paper by Mantel and Haenszel (43).

Advantages and limitations of retrospective studies   The backward look in epidemiologic research has important advantages to commend it. Except for studies of relatively rare diseases in which a long time may be needed to collect cases, both the patient and control groups can be chosen fairly quickly. Because of this, and because information concerning exposure to suspect factors can be quickly obtained in most cases, results are usually rapidly available. Finally, retrospective studies are often quite inexpensive.

Of course, limitations of the method must be recognized. These include the possibility of several important sources of bias. The common restriction of the disease group to patients of one clinic or hospital may lead to selection of patients with a particular form or severity of the disease or differing otherwise (for example, by race or social class) from all patients with the disease. The equally common practice of forming the control group from patients with other diseases (to which the suspect determinant may also have contributed) entails the additional risk of overestimating the prevalence of exposure among all comparable persons free of the disease. Often, as when ascertaining smoking or other personal habits, studies are limited to persons still living with the disease. The amount of bias so introduced is unknown but may be large when, as with coronary heart disease, many attacks are fatal. A study of the relation of smoking to Parkinson's disease (PD) suggests how bias arising from the latter two practices may lead to a spurious association. The study groups were formed from 198 living PD patients in Veterans Administration hospitals and 198 matched control patients. Significantly more control patients than PD patients were smokers. The investigators suggest two explanations for this finding: (1) a high proportion (45 per cent) of the control patients had been admitted for diseases (lung cancer, ulcer, heart disease, and so on) to which smoking is believed to contribute; and (2) mortality from other diseases caused by smoking may have selectively reduced the number of living PD patients who do smoke (44). Still another source of bias exists when the information concerning exposure is not a matter of record and must be obtained by interview. Information so obtained is subject to errors resulting from memory failure (which increases with the time span covered) or to faulty interpretation of the questions by the persons interviewed and of the answers by the interviewer.

Finally, although indirect estimates of relative risk may be possible, the retrospective approach does not permit a direct estimate of the contribution to disease occurrence made by the suspect factor. Direct answers cannot be given to such questions as "How much does smoking increase the likelihood that I will get lung cancer?" or, the most pressing question for the expectant mother suffering from German measles, "What is the probability that my baby will suffer from a serious defect?" Although the limitations just outlined are substantial, their existence should not diminish the importance of the method of looking backward. As illustrated in the stories of lung cancer and congenital cataracts, this method often constitutes the vital first step in resolving major disease problems.

12-8   The Prospective (Cohort) Approach

Study design   Having found that heavy cigarette smoking is significantly more common among lung cancer patients than among comparable non-patients, we face the problem of obtaining a direct estimate of just how much cigarette smoking does increase the risk of developing lung cancer. The basic method is to observe how frequently the disease develops in otherwise comparable groups of smokers and nonsmokers formed from presently healthy persons. The key features of the design of such a prospective study are: (1) choice for study of population segments which, on the basis of existing knowledge, will efficiently reflect any real difference in disease occurrence (males thirty-five years and older would be indicated for lung cancer); (2) use of appropriate sampling procedures in selecting exposed and unexposed groups so that the results can be generalized to the population sampled and also to maximize the comparability of the study groups with respect to possibly important variables other than those under study; (3) availability of reliable methods for recognizing disease when it develops: and (4) provision for continuing observation for whatever period may be required.

Comparability of study groups   One approach to maximizing comparability of the population samples to be studied is to use the method of matching, essentially as described for retrospective studies. One type of example could be the influence of some potentially adverse factor (e.g., rubella) on the outcome of pregnancy. In this example we would select within the total population of pregnant women, seeking first those who had been subjected to the suspect influence and, for each exposed woman found, further seeking one or more unexposed women in the same stage of pregnancy, of the same age, parity, social class, race, and area of residence and, perhaps, attending the same prenatal clinic. The choice of variables is dictated by their known or reasonably possible association with abnormal outcome. With such matching, any excess in fetal Joss or other abnormal outcome of pregnancy might be attributed to the suspect influence; the frequency of such outcome could further be related to the stage of gestation when exposure occurred.

An alternative to matching, when the population samples are large enough to warrant it, is to use adjustment procedures (as described in Chapter 7 for age, race, and sex) to take account of differences resulting from important other variables. Rates for disease occurrence in subgroups of the control population, defined by age, sex, and other variables considered important, are applied to the corresponding subgroups of the exposed population to determine how much disease would be "expected" in the absence of exposure. The ratio of disease (morbidity or mortality) observed to that "expected" then provides a measure of the effect of the factor under study. Based on data from the study by Dorn (45) of United States military veterans, the design of which is described in the following section, mortality ratios were employed to visualize the influence on deaths from all causes of different methods and levels of smoking, as shown in Figure 12-8. Mortality of those who never smoked was taken as 1.0. Current consumption of twenty or more cigarettes per day was associated with obvious excess mortality and the ratio approached 2.0

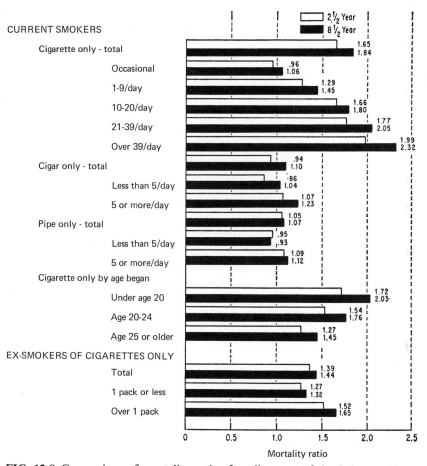

FIG. 12-8 Comparison of mortality ratios for all causes of death by smoking category—2½- and 8½-year follow-up. (Harold A. Kahn. The Dorn study of smoking and mortality among U.S. veterans: Report on eight and one-half years of observation. National Cancer Institute Monograph 19: *Epidemiological Approaches to the Study of Cancer and Other Chronic Diseases.*)

with two or more packs daily after 2½ years of follow-up and reached 2.3 when follow-up was extended to 8½ years. Little or no effect can be seen when smoking was restricted to pipes or cigars.

The representativeness of study groups   The requirement that the exposed and unexposed samples to be studied be representative of the corresponding segments of the general population sampled poses another problem. Theoretically, we could identify each member of the population, characterize him as exposed or not, and then choose a sample from each segment on a random basis. The practical difficulty of locating and interrogating every member of a large population usually precludes this approach. Although very large proportions of the populations of the communities were both identified and brought under observation in the Tecumseh and Framingham studies described in the section on Surveillance, both study communities were of only modest size.

A more feasible approach would be to draw a single sample from a broad segment of the population in which disease is known to occur and, on the basis of information subsequently developed, break it into the desired comparison groups for continuing observation. This conceptual approach was employed by Hammond and Horn who, under the aegis of the American Cancer Society, sought to study the relation of smoking to lung cancer in a large sample of the white male population of the United States in the 50–69-year age group (46). These investigators recruited 22,000 volunteer workers for their field staff, each of whom was instructed to choose ten eligible men whom she knew well and would be able to trace and whom she could induce to complete a questionnaire on smoking habits. As the basis for follow-up, the volunteers were asked to report each year deaths that had occurred in her group. For each death, the corresponding death certificate was obtained and, whenever cancer was mentioned, further information was sought from the physician, hospital, or tumor registry. Although relatively inexpensive and very successful in recruiting the desired large sample, this study is open to serious criticism because of the impossibility of precisely defining the sampling method used (each of the 22,000 volunteers recruited her study subjects in her own unspecified way). Because of this defect, the validity of the results cannot be properly assessed.*

The drawing of probability samples from large civilian populations is so difficult and costly that few prospective studies attempt it. An alternative is to study large specialized populations for which an accurate listing of the members exists. This was the case with two other well-known studies of smoking and lung cancer in which the investigators sought to use entire populations defined by profession or former military service. Doll and Hill, in an effort to assure comparability with respect to other important factors and to subsequent detection of disease, recruited their sample from a specialized and highly homogeneous population, namely British physicians thirty-five years of age or older (48, 49). Their basic

---

*In 1959 Hammond initiated a new and much larger study of the relation of smoking to health based on the continuing observation of more than a million men and women representing virtually all segments of the population (47). This time 68,116 volunteers were used, their selection being governed by their access to specific population segments. Each volunteer was asked to enroll ten families, each with at least one person over the age of forty-five, and then request all members of these families over the age of thirty to fill out a confidential questionnaire. Once again, follow-up was based on deaths as ascertained by annual checking of the enrolled families. Although subject to the same basic criticism as the earlier study of older men, this new study offers greater possibilities for comparisons between sizeable population segments defined by age, sex, urban or rural residence, and other attributes with respect to the relation between smoking and mortality experience.

method involved a mailed questionnaire concerning smoking habits, to which a disappointingly low proportion (66 per cent) replied, and a follow-up based on systematic notifications of physicians' deaths from the Registrar-General, the General Medical Council, and the British Medical Association, supplemented by further information from the physicians who certified the deaths. Perhaps the best study was that conducted by Dorn who utilized United States Government life insurance policy holders as his study group and, like Doll and Hill, depended on a mailed questionnaire to elicit smoking history (45). Two mailings resulted in nearly 250,000 usable replies, about 85 per cent of the population covered in the study. Follow-up in this instance was particularly simple and efficient, death certificates and supplementary information being obtained through the Veterans Administration.

The three prospective lung cancer studies here described were alike in that the sample populations could be formed into several comparison groups based on the fact, type, amount, and duration of smoking and, for former smokers, the time elapsed since stopping. Thus, in all three studies, account could be taken of both the fact and degree of exposure as reflected in the manner, amount, and duration of smoking. The clear and consistent relation between degree of exposure and risk and the indication of decreasing risk with increasing time since exposure was terminated go well beyond simple association between smoking and excess lung cancer mortality in supporting the commonly held conviction that cigarette smoking is a major cause of lung cancer.

Recognition of disease   So far we have ignored the problem of the reliability and completeness of disease recognition, which vary substantially with the specific disease in question. This can be illustrated readily within the framework of exploring the influence of smoking on health. It should be noted that the three prospective studies cited for their observations relating to lung cancer also examined the relation of smoking to many other specific causes of death and to death from all causes. Because lung cancer is almost always lethal, and rather rapidly so at that, detection of disease in the study groups could be left with reasonable confidence to a scrutiny of deaths, the recording of which in the three studies was essentially 100 per cent. Proper assignment of the cause of death could be made for lung cancer with great reliability when tumor tissue from biopsy or postmortem could be examined microscopically and, without such confirmation, fairly confident diagnosis could be made from chest X ray. Our principal problem, hence, rests chiefly with deaths that occurred without adequate medical attendance. The extreme disability caused by lung cancer prior to death makes it very unlikely that patients would die without having had medical attendance.

Use of mortality data, as in the three studies cited, to reflect the relation between smoking and coronary heart disease is less satisfactory than with lung cancer, for two main reasons. First, the possibility of inaccurate assignment of cause of death is increased by the fact that death not infrequently occurs with such suddenness that the terminal illness was not medically attended. Second, even properly assigned heart disease deaths only partially reflect the total disease occurrence, because many persons with heart disease die of other causes or have one or more attacks prior to that which results in death. These difficulties may not be too serious if we can safely assume that the ratio between deaths assigned to coronary heart disease and the true existence of disease is the same in each of the comparison groups.

Length of observation   The foregoing studies also are of interest with respect to the possibility of and the need for prolonged observation. The possibility for maintaining observation indefinitely is greatest for the Doll and Hill and the Dorn studies, because the nature of the study groups is such that few deaths will go undetected. However both the original Hammond and Horn study and the more recent larger study by Hammond also have the possibility for long-continued, effective observation. Relatively prolonged periods of smoking are presumably required to influence the occurrence of diseases such as lung cancer and emphysema, if not coronary heart disease. Because many of the smokers included in these studies had already been exposed for extended periods of time, all yielded data of interest after only a few years of observation. However, as the data from the Dorn study presented in Figure 12-8 indicate, extension of observation from $2\frac{1}{2}$ to $8\frac{1}{2}$ years resulted in a consistent increase for smokers of all classes in mortality ratios for all causes of death and, hence, in an increased (and probably more accurate) estimate of the over-all risk attributable to smoking. Such extension of observation also should result in more reliable estimates of the contribution of smoking to deaths attributable to specific diseases, particularly to those of lesser frequency. In the Framingham and Tecumseh studies the factors of interest are numerous and, presumably, have come into play at differing stages in life. Hence, it can hardly be assumed for any of these studies that continuation of observation will yield no new information although, obviously, this yield will decrease progressively with time.

Fortunately, many worthwhile prospective studies do not require long periods of observation. Most infections are of fairly short duration and their outcome is soon evident. Thus, in evaluating the pathogenic potential of specific infectious agents, individual infected persons, once identified, need be observed for only a few weeks. Also, observation in studies of the abnormal outcome of pregnancy need continue beyond termination of pregnancy only for a time sufficient to insure that all significant congenital defects will have been detected.

Follow-up of previously existing populations   Even when a disease requires a long time to develop, prospective studies can sometimes be conducted without a lengthy period of waiting for disease to occur. To do this requires finding a population that existed at some time in the past and whose subsequent experience can be traced to the present.* Finding and exploiting such populations may require both great good fortune and great ingenuity. The information concerning exposure must be a matter of record, so that the exposed and unexposed members of the population can be identified. Although it obviously would be helpful if the subsequent occurrence of disease were also a matter of record, this is not essential if there is some method for *follow-up*. Obvious candidate populations for such study include life insurance policy holders, certain industrial groups, and members of the armed forces, for all of whom health histories are taken and physical examinations made at time of entrance into the candidate population. For life insurance policy holders and military personnel, through the Veterans Administration and government insurance policy records, follow-up of mortality experience is relatively simple. Even morbidity experience for some diseases can be ascertained for military veterans on the basis of utilization of veterans' hospitals. Other possible populations include organized professional groups such as physicians, members of large medical care plans such as the Health Insurance Plan of Greater New York, and college students. Follow-up of students is particularly possible because colleges and universities, with mercenary motivation, make a continuing effort to keep track of their alumni.

The utility of previously existing populations is governed by the extent to which information concerning exposure was originally elicited and subsequently retained. Among life insurance policy holders, for example, one should be able to explore the relation between obesity or blood pressure and coronary heart disease mortality and, possibly, to demonstrate familial predisposition to disease. Studies of physicians' groups have yielded important information concerning the relation between professional exposure to irradiation and the incidence of leukemia. Finally, the membership of a large medical care plan should afford excellent opportunities for identifying populations of many types including, as one example, pregnant women who could be followed through records with respect to the outcome of their pregnancies.

Advantages and limitations   An effort has been made in the foregoing sections to point out the advantages and limitations of prospective studies, but a brief recapitulation may be helpful. The advantages are indeed

---

*Follow-up studies in a previously existing general population are rendered impractical by two problems which, as noted on pp. 292–93, also affect follow-ups in long continuing studies of present populations. These problems are population mobility and, for any given individual, the multiplicity and geographic diversity of records containing relevant health information from birth to death. An NCHS report (Vital and Health Statistics, Ser. 4, No. 7, March, 1968) stresses the need for improved methods of *record linkage* as a partial solution to these problems and provides an excellent selected bibliography on the subject.

important. Disease occurrence can be expressed as incidence rates and the difference between rates in exposed and unexposed groups provides a direct measure of the risk attributable to exposure to the suspect disease determinant. Since the comparison groups are formed before disease develops, certain forms of bias can be minimized. Information concerning exposure is usually current at the time elicited and so is less subject to misclassification. One important limiting factor is the difficulty of selecting comparison groups which are representative of the exposed and unexposed segments of a general population. The common use of nonrepresentative but available populations means that, technically, the results obtained relate only to the population studied and their generalization to wider populations becomes a matter of epidemiologic or biologic (not statistical) judgment. It is reasonable, for example, to assume that, if smoking is bad for physicians, it also is bad for nonphysicians. The other principal drawbacks relate to studies (chiefly of chronic diseases) involving large numbers of people followed over long periods of time. These are usually very costly. The time may be so long that no single investigator can reasonably expect to see them to their conclusion. Also, at least within the United States, population mobility is such that tracing study members for continued observation may become very difficult. Use of previously existing populations affords a way to reduce both the cost and the time required in the study of some problems.

12-9 Association and Causation

This chapter must be concluded by reminding ourselves that significant association, though essential to, does not imply a biological cause-and-effect relationship, because there may be an unsuspected third factor (or set of factors) which constitutes the bridge between the conditions shown to be associated. One example of this is endemic goiter, the frequency of which increases with altitude. The bridge in this case is iodine content in the food; goiters result from low iodine content which, in turn, is more frequent at high altitude. The most convincing evidence for a causal relation comes from association demonstrated experimentally that can be reproduced in succeeding experiments.

Unfortunately, in many instances of suspected causal relations meaningful experimentation is very difficult or even impossible. For example, the role of viruses in inducing cancers of various types in man is regarded as highly probable, because by experimentation we are able to show beyond question that specific viruses do induce analogous cancers in experimental animals. So far no specific virus has been meaningfully related to any human cancer. However, even when it becomes possible to show association between a viral infection and the development of cancer in man, the direct experiment (deliberate induction of cancer in man) remains unthinkable. Although the indirect experiment, perhaps prevention by a specific vaccine, is not precluded, the results would be available only after some time. As another example, the problem of possible genetic contributions to human disease can be attacked only by a search for associations in observational studies, at least in the light of our present knowledge.

The pressing problem of the relation of smoking to health, which has been abundantly illustrated in previous sections, has not so far lent itself to meaningful experimentation. Faced with need to make recommendations for action, an advisory committee to the Surgeon General of the United States Public Health Service came to the conclusion that a causal relation does exist between cigarette smoking and lung cancer. They considered all of the available evidence in the light of a number of criteria which, in fact, have general application and are listed in the following paragraph taken from the Committee's report (50).

CAUSAL SIGNIFICANCE OF THE ASSOCIATION.—As already stated, statistical methods cannot establish proof of a causal relationship in an association. The causal significance of an association is a matter of judgment which goes beyond any statement of statistical probability. To judge or evaluate the causal significance of the association between cigarette smoking and lung cancer a number of criteria must be utilized no one of which by itself is pathognomonic or a *sine qua non* for judgment. These criteria include:

(a) The consistency of the association
(b) The strength of the association
(c) The specificity of the association
(d) The temporal relationship of the association
(e) The coherence of the association.

In the following pages of the report each of these phrases is defined. The definitions are summarized here.

Consistency   Consistency implies that diverse methods of approach in the study of an association will provide similar conclusions.

Strength   The most direct measure of the strength of the association between smoking and lung cancer is the ratio of the lung cancer rates for smokers to the rates for nonsmokers, provided these two rates have been adjusted for the age characteristics of each group.

Specificity   The concept of specificity cannot be entirely dissociated from the concept inherent in the strength of the association. It implies the precision with which one component of an associated pair can be utilized to predict the occurrence of the other, that is, how frequently the presence of one variable (for example, lung cancer) will predict, in the same individual, the presence of another (for example, cigarette smoking).

Temporal relationship of associated variables   In chronic diseases, insidious onset and ignorance of precise induction periods automatically present problems on which came first—the suspected agent or the disease. In any evaluation of the significance of an association, exposure to an agent presumed to be causal must precede, temporally, the onset of a disease it is purported to produce.

Coherence   A final criterion for the appraisal of causal significance of an association is its coherence with known facts in the natural history and biology of the disease.

12-10   Summary

The goals of epidemiologic research include determination and characterization of the primary agent (if such exists), definition of transmission and reservoir mechanisms, discovery and evaluation of contributory factors, and development and evaluation of preventive measures. A major current interest is in assessing the disease potential of agents not yet associated with disease.

Epidemiologic research can be classified by setting (laboratory or field) and by approach (experimental or observational). Observational studies may be further classified by purpose (descriptive or analytic) and by nature (survey, continuing surveillance, retrospective, or prospective).

Important objectives of laboratory studies include experimental reproduction of a disease, use of experimental disease to study factors important to host resistance and susceptibility, elucidation of epidemiologically important properties of disease agents, search for leads as to the natural history of disease (including testing suspect vertebrate and invertebrate hosts for susceptibility), and the development of preventive measures.

Experimental epidemiology, whether in laboratory animals or in man, involves determining by direct experiment the influence of potential disease determinants on disease occurrence in comparable population samples. These determinants may include host genetic factors, proportion of host susceptibles, dietary factors or other environmental influences, suspect agents of disease, and vaccines or other possible preventive measures. Vaccine trials are a common form of experiment in human populations. With appropriate simulation of probability models, experiments using theoretical populations also can be done with the aid of a computer.

Observational studies differ from experimental studies most importantly in that the investigator observes events in their natural setting and does nothing to influence their occurrence. Surveys are the simplest, but are an important form of such studies. Commonly, they represent efforts to describe the impact of disease agents on man, for example, prevalence of current infection, seroimmunity, or subclinical diseases, and are cross-sectional in nature. Longitudinal surveys (or continuing surveillance) are a means for describing the dynamics of disease agents or contributing factors.

Analytic studies are those which explore the possible association between a suspect determinant (cause or contributing factor) and disease. These may be carried out by beginning with disease and looking backward (retrospective) or with exposure to a suspect factor and looking forward (prospective).

Prospective studies constitute the direct approach to the question, Does exposure increase risk of disease (and how much)? They are simple in concept. Groups free of disease, exposed and unexposed but otherwise comparable, are identified and observed for disease experience. The difficulties are practical: difficulty in selection of exposed and unexposed groups that are representative of large populations from which they are drawn, expense, and, especially for chronic diseases, prolonged period of observation. Sometimes the time requirement can be greatly shortened by identifying a population that existed in the past and whose experience until the present can be ascertained.

Retrospective studies are an indirect approach to the question of exposure versus increased risk. Persons with disease and comparable healthy controls are investigated for prior exposure to the suspect factor. Composition of the control group is crucial, and it is usually chosen on the basis of its similarity to the study group. Retrospective studies are inexpensive, usually quick, and commonly used for identifying suspect factors. The results provide direct measures only of the frequencies of exposure (exposure rates) in the diseased and healthy groups. In some instances, however, the exposure rates can be used to estimate the relative risk of disease attributable to the suspect determinant.

Associations discovered by analytic studies are consistent with, often suggestive of, but never proof of a causal relation. Biologic plausibility and repeated demonstration strengthen the presumption of causal relation but "scientific proof" is provided only by experimental demonstration of the association.

GLOSSARY

Natural history (of a disease)   Comprehensive account of nature of agent, its sources and distribution, mechanisms of reservoir and transmission, and its impact on man; in other words, what many mean by *the* epidemiology of a disease.

Screening (methods)   Methods for rapid qualitative (not quantitative) testing, e.g., for serum antibody, sugar in urine, or cancerlike cells in cervical smears.

Selective inbreeding   Inbreeding, with mice, means brother–sister matings which, if practiced through enough generations, yield a genetically homogenous population. The process becomes selective when, with each generation, breeding mice are selected for some desired characteristic, e.g., resistance to mouse typhoid.

REFERENCES

1. Eaton, Monroe D., Meiklejohn, G., and von Herick, W. Studies on the etiology of primary atypical pneumonia. A filterable agent transmissible to cotton rats, hamsters, and chick embryos. *J. Exp. Med.* **79**:649–668, 1944.

2. Foy, Hjordis M. *et al.* Epidemiology of *Mycoplasma pneumoniae* infection in families. *J. Amer. Med. Ass.* **197**: 859–866, 1966.

3. Carson, Rachel. *Silent Spring.* Boston: Houghton Mifflin Company, 1962.

4. Enders, John F., Weller, T. H., and Robbins, C. F. Cultivation of the Lansing strain of poliomyelitis virus in cultures of various human embryonic tissues. *Science* **109**: 85–87, 1949.

5. Theiler, M., and Smith, H. H. Effect of prolonged cultivation *in vitro* upon pathogenicity of yellow fever virus. *J. Exp. Med.* **65**:767–786, 1937.

6. Chanock, Robert M. Mycoplasma infections of man. *New Eng. J. Med.* **173**:1199–1206, 1257–1264, 1965.

7. Wheeler, Charles M. Control of typhus in Italy 1943–1944 by use of DDT. *Amer. J. Public Health* **36**:119–129, 1946.

8. Cox, H. R. Use of yolk sac of developing chick embryo as medium for growing rickettsiae of Rocky Mountain spotted fever and typhus groups. *Public Health Rep.* **53**:2241–2247, 1938.

9. Gallardo, F. Perez, and Fox, John P. Infection and immunization of laboratory animals with *Rickettsia prowazekii* of reduced pathogenicity. *Amer. J. Hyg.* **48**:6–21, 1948.

10. Stamler, Jeremiah. Current status of the dietary prevention and treatment of atherosclerotic coronary heart disease. *Progr. Cardiovasc. Dis.* **3**:56–95, 1960.

11. Greenwood, Major, Hill, A. Bradford, Topley, W. W. C., and Wilson, J. *Experimental Epidemiology.* Medical Research Council, Special Report Series No. 209. London: His Majesty's Stationery Office, 1936.

12. Webster, Leslie T. Experimental epidemiology. *Medicine* **25**:77–109, 1946.

13. Andrewes, C. H., and Allison, A. C. Newcastle disease as a model for studies of experimental epidemiology. *J. Hyg. (Camb.)* **59**:285–293, 1961.

14. Schulman, J. L., and Kilbourne, E. D. Experimental transmission of influenza virus infection in mice. I. The period of transmissibility. *J. Exp. Med.* **118**:257–266. 1963. II. Some factors affecting the incidence of transmitted infection, *ibid.*, 267–275. III. Differing effects of immunity induced by infection and by inactivated influenza virus vaccine on transmission of infection. *ibid.* **125**: 467–478, 1967. IV.

Relationship of transmissibility of different strains of virus and recovery of airborne virus in the environment of infector mice. *ibid.* 479–488.

15. Schneider, Howard A. Nutrition of the host and natural resistance to infection. II. The dietary effect as conditioned by the heterogeneity of the test pathogen population. *J. Exp. Med.* **84**:305–322, 1946.

16. Krugman, Saul. Studies on the natural history of infectious heptatis. *New Eng. J. Med.* **261**:729–734, 1959.

17. Krugman, Saul, and Ward, Robert. Infectious hepatitis. Current status of prevention with gamma globulin. *Yale J. Biol. Med.* **34**:329–339, 1961/2.

18. Roden, A. T. Variations in the clinical pattern of experimentally induced colds. *J. Hyg. (Camb.)* **61**:231–246, 1963.

19. Fox, John P., Jordan, Martha E., and Gelfand, Henry M. Immunization of man against epidemic typhus by infection with avirulent *Rickettsia prowazekii* strain E. IV. Persistence of immunity and a note as to differing complement-fixation antigen requirements in post-infection and post-vaccination sera. *J. Immun.* **79**:348–354, 1957.

20. Fox, John P., Montoya, Juan, Jordan, Martha E., and Espinosa, Max. Immunization of man against epidemic typhus by infection with avirulent *Rickettsia prowazekii* (strain E). *Amer. J. Hyg.* **61**:183–196, 1955.

21. Abbey, Helen. An examination of the Reed–Frost theory of epidemics. *Hum. Biol.* **24**:201–233, 1952.

22. Elveback, Lila R., Ackerman, Eugene, Young, Greg, and Fox, John P. A stochastic model for competition between viral agents in the presence of interference. 1. Live virus vaccine in a randomly mixing population, Model III. *Amer. J. Epidem.* **87**:373–384, 1968.

23. *Snow on Cholera.* being a reprint of two papers by John Snow together with a biographical memoir by B. W. Richardson and an introduction by Wade Hampton Frost. New York: The Commonwealth Fund, 1936. pp. 77–92.

24. Hyge, Tage V. The efficacy of BCG vaccine. *Acta Tuberc. Scand.* **32**:89–107, 1956.

25. Paul, John R. The story to be learned from blood samples. *J. Amer. Med. Ass.* **175**:601–605, 1961.

26. Paul, John R., Riordan, John T., and Melnick, Joseph L. Antibodies to three different antigenic types of poliomyelitis virus in sera from North Alaskan Eskimos. *Amer. J. Hyg.* **54**:275–285, 1951.

27. Clarke, Delphine H., and Casals, Jordi. Arboviruses; Group B, in *Viral and Rickettsial Infections of Man*, 4th ed. Frank L. Horsfall and Igor Tamm, eds. Philadelphia: J. B. Lippincott, 1965. pp. 606–658.

28. Kent, Gerald T., and Leonards, Jack R. Analysis of tests for diabetes in 250,000 persons screened for diabetes using finger blood after a carbohydrate load. *Diabetes* **17**:274–280, 1968.

29. Papanicolaou, G. N., and Trout, H. F. *Diagnosis of Uterine Cancer by the Vaginal Smear.* New York: The Commonwealth Fund, 1943.

30. Smith, Hugh H. Controlling Yellow Fever, in *Yellow Fever.* George K. Strode, ed. New York: McGraw-Hill, 1951, pp. 588–596.

31. Lidwell, O. M., and Sommerville, T. Observations on the incidence and distribution of the common cold in a rural community during 1948 and 1949. *J. Hyg. (Camb.)* **49**:365–381, 1951.
    Brimblecombe, F. S. W. *et al.* Family studies of respiratory infections. *Brit. Med. J.* **1**:119–128, 1958.

32. Dingle, John H., Badger, George F., and Jordan, William S. *Illness in the Home.* Cleveland: Press of Western Reserve University, 1964.

33. Gelfand, Henry M., LeBlanc, D. R., Fox, J. P., and Conwell, D. P. Studies on the development of natural immunity to poliomyelitis in Louisiana. II. Description and analysis of episodes of infection observed in study group households. *Amer. J. Hyg.* **65**:367–385, 1957.

34. Fox, John P. *et al.* The Virus Watch program: A continuing surveillance of viral infections in metropolitan New York families. Papers I, II, III. *Amer. J. Epidem.* **83**:389–454, 1966.

35. Fox, John P. *et al.* The Virus Watch program: A continuing surveillance of viral infections in metropolitan New York families. VI. Observations of adenovirus infections: virus excretion patterns; antibody response; efficiency of surveillance; patterns of infection; and relation to illness. *Amer. J. Epidem.* **89**:25–50, 1969.

36. Francis, Thomas, Jr., and Epstein, Frederick H. Survey Methods in General Populations Tecumseh, Michigan, in *Comparability in International Epidemiology.* Roy M. Acheson, ed. Princeton, N.J.: Milbank Memorial Fund, 1965, pp. 333–342.

37. Dawber, Thomas R., Kannel, William B., and Lyell, Lorna P. An approach to longitudinal studies in the community: The Framingham Study. *Ann. N.Y. Acad. Sci.* **107**:539–556, 1963.

38. Wynder, Ernest L., and Graham, Evarts A. Tobacco smoking as a possible etiologic factor in bronchiogenic carcinoma. *J. Amer. Med. Ass.* **143**:329–336, 1950.

39. Gregg, N. McAlister. Congenital cataract following German measles in the mother. *Trans. Ophthal. Soc. Aust.* **3**:35–46, 1941.

40. Doll, Richard, and Hill, A. Bradford. A study of the aetiology of carcinoma of the lung. *Brit. Med. J.* **2**:1271–1286, 1952.

41. Hill, A. Bradford, and Knowlden, J. Inoculation and poliomyelitis. *Brit. Med. J.* **2**:1–6, 1950.

42. Woolf, Barnet. On estimating the relation between blood groups and disease. *Ann. Hum. Genet.* **19**:251–253, 1955.

43. Mantel, Nathan, and Haenszel, William. Statistical aspects of the analysis of data from retrospective studies of disease. *J. Nat. Cancer Inst.* **22**:719–748, 1959.

44. Nefzger, M. Dean, Quadfasel, Fred A., and Karl, Virginia C. A retrospective study of smoking in Parkinson's Disease. *Amer. J. Epidem.* **88**:149–158, 1968.

45. Kahn, Harold A. The Dorn Study of Smoking and Mortality Among U.S. Veterans: Report on Eight and One-Half Years of Observation. National Cancer Institute Monograph 19. *Epidemiological Approaches to the Study of Cancer and Other Chronic Diseases.* William Haenszel, ed. Washington, D.C.: U.S. Department of Health, Education, and Welfare, 1966, pp. 1–125.

46. Hammond, E. Cuyler, and Horn, Daniel. Smoking and death rates— report on forty-four months of follow-up of 187,783 men. *J. Amer. Med. Ass.* **166**:1159–1172; 1294–1308, 1958.

47. Hammond, E. Cuyler. Smoking in Relation to the Death Rates of One Million Men and Women. National Cancer Institute Monograph 19. *Epidemiological Approaches to the Study of Cancer and Other Chronic Diseases.* William Haenszel, ed. Washington, D.C.: U.S. Department of Health, Education, and Welfare, 1966, pp. 127–170.

48. Doll, Richard, and Hill, A. Bradford. Mortality in relation to smoking. 10 years observation of British doctors. *Brit. Med. J.* **1**:1399–1410; 1460–1467, 1964.

49. Doll, Richard, and Hill, A. Bradford. Mortality of British Doctors in Relation to Smoking: Observations on Coronary Thrombosis. National Cancer Institute Monograph 19. *Epidemiological Approaches to the Study of Cancer and Other Chronic Diseases.* William Haenszel, ed. Washington, D.C.: U.S. Department of Health, Education, and Welfare, 1966, pp. 205–268.

50. Advisory Committee to the Surgeon General of the Public Health Service. *Smoking and Health.* P.H.S. Publication No. 1103. Washington, D.C.: Public Health Service, 1964, pp. 182–189.

Additional Suggested Readings

1. Cochran, H. A., and Buck, N. F. A mortality study of an insured diabetic population. *Proc. Med. Sect. Amer. Life Convention* **49**:145–184, 1961.

2. Cornfield, J. A Statistical Problem Arising from Retrospective Studies. *Third Berkeley Symposium,* 135–148, 1956.

3. White, C., and Bailar, J. C. Retrospective and prospective methods of studying association in medicine. *Amer. J. Public Health* **46**:35–44, 1956.

4. Lilienfeld, A. Epidemiological methods and inferences in studies of noninfectious diseases. *Public Health Rep.* **72**:51–60, 1957.

5. Yerushalmy, J., and Palmer, C. E. On the methodology of investigations of etiologic factors in chronic diseases. *J. Chronic Dis.* **10**:27–40, 1959.

13

The Practice of Epidemiology

D. R. Peterson, M.D., M.P.H.*

13-1 Epidemiology as the Public Practice of Medicine

The practice of epidemiology involves application of theory, methods, and established epidemiologic facts to circumstances of ordinary community life. In this case, a community may be thought of as any existing definable population ranging in number from a relatively few individuals to the citizens of an entire nation. Because epidemiology is fundamentally a medical discipline, it is not surprising that most practicing epidemiologists are physicians; a few are dentists, veterinarians, or persons from other allied professions. In the United States they work primarily under the aegis of local, state, or national government. A few are employed at the international level, and others work for nongovernmental health agencies, hospitals, or industrial corporations.

Since practicing epidemiologists concern themselves with communities of one sort or another, the practice of epidemiology can be construed as a public practice of medicine (or dentistry or veterinary medicine, and so on). This concept contrasts with private practice in which individual patients are the central concern of the practitioner.

*This final chapter is a solicited contribution from an active and effective practitioner of epidemiology in his post as epidemiologist for the Seattle–King County Health Department. The authors are particularly grateful to Dr. Peterson for providing this authoritative insight into the practice of epidemiology.

In public practice, therefore, the "patient" is an entire community or a recognizable segment thereof. This "patient" is "diagnosed" by epidemiologic examination and "treated" through organized community effort aimed either at preventing disease or lessening its impact. In contrast, the patient of the private medical practitioner is diagnosed by conventional medical means and treated by whatever modality is indicated to improve that particular individual's state of health. In actual fact, this contrast is not as sharp as is drawn here for descriptive purposes. Indeed, public and private medical practices are complementary. Epidemiologists rely on their colleagues in private practice to diagnose and report cases of disease of epidemiologic interest and to develop ever better methods of diagnosis. Practicing physicians rely on epidemiolgists to identify actual or potential epidemics, to ferret out the cause, if possible, and to suggest remedies when indicated. The epidemiologist may also provide consultation to practicing physicians in difficult or unusual cases or in matters pertaining to immunization. He may do this directly on request and by regularly providing his colleagues in private practice with information on disease occurrence in their community. Such information may lead to establishing a diagnosis in an individual patient that otherwise would not have been suspected.

In a recent instance, for example, single reports from individual physicians scattered over a wide area indicated that an unusual syndrome was occurring among young children and some of their mothers. The illness was characterized by small vesicles on the palms, soles, and buccal mucous membranes. Virologists in the same area concurrently reported a number of enterovirus isolations including many coxsackieviruses from a variety of different syndromes. This preliminary information, coupled with that from a recent publication describing a similar occurrence elsewhere and implicating coxsackievirus, suggested that these unusual cases were self-limiting enterovirus infections. As the epidemic continued, more and more physicians requested advice. The "big-picture" perspective permitted the epidemiologist to suggest to them what a possible diagnosis might be.

The diagnosis of true influenza in individual patients is notoriously unreliable, because the symptoms are common to many viral diseases not caused by the influenza virus. However, when the epidemiologist identifies high absence rates in schools and industry that are characteristic of influenza, he can advise his colleagues in private practice with some assurance concerning individual patients.

As certain diseases become rare, the epidemiologist is often the only physician in a community who follows literature on the disease in question. Cases of smallpox, diphtheria, rabies, and many parasitic diseases are in this category. Syphilis is almost so, because so few cases occur that physicians do not find it profitable to keep abreast of new developments. As a repository of information on the more esoteric diseases, some of which were once common but now occur only as sporadic events, the practicing epidemiologist can be a unique community resource.

The way in which a physician serves his patient may be as important or more important than what he does on the patient's behalf. This art of practice is as essential in public practice as in private practice, particularly since the epidemiologist is occasionally a public figure subject to scrutiny by the press, the medical community, and other critics.

13-2 The Epidemiologic Team and Its Direction

In the not too distant past private medical practice was essentially a one-man operation. Then helpers (nurses, laboratory technicians, and others) and, subsequently, colleagues with special interests and training became his regular associates. Today, the team approach to individual patients in hospitals, clinics, and group offices utilizing a variety of medical and paramedical specialists is the rule. From the beginning, by its very nature epidemiologic practice has been a team effort, with only occasional exception. Co-workers include nurses, sanitarians, engineers, microbiologists, chemists, health educators, biostatisticians, demographers, clerks, and a variety of other specialists with talents appropriate to the task of dealing with communities of people. The practicing epidemiologist, therefore, must also be an administrator in order to manage this retinue and coordinate their efforts toward a desired end. Not infrequently his role also includes that of educator—either of his own staff or of others who desire or require a practical epidemiologic perspective.

The amount of administrative responsibility involved varies widely. Generally, at lower government echelons there is less of this type of responsibility than at higher ones. For example, at the national level in the United States epidemiologic practice is concentrated in two relatively large program areas of the Public Health Service. One of these is the National Communicable Disease Center, with headquarters in Atlanta, Georgia. The other includes several of the National Institutes of Health in Bethesda, Maryland, which are concerned primarily with noncommunicable diseases. These operations, jurisdictionally broad in scope, require a great deal more organizational and administrative concern on the part of those employed than a metropolitan area, for example, with one physician epidemiologist, a public health nurse, a clerk, and perhaps, a specialist in environmental health. Nongovernmental sponsors with specific and generally narrow interests have similar modest demands for manpower and their supervision.

13-3   Epidemiologist as Persuader, Politician, and Publicist

Directing activities of personnel, important as it is, is probably secondary in importance to maintaining close ties with the community. Because both data collection for epidemiologic diagnosis and the organized effort that solution demands are, by their nature, collaborative enterprises, the epidemiologist must know his community intimately. He must rely on friends and associates in various walks of life, as well as colleagues for advice and counsel; he must also be sensitive to the power structure of his community. At varying times and for varying reasons he must persuade those in executive, legislative, or judicial positions to exercise their power on his recommendation. Support from a variety of voluntary organizations, some with only indirect commitments to health conservation, is often vital to a successful public prescription. Support is often solicited from agricultural agencies and trade unions, for example. Finally, it is the epidemiologist's responsibility to reveal his findings and their judicious interpretation to the public he serves so that the community ultimately benefits. Although this function is performed in a variety of ways that need not be gone into here, one requires comment—the epidemiologist's relationship with mass communication media such as the press, radio, and television. Intimidation by any of these is tantamount to failure. Their support is no guarantee of success, but it can be of considerable help.

13-4   Surveillance, or Taking the Pulse of the Community

Disease surveillance is the practicing epidemiologist's primary occupation; it pervades and keynotes all his activity. Monitoring disease occurrence for endemic prevalence and epidemic incidence sets the stage for whatever subsequent role he chooses to play. Disease surveillance, then, is a finger on the pulse of the community by which the practicing epidemiologist senses when to act. The backbone of surveillance is some sort of formal system for data collection, tabulation, and evaluation. Basic surveillance data is usually derived from that unit of government closest to the data source—local government. The data flow chart (Figure 13-1) depicts one such operation that, over the years, has proven reasonably satisfactory for dealing with communicable diseases. Modifications of the schema will likely also suffice to monitor noncommunicable diseases as the practice of epidemiology moves into this sphere at the local level. Physicians specializing in occupational medicine who maintain epidemiologic

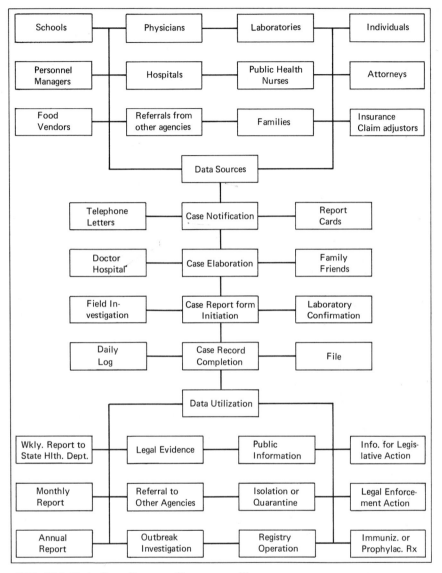

FIG. 13-1 Data flow diagram, disease surveillance.

surveillance on a work force would employ a schema different in detail but essentially the same in design.

Further insight into community disease surveillance is provided by the diagram titled "Contingencies of Reporting" (Figure 13-2). In this diagram the possible actions of a person with a particular illness are arrayed in a logical sequence that produces a cascade of contingencies, that is, each

CONTINGENCIES OF MORBIDITY REPORTING

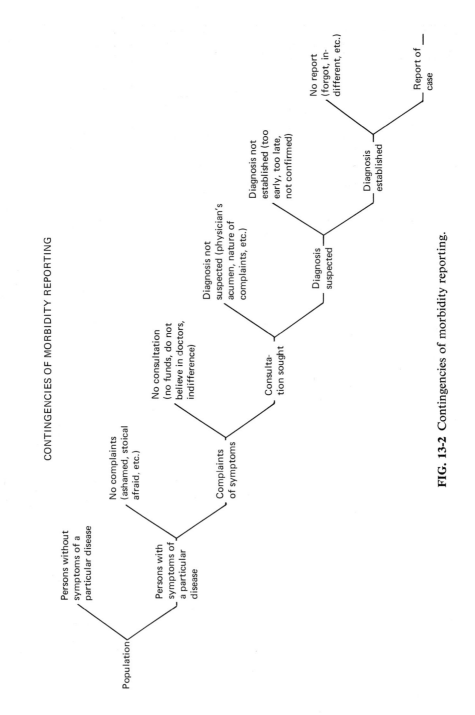

FIG. 13-2 Contingencies of morbidity reporting.

positive action is contingent on the series of actions which preceded it. By recognizing this principle, it is possible to intercept the sequence at the appropriate point and tap information. For example, if the disease is one which is not followed by serious complications and typically produces only mild symptoms of short duration, it would be folly to expect physicians to report. They would see few, if any, such cases. A survey would be a more appropriate method for measuring the incidence of mild gastroenteritis, warts, mild hearing loss, or a similar phenomenon. However, individual reports from physicians sometimes provide a clue to an epidemic of mild disease which would be missed by reliance solely on a survey system. Reasonably good information on diseases such as epidemic influenza can be gotten indirectly by monitoring absenteeism in schools and industries. Although the clinical diagnosis of sporadic influenza is notoriously unreliable, the consequences of its epidemic spread are highly predictable. Measles is usually obvious to the mother of a child so afflicted. Excuses of absence from school giving measles as the reason provide a basis for surveillance. Such reports circumvent the loss that would doubtless accompany the following of the contingency principle to its conclusion. Collection of epidemiologic information, therefore, is a matter of selecting sources that will produce data of maximal usefulness.

Experience reveals that any surveillance system, whether mandated by law or based entirely on voluntary cooperation, falls far short of a complete revelation of what occurs in a community. Experience also shows that informal intelligence produces leads worth following. The term "informal intelligence" is used here to designate information that comes to the epidemiologist by a variety of routes: casual conversations with medical colleagues, inquiries and complaints from the public, serendipitous laboratory discoveries, overheard chance remarks in elevators and other such places, newspaper reports, research findings, or special inquiries initiated by the epidemiologist himself. Occasionally a "crank" caller turns out to be someone, upset by bureaucratic referrals from one office to another, who has valuable information to impart. Thus, both formal and informal surveillance constitute the core of the practicing epidemiologist's concern.

Obviously, however, much disease is undetected even under the best of circumstances. The iceberg concept is an everyday fact of life. Armed with data of uncertain quantity, the practicing epidemiologist must attempt, when possible, to ascertain its quality as indicated in the flow diagram (Figure 13-1). This may require a few phone calls to physicians, a visit to a school, consultation with an academic colleague, additional laboratory tests, or expectant waiting for other cases to appear. Here, again, something less than 100 per cent efficiency is the rule. Surveillance, then, is a necessary tool for roughing out the dimensions of community health problems. The products, if the tool is used consistently, are trends rather than absolute measures of incidence or prevalence. Alternately, an alert surveillance posture will often produce evidence of considerable public health significance from detailed epidemiologic investigation of only a few cases, and sometimes of a single case. Thus, "dearthy" as well as "dirty" data are the stuff of surveillance at the grassroots level. Epidemiologists at all succeeding levels of government, by collation of data from lower echelons, are faced with the even more complex situation of compounding the problems already described. Despite such disparagement, surveillance works when people work at it. It is the basic minimum activity that a community must support for its own defense against the spread of disease, just as it supports activities to combat fire or crime.

13-5 Epidemiologic Detective

Investigations of outbreaks discovered through disease surveillance provide many of the elements, including the excitement which attends a typical police detective operation, in which an attempt is made to reconstruct the crime for clues to the identity of the villain. Both disease outbreak investigation and criminal investigation are "after the fact" and therefore retrospective. The chief difference is in perspective. Although the police detective may be aware of population determinants of criminal behavior, he must focus on identification of a particular culprit so as to bring him to justice. The medical detective, on the other hand, is relatively less concerned with the final disposition of the cause of a particular outbreak than he is with how occurrences can be prevented or minimized in the future.

The method of processing a particular meat product called head cheese, made largely from pork and gelatin, came under scrutiny because several one- and two-person outbreaks of salmonellosis were investigated carefully. In particular, investigation included scrupulous documentation of food histories, collection of appropriate specimens for bacteriologic analysis, and sanitary inspection of the production facilities. The chain of evidence obtained was sufficiently strong that substantial out-of-court settlements resulted when litigation was initiated. The basic fault was found to be inattention to sanitary practice; cooked meat was ground in machines previously used for raw meat without adequate cleaning in between. Head cheese contains so much gelatin that no final heat treatment, which would obviate contamination, is given. Hence, among all the luncheon meats, this particular meat product is most likely to provide a vehicle for salmonella transmission. Considering the many years that commercially prepared head cheese has been available, it is indeed remarkable that problems with it have been recognized only recently. Doubtless many infections occurred which were not reported or, if reported, were not investigated with this possibility in mind. Thus, the bulk of the cases, like the submerged portion of an iceberg, is hidden from view, and we detect only a few cases which correspond to the tip of the iceberg that is visible.

Another example involved two elderly ladies who had eaten cheese sandwiches on two occasions and developed identical illness which resembled staphylococcal intoxication. This episode initiated investigation with far-reaching consequences. The uneaten portion of cheese was found to contain coagulase positive staphylococci, as did a high proportion of packages of the same lot number obtained from the same supermarket in which the cheese was originally purchased and from other retail outlets. Since this was a commodity in interstate commerce, federal as well as state studies were initiated and all corroborated the initial findings of contaminated cheese. These two old ladies provided the charge that set off a whole series of explosions, ultimately resulting in a serious review of cheese-making practices and control legislation in the state in which the cheese was manufactured.

13-6 Feasibility and Compromise

A frequent dilemma for the practicing epidemiologist involves deciding what is feasible in the light of theoretical desirability. His work is seldom a model of scientific rigor, but rather a compromise lending an element of uncertainty, perhaps, to final conclusions. It is here that the flexibility of the epidemiologic approach becomes most apparent; the discipline permits admission of evidence of many descriptions.

A classical case in point was that of Goldberger's investigation of pellagra (1). He decided, on the basis of traditional epidemiologic data, that diet rather than infection was implicated causally in pellagra. He then performed a series of experiments with groups in prison and orphanages to confirm his initial impression. Those on a severely restricted diet developed pellagra and those on a more generous diet did not. If more generous feeding with meat, milk, and vegetables was started soon enough, those with pellagra recovered. These crucial experiments were later confirmed when the missing ingredient in the restricted diet was found to be the vitamin niacin.

A recent example in the writer's experience involved an outbreak of salmonellosis on a college campus. It was hoped that data generated from this readily accessible population would clearly spell out the vehicle of infection so that the college authorities could take action to forestall a recurrence. In all, 326 students and faculty became ill, an attack rate of 28.5 per cent. Complete food histories were obtained from 1,142 out of a total of 1,810 persons. Analysis of these data, as well as data on a variety of other possible factors that might have been associated with risk of illness, gave no statistical clues by which one could explain the epidemiogenesis of the outbreak. However, before the epidemic was more than a few cases old, a sanitary field investigation was conducted which revealed that the processing of precooked, boned chicken and its subsequent handling in the college kitchen could have been the source. Selective sampling of leftover chicken, undistributed chicken in the plant warehouse where it was processed, and from the product in interstate transit revealed contamination with *Salmonelleae*. Furthermore, the leftover chicken produced the same serotype as was found in the patients' stools. This experience emphasizes the eclectic nature of the practice of epidemiology—taking advantage of whatever information bears on the problem under investigation. Being on the scene of an outbreak as promptly as possible enhances the opportunity to take advantage of the flexible approach. In practice the exercise of "shoe leather epidemiology" and "peppy epi," as it is known in venereal disease control work, is an indispensable element to successful investigation.

However valuable intelligent field investigation may be, it cannot be done blindly. Sometimes samples for laboratory analysis are collected indiscriminately and in large numbers in the pious hope that something will come to light. Aside from the expense in time, money, and effort involved in such a shotgun approach, it seldom works. Chances of success are greater when initial field studies start with epidemiologic definition of the outbreak, even though the data are incomplete and inexact. Simple, temporal distribution of case onsets roughly outlines the epidemic curve; from this the likelihood of a point source outbreak can be inferred. Use of this information together with age and sex distributions, food and occupational histories, and so on, applied selectively to fit each circumstance, is comparable to shooting at a solution with a rifle instead of a blunderbuss. Preliminary epidemiologic data then, however scanty, is a requisite precondition to a working, epidemiologic diagnosis. This rationale is the same as that employed in private medical practice in which the history and physical examination suggest a diagnosis or at least a number of probable ones. Laboratory tests, a test of time, and/or responses to a trial of medication ultimately establish the diagnosis.

13-7 Measuring Results

The practicing epidemiologist, more often than his academic colleague, is concerned with evaluation of control efforts. It is not difficult to see how a vaccine field trial, which is an evaluation of a control method, fits the epidemiologic mold. It is perhaps harder to see attempts to evaluate administrative practices or legal requirements in the same light. Nonetheless, evaluation studies are a matter of practical importance. In simplest terms this may be only a matter of documenting a decreased incidence of some disease or condition coincident with institution of control. It may, on the other hand, involve a detailed scrutiny of the population to see if change results and what the ramifications of change might be. Although the efficacy of immune serum globulin for prevention of symptoms of infectious hepatitis under controlled conditions is well documented, the writer had grave doubts about this under conditions of everyday living in his community. Only after evaluation under those circumstances showed its utility, were thoughts abandoned of discontinuing an established program for making immune globulin available to household contacts of the disease.

Indirectly, disease surveillance itself is an evaluative tool of the practicing epidemiologist. For example, foodborne epidemics that occur with increasing frequency suggest that sanitary controls need attention. A sudden spurt of pertussis incidence suggests, though it does not prove, that immunization effort has been lagging. Once baseline trends are established for a high-incidence disease such as coronary artery disease, we may be able to evaluate, at least in a crude way, the impact of education concerning factors of risk that have a role in the genesis of this disease. Something of this sort is currently underway with respect to lung cancer and smoking, for example.

13-8   Control Activities

The prescription for control usually involves an attack on many fronts. Since this prescription deals with organized effort, the practicing epidemiologist may fill his prescription blank with notes on proposed legislation, or with arguments mustered to oppose legislation or replace outmoded or unnecessary statutes. In another situation he may find himself as a public functionary in a promotional endeavor aimed at broad public compliance, such as a community-wide measles immunization program. His lot is also to appear as an expert witness or friend of the court in matters of legal dispute. Most commonly, his responsibility is to assure himself that everyday disease control efforts are relevant to the current or future state of affairs. This implies a constant shifting of work assignments of his staff and other support personnel to assure productivity of effort. It is all too human to persist in some pursuit only because it has been done X number of years. For example, a decision to abandon routine surveillance of throat smears for *Corynebacterium diphtheriae* numbering about 100,000 per year, when no carriers had been found over a five-year period, netted the laboratory one full-time employee without creating a new position. Another case involved pitting the value of diagnostic virology service to practicing physicians against the value of epidemic intelligence so derived. When, on balance, it was decided to discontinue the service, the virologists were assigned to more cogent tasks involving their skills. Epidemiologic prescription writing need not follow a prescribed course, but should fit the community to which it is addressed. Furthermore, there are constant opportunities for innovations and observational experiments to challenge any creative streak the epidemiologist in practice may possess.

13-9 A Prospective Look

This chapter has dealt with everyday application of epidemiology as a public practice of medicine for the community, as contrasted with private medical practice for individuals. The types of applications cited are drawn largely from the local level of government, because it is here that most data used by higher echelons for surveillance are derived. This emphasis is not intended to deprecate those working under other auspices, but simply to provide a convenient foundation for dealing with the subject.

What of the future of epidemiologic practice? The tendency of man around the globe to congregate in or around urban centers becomes increasingly apparent, even as his total numbers increase at a phenomenal rate. The increase of population by itself suggests that more epidemiologists will find their professional niche in practice as well as in research or teaching. Aside from the increase of population, the concentration of people which attends urbanization will bring a physical environment that is more complex, a social environment that is more involved, and a mental environment that is more intense. Coupling these observations with those of Dr. Acheson under the heading "New Horizons in Epidemiology," we see that we have only begun to appreciate the role of epidemiology in its practical application in public health.

Epidemiology is a burgeoning science. Generations of philosophers and physicans have realized that certain patterns of living have been associated with promotion of certain diseases. In former times in the Western World such diseases were contagious and nearly always the single quality shared by communities in which they occurred was poverty. A very few diseases, such as gout, and perhaps diabetes, were considered to be a consequence of riches and the surfeit which often accompanies them. It is only since the Second World War that it has become clear that *all* disease stems directly or indirectly from the patterns of men's lives. . . . The realization of the immense complexity in the balance between health and disease has stimulated efforts to meet the need for broadening the horizons of epidemiology from single-minded concentration on studying contagions. It is now concerned with all health and illness in population groups and with the factors—including health services—which affect them. . . .
(2)

REFERENCES

1. Terris, Milton, ed. *Goldberger on Pellagra.* Baton Rouge: Louisiana State University Press, 1964.
2. Acheson, R. M. The need for comparability in international epidemiology. *Milbank Mem. Fund Quart.* **43**:(No. 2, Part 2), 11–16, 1965.

Index

Note: Page references to illustrations are printed in boldface type.

alcohol, 206, 253–56
sex, 196
socioeconomic status, 204
Climate, 95–99
Clinical impression of disease, 294
Clinical response, range of, 186–87
Clinical syndrome, 186, 207
clue to disease causation, 187
factors affecting development, 33,
188
Cohort, age profile of disease, 191–
192
analysis, death rates, 261–63
of related persons, 197
studies, 269, 299–306
Communicable disease, 25, 28
Communicability, 16, 57
Community, epidemiologic area, 14–
15, 315–17
as "patient," 316
Comparative data, 210–11
Computer-simulated populations,
280–84
Confidence interval, 176–78, 181,
273
Congenital infection, 60
Congenital malformations, death
rates, 225
defined, 237
rubella, 7–9, 165–66
Contact, direct, 63
indirect, 63
Contagion, 21, 29
Contingencies of disease reporting,
319–22
Continuing source outbreak, 246–47
Control (of disease), activities in
community, 325–26
cholera, 2–3, 24–25
development of methods, 270–72
epidemic typhus, 272
goal of epidemiology, 2
influenza, 52
yellow fever, 10
Control groups, matching, 293
placebo vs. observed, 10, 162, 272–
273

polio vaccine trials, 10
randomization in formation of,
162, 164–65, 272–73
rubella studies, 7, 8
selection, 294
use of volunteers, 162–63
Conveyance of disease agents, 63–64
Coronary heart disease, obesity and
activity, 163
serum cholesterol, 171
study of, 291
Cowpox, 2, 24
Cox, H., 272
Crookshank, Dr., fable of, 32
Crude death rates, 128, 132
Curiosity, epidemiologic, 1
Cutter polio vaccine episode, 243–44
Cyclic variation, infectious disease,
251

Data sources, national, 217
Death certificate, 118–21
Death rates, age-specific, 129–32
cause-specific, 128, 139–47
color-specific, 128–29
crude, 128
sex-specific, 129
Death Registration Area, 118
Demographic base map, 221–23
Demography, 12
Detecting power of a test, 178–80,
181
Determinants of disease occurrence, 1
Devonshire colic, 28
Diabetes, screening, 288
Diagnosis, comparability over time,
257
importance in research, 10, 303–
304
Dietary patterns and disease, 84–85
Disease, epidemiologic description, 6,
185, 188
epidemiologic surveillance, 318–22
following infection, 70
manifestations, 45, 186–88
methods for prevention, 2
recognition, 10, 187–88, 303–304